# Veterinary Dentistry and Oral Surgery

*Editor*

ALEXANDER M. REITER

# VETERINARY CLINICS OF NORTH AMERICA: SMALL ANIMAL PRACTICE

www.vetsmall.theclinics.com

January 2022 • Volume 52 • Number 1

**ELSEVIER**

1600 John F. Kennedy Boulevard • Suite 1800 • Philadelphia, Pennsylvania, 19103-2899
http://www.vetsmall.theclinics.com

VETERINARY CLINICS OF NORTH AMERICA: SMALL ANIMAL PRACTICE Volume 52, Number 1
January 2022 ISSN 0195-5616, ISBN-13: 978-0-323-84920-3

Editor: Stacy Eastman
Developmental Editor: Axell Ivan Jade Purificacion

*Veterinary Clinics of North America: Small Animal Practice* (ISSN 0195-5616) is published bimonthly by Elsevier Inc., 360 Park Avenue South, New York, NY 10010-1710. Months of issue are January, March, May, July, September, and November. Business and Editorial Offices: 1600 John F. Kennedy Blvd., Ste. 1800, Philadelphia, PA 19103-2899. Customer Service Office: 3251 Riverport Lane, Maryland Heights, MO 63043. Periodicals postage paid at New York, NY and additional mailing offices. Subscription prices are $369.00 per year (domestic individuals), $980.00 per year (domestic institutions), $100.00 per year (domestic students/residents), $465.00 per year (Canadian individuals), $1029.00 per year (Canadian institutions), $503.00 per year (international individuals), $1029.00 per year (international institutions), $100.00 per year (Canadian students/residents), and $220.00 per year (international students/residents). To receive student/resident rate, orders must be accompanied by name of affiliated institution, date of term, and the *signature* of program/residency coordinator on institution letterhead. Orders will be billed at individual rate until proof of status is received. Foreign air speed delivery is included in all *Clinics* subscription prices. All prices are subject to change without notice. **POSTMASTER:** Send address changes to *Veterinary Clinics of North America: Small Animal Practice*, Elsevier Health Sciences Division, Subscription Customer Service, 3251 Riverport Lane, Maryland Heights, MO 63043. Customer Service (orders, claims, online, change of address): Elsevier Periodicals Customer Service, Elsevier Health Sciences Division Subscription **Customer Service 3251 Riverport Lane Maryland Heights, MO 63043. Tel: 1-800-654-2452 (U.S. and Canada); 314-447-8871 (outside U.S. and Canada). Fax: 314-447-8029. E-mail: journalscustomerservice-usa@elsevier.com (for print support); journalsonlinesupport-usa@elsevier.com (for online support).**

*Reprints.* For copies of 100 or more of articles in this publication, please contact the Commercial Reprints Department, Elsevier Inc., 360 Park Avenue South, New York, NY 10010-1710. Tel.: 212-633-3874; Fax: 212-633-3820; E-mail: reprints@elsevier.com.

*Veterinary Clinics of North America: Small Animal Practice* is also published in Japanese by Inter Zoo Publishing Co., Ltd., Aoyama Crystal-Bldg 5F, 3-5-12 Kitaaoyama, Minato-ku, Tokyo 107-0061, Japan.

*Veterinary Clinics of North America: Small Animal Practice* is covered in *Current Contents/Agriculture, Biology and Environmental Sciences, Science Citation Index, ASCA, MEDLINE/PubMed (Index Medicus), Excerpta Medica,* and *BIOSIS.*

# Contributors

## EDITOR

**ALEXANDER M. REITER, Dipl Tzt, Dr Med Vet**
Diplomate, American Veterinary Dental College; Diplomate, European Veterinary Dental College; Founding Fellow AVDC-OMFS, Professor of Dentistry and Oral Surgery, Head of the Dentistry and Oral Surgery Service, Department of Clinical Sciences and Advanced Medicine, School of Veterinary Medicine, University of Pennsylvania, Philadelphia, Pennsylvania, USA

## AUTHORS

**JAMIE G. ANDERSON, DVM, MS**
Diplomate, American Veterinary Dental College; Diplomate, American College of Veterinary Internal Medicine; Adjunct Professor, Department of Oral Medicine, School of Dental Medicine, University of Pennsylvania, Philadelphia, Pennsylvania, USA

**KRISTIN M. BANNON, DVM**
Fellow Academy of Veterinary Dentistry, Diplomate, American Veterinary Dental College; Practical Veterinary Dentistry, Algodones, New Mexico, USA

**MARY L. BERG, BS, LATG, RVT, VTS (Dentistry)**
Beyond the Crown Veterinary Education, Lawrence, Kansas, USA

**ANA C. CASTEJÓN-GONZÁLEZ, DVM, PhD**
Diplomate, American Veterinary Dental College; Diplomate, European Veterinary Dental College; Department of Clinical Sciences and Advanced Medicine, School of Veterinary Medicine, University of Pennsylvania, Philadelphia, Pennsylvania, USA

**CURT COFFMAN, DVM**
Diplomate, American Veterinary Dental College; Arizona Veterinary Dental Specialists, Scottsdale, Arizona, USA

**ERIC M. DAVIS, DVM**
Animal Dental Specialists of Upstate New York, Fayetteville, New York, USA

**JEANETTE M. ELIASON, CVT, RDH, VTS (Dentistry)**
The University of Pennslyvania - School of Veterinary Medicine, Levittown, Pennsylvania, USA

**STEPHANIE GOLDSCHMIDT, BVM&S**
Diplomate, American Veterinary Dental College; Assistant Professor, Dentistry & Oral Surgery, University of Minnesota, St Paul, Minnesota, USA

**COLIN HARVEY, BVSc, FRCVS**
Diplomate, American College of Veterinary Surgeons; Diplomate, American Veterinary Dental College; Owner, Colin Harvey LLC, Cherry Hill, New Jersey; Professor Emeritus, School of Veterinary Medicine, University of Pennsylvania, Philadelphia, Pennsylvania, USA

**PHILIPPE HENNET, DV**
Diplomate, American Veterinary Dental College; Diplomate, European Veterinary Dental College; Oromaxillofacial Dentistry and Surgery Unit, ADVETIA Centre Hospitalier Vétérinaire, Vélizy-Villacoublay, France

**BRIAN HEWITT, DVM**
Diplomate, American Veterinary Dental College; Cheyenne West Animal Hospital, Las Vegas, Nevada, USA

**NAOMI HOYER, DVM**
Diplomate, American Veterinary Dental College; Assistant Professor, Dentistry & Oral Surgery, Colorado State University, Fort Collins, Colorado, USA

**STEPHEN JURIGA, DVM**
Diplomate, American Veterinary Dental College; Veterinary Dental Center, Aurora, Illinois, USA

**CHARLES LOTHAMER, DVM**
Diplomate, American Veterinary Dental College Clinical Assistant Professor, University of Tennessee College of Veterinary Medicine, Knoxville, Tennessee, USA

**BRENDA L. MULHERIN, DVM**
Diplomate, American Veterinary Dental College; Clinical Professor, Department of Veterinary Clinical Sciences, College of Veterinary Medicine, Iowa State University Lloyd Veterinary Medical Center, Ames, Iowa, USA

**ALEXANDER M. REITER, Dipl Tzt, Dr Med Vet**
Diplomate, American Veterinary Dental College; Diplomate, European Veterinary Dental College; Founding Fellow AVDC-OMFS, Professor of Dentistry and Oral Surgery, Head of the Dentistry and Oral Surgery Service, Department of Clinical Sciences and Advanced Medicine, School of Veterinary Medicine, University of Pennsylvania, Philadelphia, Pennsylvania, USA

**CHRISTOPHER J. SNYDER, DVM**
Diplomate, American Veterinary Dental College; Clinical Professor, University of Wisconsin-Madison, School of Veterinary Medicine, Madison, Wisconsin, USA

**JASON W. SOUKUP, DVM**
Diplomate, American Veterinary Dental College; Dentistry and Oromaxillofacial Surgery, Department of Surgical Sciences, University of Wisconsin-Madison, School of Veterinary Medicine, Madison, Wisconsin, USA

**SHARON STARTUP, DVM**
Animal Dental Services, Mount Pleasant, South Carolina, USA

**GRAHAM P. THATCHER, DVM**
Diplomate, American Veterinary Dental College; Founding Fellow, Oromaxillofacial Surgery, Department of Surgical Sciences, University of Wisconsin-Madison, School of Veterinary Medicine, Madison, Wisconsin, USA

**ANSON J. TSUGAWA, VMD**
Diplomate, American Veterinary Dental College; Dog and Cat Dentist, Culver City, California, USA

**LENIN A. VILLAMIZAR-MARTINEZ, DVM, MS, PhD**
Diplomate, American Veterinary Dental College; North Carolina State University College of Veterinary Medicine, Department of Clinical Sciences, Raleigh, North Carolina, USA

**J. SCOTT WEESE, DVM, DVSc**
Ontario Veterinary College, University of Guelph, Guelph, Ontario, Canada

# Contents

Veterinary practices should consider designing and equipping a dedicated space to provide companion animal dental and oral surgical care. A single or multi-table dental suite design will allow organized and efficient delivery of dental care. Each workstation should be equipped with a procedural table that will allow for drainage, shadow-free procedural lighting, an anesthetic machine with monitoring, thermal support, anesthetic scavenger system, dental radiographic equipment, and an air-driven dental delivery system. Lift tables, dental-specific seating, swivel handpieces, and headlamp/surgical loupe lighting should also be considered to improve ergonomics.

Communication is the basis of any relationship. Communication can help strengthen the relationship between veterinarians, their clients, and their colleagues throughout the profession. Different models of communication have been demonstrated including the directive model, consumerism model, and relationship-centered model. When veterinarians refer to a specialist, they view the referral as an extension of the care they provide. Therefore, developing a relationship with the specialist is an important facet of patient care. Creating an appropriate veterinary–client–patient relationship (VCPR) helps the patient receive the best care possible. This needs to be considered when offering telemedicine or teledentistry to clients or referring veterinarians.

It is important to remember that dentistry is one area of the veterinary practice that veterinary technicians/nurses/hygienists can take ownership of and drive the dental program forward under the supervision of a veterinarian. With proper training they can perform all skills except diagnosis and surgery. The veterinary technician/nurse/hygienist should educate the client about the dental procedure, perform a thorough oral examination and report findings on the dental chart, take dental radiographs, perform dental scaling and polishing, administer nerve blocks, administer perioceutics, maintain instruments and equipment, and provide discharge and home care instructions to the pet owner.

The main objective of oral and maxillofacial (OMF) tumor resection is to get local control of the disease. Many OMF tumors can be cured with wide or radical surgery, whereas others might only achieve temporary local control of the disease by removing gross disease, infection and the source of pain, thereby improving the quality of life of the patient while keeping masticatory function. The standard of care on managing OMF tumors includes the diagnosis and identification of the local and distant extension of the disease to establish an appropriate treatment plan tailored for each patient. In this article, we provide a practical review of the current information related to staging, biopsy, and main surgical techniques for OMF tumor removal.

Maxillofacial trauma is a common presentation in veterinary medical practice. Accurate assessment, diagnostics, pain management, and finally repair are tenants to treatment. In addition to typical tenants for fracture repair, the restoration of occlusion and return to function (eating, drinking, grooming) are unique to trauma management in these patients. Options for repair include conservative management (tape muzzles), noninvasive repair techniques (interdental wiring and composite splinting), and invasive repair techniques (interfragmentary wiring and plate and screw fixation).

# VETERINARY CLINICS OF NORTH AMERICA: SMALL ANIMAL PRACTICE

**FORCOMING ISSUES**

*March 2022*
**Soft Tissue Surgery**
Nicole J. Buote, *Editor*

*May 2022*
**Hot Topics in Small Animal Medicine**
Lisa Powell, *Editor*

*July 2022*
**Small Animal Orthopedic Medicine**
Felix Duerr and Lindsay Elam, *Editor*

**RECENT ISSUES**

*November 2021*
**Diagnostic Imaging: Point-of-Care Ultrasound**
Gregory R. Lisciandro, Jennifer M. Gambino, *Editors*

*September 2021*
**Effective Communication in Veterinary Medicine**
Christopher A. Adin, Kelly D. Farnsworth, *Editors*

*July 2021*
**Working Dogs: An Update for Veterinarians**
Maureen A. McMichael, Melissa Singletary, *Editors*

---

**SERIES OF RELATED INTEREST**

*Veterinary Clinics of North America: Exotic Animal Practice*
https://www.vetexotic.theclinics.com/

---

**THE CLINICS ARE NOW AVAILABLE ONLINE!**
Access your subscription at:
www.theclinics.com

# Preface

# It's not Just Dentistry, It's Dentistry *and Oral Surgery*!

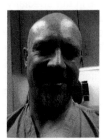

Alexander M. Reiter, Dipl Tzt, Dr Med Vet
*Editor*

When I completed my residency at the University of Pennsylvania School of Veterinary Medicine (Penn Vet) in 2000, I felt comfortable performing a number of dental and oral surgical diagnostic and therapeutic procedures in dogs and cats. They included oral examination, dental radiography, nerve blocks, dental cleaning, periodontal surgery, tooth extraction, endodontic treatment, restorations and prosthodontic crowns, oral tumor resections, jaw fracture repair, palate defect surgery, temporomandibular joint procedures, and regional lymph node and salivary gland resections. But the name of our hospital service at that time was still the "Dental Service." In 2006, I reached out to Penn Vet's leadership and proposed a name change. *"Changing the service name by adding '... and Oral Surgery' will demonstrate the actual work done in our service and provides more opportunities for the service personnel to be recognized as experts in their specialty."* From that time on, our service was known as the Dentistry and Oral Surgery Service!

I want to thank Elsevier for the opportunity to be the guest editor of this issue of *Veterinary Clinics of North America: Small Animal Practice*. We have come a long way. Small animal dentistry issues of *Veterinary Clinics of North America: Small Animal Practice* have been published in 1986, 1992 (feline), 1998 (canine), 2005, and 2013. Conditions impacting the health of the masticatory apparatus can affect many tissues and structures of the mouth, pharynx, upper neck, and surrounding areas. They include teeth, periodontal tissues, jaw bones, facial bones, oral mucosa, tongue, palate, lips, cheeks, palatine tonsils, temporomandibular joints, masticatory muscles, regional lymph nodes, salivary glands, and skin of the face and upper neck. When I was asked to serve as guest editor of this issue of *Veterinary Clinics of North America: Small Animal Practice*, my wish that the topic be called "Dentistry and Oral Surgery" was granted without hesitation. Diplomates of the American Veterinary Dental College (AVDC) are recognized as leaders in their specialty, and those that excel in oral and

Vet Clin Small Anim 52 (2022) xi–xii
https://doi.org/10.1016/j.cvsm.2021.10.001
0195-5616/22/© 2021 Published by Elsevier Inc.

**vetsmall.theclinics.com**

maxillofacial surgery (OMFS) may become Fellows of AVDC-OMFS. It is my hope that this collection of articles will help update all veterinary professionals so that they can offer the very best recommendations and latest treatment options for their patients.

I have chosen Drs Juriga and Startup to provide advice on how to design and equip a modern dentistry and oral surgery suite. Drs Mulherin and Bannon discuss the importance of communication, establishing a veterinary-client-patient relationship, and aspects of teledentistry. Mary Berg and Jeanette Eliason highlight the role veterinary technicians and dental hygienists play on a daily basis in our specialty field. Drs Villamizar-Martinez and Tsugawa cover routine and advanced diagnostic imaging to understand oral and maxillofacial anatomy and pathology. Drs Davis and Weese explain the oral microbiome in dogs and cats and critically discuss the use of antimicrobial therapy in dental and oral surgical patients. Dr Harvey offers an insight about the evidence of the relationship between periodontal infection and systemic and distant organ disease. Drs Goldschmidt and Hoyer report about the management of dental and oral developmental conditions in dogs and cats. Drs Anderson and Hennet share with us their views on the diagnosis and treatment of severe oral inflammatory conditions. Drs Hewitt and Coffman provide an update on endodontic, restorative, and prosthodontic therapy. Drs Thatcher and Soukup discuss emerging topics of virtual surgical planning and 3D printing in dentistry and oromaxillofacial surgery. Dr Castejon-Gonzalez and I describe the management of oral and maxillofacial tumor patients from biopsy to surgical resection. Drs Snyder and Lothamer explain patient triage, first aid care, and the management of oral and maxillofacial trauma.

I thank these exceptional authors for sharing their experience, expertise, and contributions to this issue. The reader will greatly benefit from the wealth of knowledge that is expressed in these well-written articles.

Alexander M. Reiter, Dipl Tzt, Dr Med Vet
Department of Clinical Sciences and
Advanced Medicine
School of Veterinary Medicine
University of Pennsylvania
MJR-VHUP #3111
3900 Delancey Street
Philadelphia, PA 19104, USA

*E-mail address:*
reiter@vet.upenn.edu

# Designing and Equipping a Modern Dentistry and Oral Surgery Suite

Stephen Juriga, DVM[a],*, Sharon Startup, DVM[b]

## KEYWORDS

- Room design • Dental X-ray • Veterinary dental suite • Anesthesia for dentistry
- Dental table • Ergonomics

## KEY POINTS

- Dental services require a dedicated space designed and equipped specifically for dentistry and oral surgery.
- The size and design of the space must consider the workstation(s), cabinetry, equipment, and space for support staff needed to provide excellent care.
- Anesthesia with intubation, physiologic support (IV fluid administration, warmth), and monitoring by a dedicated, trained team member is necessary to perform a Comprehensive Oral Health Assessment and Treatment (COHAT).
- Intraoral radiography is an essential diagnostic tool that should be used in every dental procedure.
- Improved ergonomics, improved workflows, and team and patient staff safety are a priority.

When designing a veterinary practice, ideally the dental suite is a new build and can be organized without compromise in terms of space for ideal workflow, equipment needs, and equipment placement. The benefit to patients and the revenue produced in a well-run dentistry practice more than warrant the additional effort to design a functional space. The best design and equipment equates to the best care and the best productivity.

However, the layout of the dental suite is often an afterthought, and multiple compromises with the space are made. This can be seen in university practices, large multi-specialty referral centers, and private practices alike. The popularity of dentistry within these practices has grown exponentially in recent years. The surge of interest in dentistry underlies the importance of appropriate design and space organization to maximize care.

[a] Veterinary Dental Center, 345 Sullivan Road, Aurora, IL 60506, USA; [b] Animal Dental Services, 985 Johnnie Dodds Boulevard, Mount Pleasant, SC 29464, USA
* Corresponding author.
E-mail address: stephenjuriga@yahoo.com

Vet Clin Small Anim 52 (2022) 1–23
https://doi.org/10.1016/j.cvsm.2021.09.001          vetsmall.theclinics.com

The space necessary for an effective dental suite depends on its separation from other services. In many cases, the dental suite is seen as a multi-use space. However, as practitioners of all types, from dental specialists to general practitioners, become more adept and educated about dentistry and oral surgery, the design of a fully equipped and autonomous work area becomes essential. As treatment becomes more comprehensive, the length of the dental procedure and productivity per patient increase. This in turn produces more revenue per square footage. As the scope of treatment broadens, interruptions of the shared space by other services become unacceptable. A productive dental practice has little if any downtime and a multiuse space is not conducive to providing high quality, efficient care.

## EXAMINATION ROOM

Good dentistry begins in the reception area with an educated client care coordinator, available literature, and educational media. It is in the examination room whereby the oral examination begins and whereby the client's education on the subject matter expands. It is of paramount importance to have educated team members who support the practice of dentistry and are committed to the oral health of their patients.

In the examination room, information about the patient's history and the owner's commitment to their pets' ongoing oral care is obtained. A thorough oral examination is performed, and educational tools (**Box 1**) such as clear acrylic dental models and real skull models are used to educate the client. Photographs taken by a smartphone can be exported to a computer monitor to illustrate oral pathological condition that requires treatment. An atlas of intraoral photography and dental radiography can be bound or archived on the examination room computer to be reviewed with the pet owner. The value of sharing photographs and dental X-ray images for the client's understanding of their pet's dental disease and treatment cannot be over-emphasized.

The oral examination completed during the initial visit allows the doctor to formulate a preliminary diagnostic plan which should be given to the pet owner in a written format. The veterinary technician or veterinarian should then discuss preanesthetic testing, anesthesia for the dental patient, the steps of a Comprehensive Oral Health

---

**Box 1**
**Examination room supplies**

- Client handouts
- Camera or smartphone
- Skull models
  - Acrylic or bone
- Brochures
  - Benefits of oral health
  - Anesthesia[a]
- Dental report card
- Dental charts/posters
- Dental newsletter
- Photo guide to a complete dental procedure

[a] https://catfriendly.com/brochures/anesthesia.pdf.

Assessment and Treatment procedure (COHAT), and the expected workflow for the procedure day.

## DEDICATED DENTAL SPACE

The American Animal Hospital Association (AAHA) guidelines state that companion animal dental procedures require an efficient, organized, and safe work environment.[1,2] As dental procedures result in aerosolized bacteria and intraoral radiography causes radiation, hospitals need to provide a dedicated space for these procedures, preferably in a low traffic area of the hospital.[1-3] This may be a separate room or an alcove commonly found near the treatment room. Proximity to the treatment room is important, as it allows access to the doctors and other support staff. Staff and doctors dedicated to the dental procedure should not be attempting to multitask, as it interferes with the quality and efficiency of care.

Veterinarians should consider a professional design team such as an architect or design services available through equipment distributors https://www.midmark.com/docs/default-source/product-literature/animal-health/007-10268-00-comprehensive-dentistry.pdf?sfvrsn=ccb5c48_12. Considering the prevalence of dental disease and the potential caseload of practice, many architects design a dental space with room for multiple tables to allow a practice to leverage their equipment and staff for efficiency. For example, a single wall-mounted X-ray generator with a long arm can provide imaging for 2 tables if positioned correctly.

AAHA's Animal Design Strategies for Better Care recommend:

- A 9-foot minimum space width requirement allows 36″ of space on either side of the table.
- An 8-foot minimum space depth allows adequate room for a 60″ table.
- A 10′ x 17′ space should be considered for a 2-table setup.
- The space should have the adequate square footage for rolling equipment, adequate electrical outlets, countertop, and cabinet space for the materials/instrumentation used to provide comprehensive veterinary dental services.[3]

To design the dental operatory that best meets the individual practitioner's needs, it is helpful to first understand what makes up the ideal dental suite in terms of form and function. Below is a brief discussion of what and who is required for a functional dental operatory. Each of these components occupies space and requires planning in terms of square footage, design options, and equipment[4] (**Boxes 2 and 3**).

## SPACE FOR EQUIPMENT AND STAFF

Dental procedures can be lengthy and require many body and head manipulations, so it is necessary to have a dedicated anesthesia technician or anesthesiologist monitor each patient for the highest level of safety. Each anesthesia technician or anesthesiologist requires both a workspace and their own equipment. The person performing anesthesia needs to be able to move around and toward the patient on one side for monitoring. Anesthesia machines, IV stands and pumps, multiparameter monitoring devices, and a workstation for logging information need to be within the reach of the anesthetist. Hand-held tablets are often used, but these still need a work surface to be placed on, as the anesthetist needs their hands free for physical monitoring, adjustment of electrical equipment, and to assist with breathing.

In dental procedures, the use of water, air/water syringes, and length of anesthesia promotes hypothermia. To keep the patient normothermic during the procedure, a

---

**Box 2**
**Pre-planning the dental space**

- Location
- Size
  - Single or multiple tables
- Ventilation/exhaust
- Lighting
  - Ambient
  - Task (wall- or ceiling-mounted)
- Electric
  - 8 outlets/table
- Plumbing
- X-ray generator type and location
- Cabinets and countertops
- Computer station(s)
- Medical gas
  - Ceiling drop, wall mount
  - Machine mounted generator
- Active scavenger
- Space for
  - Anesthesia
  - Dental delivery system
  - Staff and workflow

---

forced warm air system and water circulating blanket must be used simultaneously. The generators of these 2 devices take up space on the floor or are attached to a countertop or attached to an IV pole.

The technician performing charting, dental radiography, scaling, and polishing, as well as the clinician performing surgery, should be seated in a chair on rollers. They must have space to travel around the head of the patient so that the operator moves whereas the patient can remain stationary. This requires that the space around the head of the table is open without encumbrances.

There should be at least 8 electrical outlets per table. Planning outlet placement to prevent wire clutter and workflow disruptions is important. Lighting is of paramount importance in dentistry because of the need to operate in the dark cavity of the mouth. High-quality surgery lights are recommended in addition to lighting integrated within surgical loupes. The lighting should be flexible to accommodate all the various views and angles needed for an oral examination and treatment.

There needs to be room for the dental delivery unit and the X-ray generator. Surfaces must be clear for surgery and dental instruments. Additionally, it is necessary to have plenty of cabinet space for anesthesia supplies such as endotracheal tubes, bags, and blood pressure cuffs. Storage for supplies such as burs, suture, needles, syringes, towels, and gloves should also be considered. A work cabinet on wheels for equipment such as dental luxators and elevators, other surgical instruments, syringes, and needles for nerve blocks can be considered.

When designing a dental suite, the authors recommend using cardboard templates of the equipment placed on the floor within the allotted square footage and staff

---

**Box 3**
**Equipping the space**

- Dental (task) lighting
  - LED ceiling-mounted
  - Headlamp light
- Dental table or tub
  - Plumbed wet table
  - Unplumbed collection style
- Dental-specific seating
- Dental X-ray generator
  - Wall, mobile, or handheld
- Digital imaging/receptor
  - DR sensor
  - CR phosphor plate
  - Film
- Computer
  - Laptop, desktop, or wall-mounted monitor
- Dental delivery equipment (mobile or mounted on an arm)
  - High-speed handpiece(s)
  - Low-speed handpiece
  - Air-water syringe
- Powered scaler
  - Ultrasonic or piezoelectric
- Suction
- Instrument table/surface

---

positioned within the area. This helps visualize and understand the best use of space, the need for space between equipment, and can help with crucial decisions around how to use floor, wall, and ceiling space.

## ROOM DESIGN

The best use of space for a dental suite has at least 2 operating stations to accommodate present and future patient load. Some examples of dental room designs are illustrated and discussed here. There are 3 basic designs with many variations of each of these for veterinary dental operatories. These 3 basic designs are the alcove/single-table room design, the multi-table room design, and the multipurpose chase design.

The single-table design may be planned in an alcove, remote area of the treatment room (**Fig. 1**) or as a separate room. The depth of the room should be at least 8 feet for the alcove design. If enclosed as a separate room, the door should be strategically placed, and it should be several feet deeper to allow staff and gurneys with patients to easily pass behind a seated staff member.

The 2-table design (**Figs. 2 and 3**) places both tables on the same wall. There should be a minimum of 5 feet of clearance between tables and adjacent walls.[4] This will allow technicians to have access to their patients and to move freely around the space. This design can be used for rooms with 1 or 2 operating tables and is often expanded to many more. This allows for plumbing (if required), electricity, and cabinetry to be run along one wall. Space should be available for up to 5 staff members, allowing for 1 anesthetist at each table, and 1 person performing dentistry at each table. For

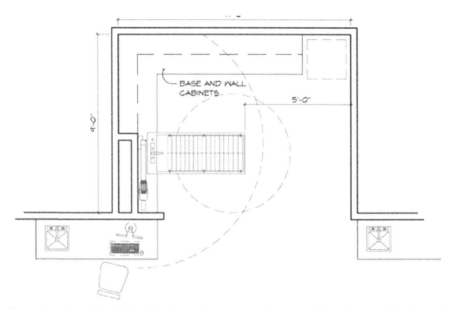

**Fig. 1.** Drawing of a single table alcove design. Note the space allotted around the head of the table in this floor plan. (*Courtesy of* Vicki J. Pollard, AIA, CVT, Ashley M. Shoults, AIA, and Animal Arts Design Studios.)

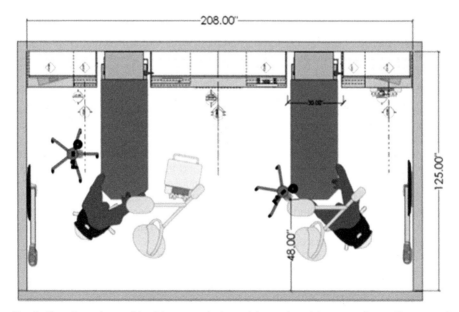

**Fig. 2.** Drawing of a multi-table room design with ample cabinetry and a wall-mounted X-ray unit for each table. (*Courtesy of* Midmark Animal Health [Versailles, Ohio]: with permission.)

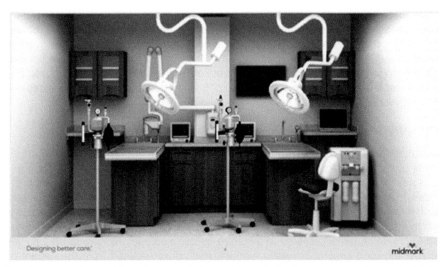

**Fig. 3.** Image of a multi-table room design with a single X-ray unit serving both tables. (*Courtesy of* Midmark Animal Health [Versailles, Ohio]: with permission.)

"four-handed" dentistry, at times there will be 3 people at one table (1 anesthetist and 2 staff performing four-handed dentistry). With either design, the X-ray generators are wall mounted, and lights are ceiling mounted, so they are out of the way of workflow. Note the ample cabinetry and countertop space in each design.

The multipurpose chase design (**Fig. 4**) allows for more freedom in the placement of plumbed or nonplumbed tables. This may serve as a multi-purpose workstation in a

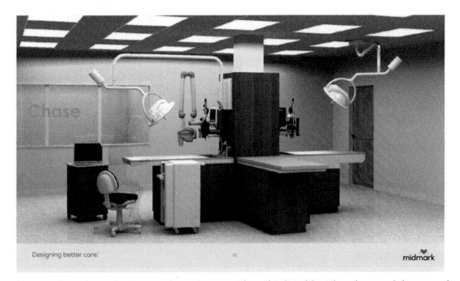

**Fig. 4.** Image of a multipurpose chase design with multiple tables placed around the central column that provides access to plumbing, electric, and allows for the mounting of anesthesia, dental X-ray, and lighting. (*Courtesy of* Midmark Animal Health [Versailles, Ohio]: with permission.)

nondedicated dental workspace which is not recommended by the authors. Dental workspaces should be dedicated and separated for the safety of the staff. One note of warning is that the length of dental procedures is unpredictable, and the next patient should never be anesthetized before the previous patient procedure is at a predictable time level to completion (ie, suturing closed or finishing a dental cleaning). To keep patients under anesthesia for the convenience of the clinician is unethical and causes unnecessary risk or harm to the patient.

## VENTILATION/EXHAUST

Ventilation (heating and cooling) must be provided in the appropriate cubic feet per minute based on the equipment and staff present in the dental space. Sufficient cooling is necessary for the heat gain calculated within the space. Heat gain per table includes, but is not limited to, a minimum of 2 staff members, patient, warm air blanket/warm water blanket, and lighting. Remember that halogen task lighting produces more heat than LED lighting. Addition of an exhaust fan above the dental table is recommended to create negative pressure to minimize aerosolized bacteria spread.[5] It also will exhaust escaped anesthetic gases, vapors, and odors released from the patient or radiosurgery/laser surgery. HVAC contractors will provide the analysis for ventilation supply and exhaust.

## AMBIENT LIGHTING

Ambient lighting provides illumination to the entire workspace. In the past, this was accomplished with fluorescent fixtures and different color temperature bulbs (measured in Kelvin). Reception and client spaces typically have incandescent or fluorescent bulbs of a warmer tone (2,800K).[6] However, it is preferable to have "whiter" color temperature similar to daylight (5,500K) in the treatment room or dental operatory.[5] This provides a consistent true "color" when monitoring mucous membranes, performing oral surgery or using photography to document pathological condition and treatment. Fortunately, LED fixtures have become the standard in construction and the preferred color temperature can be selected for the illumination of the dental space (4,100K–5,500K).

Task or operatory lighting can be mobile, ceiling, or wall mounted. Confirm the arm length reaches the table end to illuminate the oral cavity for the induction of anesthesia and procedure illumination. If possible, it is beneficial to have an exterior window in the operatory. This creates a pleasant atmosphere for the staff and depending on the tint of the windows can improve the color balance of oral tissue.

## ELECTRIC/PLUMBING

The dental space must have a minimum of 8 outlets per workstation that are strategically placed to power the dental delivery system/compressor, powered scaler, IV fluid pump, anesthetic monitor, warming devices, lift table (if included), computer, charging station for tablets, or camera. Plumbing requirements depend on whether the design will include plumbed wet table or unplumbed collection tables.

## X-RAY GENERATOR

Dental radiology has become the standard of care and is mandatory for the practice of veterinary dentistry. They can be wall mounted, mobile floor-mounted, or handheld.[4,7,8] A wall mounted X-ray generator has a retractable arm that can fold flat against the wall when not in use. When designing the dental room makes sure the placement of the unit does not interfere with cabinetry or workflow. The dental X-ray arm needs to be able to reach the head of the patient[3] and should not interfere with the work of other operators when X-ray is in use. For 2 tables, one wall- or ceiling-mounted unit could reach 2 table heads, as there are many arm lengths available (56″, 66″, 76″, and 82″).

As an alternative to a wall- or ceiling-mounted unit, a mobile floor X-ray unit mounted on a stand with rollers can be purchased. This unit can be reached multiple treatment tables. However, it has a large footprint, and room design must take this piece of equipment into consideration. Due to their bulk and size and the additional clutter they create, most practitioners prefer wall mounted units.

A handheld unit is another consideration, as it may be used at multiple tables or in other rooms in the hospital. It is the hospital's responsibility to purchase an FDA and State approved handheld device to ensure personnel safety.[9]

## CABINETRY/COUNTERTOPS

Cabinet space for all materials needed in dentistry must be considered. Some operators prefer to have instruments stored in a rolling cabinet for easy access during procedures. There must also be space for all the materials needed in anesthesia such as endotracheal tubes, blood pressure cuffs, fluids, needles, and syringes. Storage of warming blankets and towels within the suite is needed. Consider workspace needed for handheld tablets or written anesthesia logs and dental charting.

## MEDICAL GAS/SCAVENGER LOCATION

Preplanning the anesthetic machine location within the operatory will direct the location of oxygen and active anesthetic gas scavenger outlets.[3,4] Oxygen can be supplied by a ceiling drop, wall outlet, or a machine-mounted tank or oxygen generator. Alternatively, a machine-mounted tank or oxygen concentrator can be used. Active scavenger systems are recommended.[1,5] Hospitals with an existing active system may add one or more outlets depending on the capacity of their unit. Active systems have an exhaust fan mounted on an outside wall and plastic pipe routed to the desired location.

## DENTAL TASK LIGHTING

Task lighting refers to the operatory light used to illuminate the oral cavity. The ideal task light should provide sufficient illumination, should not produce shadows, and have optimal color rendition.[6] Operatory lights are equipped with either halogen or light-emitting diode (LED) and are commonly mounted to the ceiling or wall in veterinary settings. The ideal light should provide a white, shadow-free illumination (large diameter) with adjustable brightness. LED lights have low heat emission and long life. Headlamp or loupe light is a spotlight preferred by some clinicians. Studies have shown that headlamps improve ergonomics by encouraging a neutral position and reducing eye strain.[10] LED is the most popular choice, as they produce a cool, white light that lasts much longer than halogen. Light intensity and color rendering vary between products.

## DENTAL OPERATING TABLE

The clinician can choose from a plumbed wet table/tub or unplumbed collection table design.[11] Each of these tables is available in 48″ and 60″ lengths. The 48″ work length will not accommodate very large breed dogs, so it is recommended to have at least one 60″ table in the operatory. Wet tables/tubs traditionally are fixed at a height of 36″ with cabinetry beneath for storage. A better choice is a plumbed dental lift table that can adjust in height from 9″ above the floor to 44" (**Fig. 5**). This table design is self-supporting, raised and lowered by an electric motor, and has a hand sprayer.

Collection tables have become very popular because they do not require any fixed plumbing. This saves on cost and requires less space. These tables use a device under the patient's head to collect the fluids generated in a dental procedure (**Fig. 6**). They can be adjusted for height by a footswitch and electric motor, allowing the operator to accommodate their individual height, and therefore meet the needs of any staff member. Dental-specific design options provide for an integrated compressor, articulating arm(s) for an anesthetic machine, dental delivery system, work surface tray, or IV pole (ie, Olympic Advanced Dental Table and Surgiden). Moreover, these tables are designed with locking casters that allow easy repositioning of the table within the room.

## SEATING

An adjustable table and a dental-specific chair will improve ergonomics. The goal is to allow the operator to sit at the table with their forearms and wrists resting on the tabletop, with their knees under the table, and feet underneath their center of gravity. The chair should have height adjustment, support the back, and facilitate a neutral posture.[12] This can be accomplished with a dental-specific chair (**Fig. 7**) with waterfall front edges, adjustable seat height, adjustable backrest to support the lower back, and a seat that allows tipping forward to open the operators' hip angle over 90°. Another type of dental seating to consider is the saddle stool design, as it has gained popularity in human dentistry (**Fig. 8**). Saddle stool design promotes a neutral pelvic position and maintains the lumbar curve to place the clinician and assistant(s) in an ergonomically correct position[13]. Ergonomics are of paramount importance for sustaining the health of doctors and staff and for producing quality work. Physical discomfort leads to impatience which decreases work quality.[14]

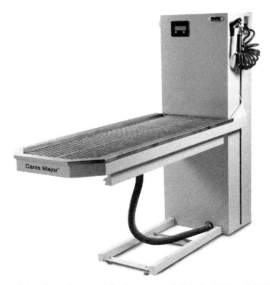

**Fig. 5.** Adjustable height dental wet table that is available in 48″ and 60″ sizes. (*Courtesy of* Midmark Animal Health [Versailles, Ohio]: with permission.)

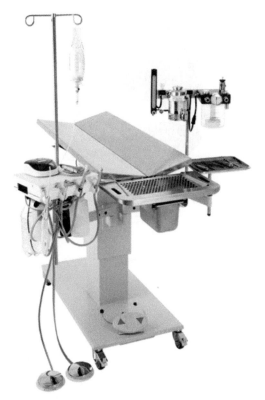

**Fig. 6.** Adjustable height collection dental table with swing arms to allow the mounting of a dental delivery system, anesthesia machine, or other equipment. (*Courtesy of* Olympic Veterinary [Mercer Island, WA] with permission.)

## DENTAL IMAGING

One of the most important decisions the practitioner must make when designing the dental operatory is what type of dental X-ray system will be used. Conventional screen-film radiography is no longer recommended and is now seldomly seen in modern veterinary practice. Unnecessary use of chemicals (developer and fixer), problems with discarding and maintaining these chemicals, the time consumption of hand or automatic processing, and inconsistency in quality make a conventional film no longer desirable. Digital systems are preferred over film-based systems, as they provide superior image quality and are available with veterinary software. Digital systems require significantly less radiation than film-based imaging, decreasing the amount of radiation which increases the safety to the patient and staff.[7] Digital systems use either a wired sensor *(digital radiography [DR or direct system])* or a phosphor plate *(computed radiography [CR or indirect system])*[4] (**Fig. 9**).

The DR system has a #2 rigid size sensor connected to a computer by a USB cord and provides an image to be viewed within 5 seconds on a computer screen. The sensor is ready within seconds for the next image and therefore can be acquired as soon as the sensor and tube head are repositioned. CR systems use a phosphor plate that is placed into a protective sleeve. Once the radiograph is taken, the phosphor plate is removed from the protective sleeve and placed into a scanner. The scanner is connected to a computer, and the image appears on a computer screen. The CR

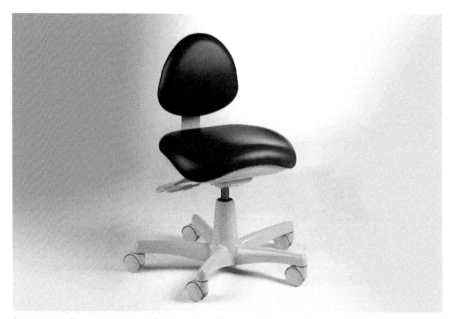

**Fig. 7.** Dental operators stool designed to allow multiple seat sizes, seat heights, and adjustability for improved comfort. (*Courtesy of* Midmark Animal Health [Versailles, Ohio]: with permission.)

plates are thin, flexible, and available in a variety of sizes (#0, #2, #4, #6 sizes) allowing imaging of larger teeth, jaw fractures, or maxillofacial tumors. When plates are fed through a scanner, the image is viewed within 20 to 30 seconds. CR plates are inexpensive to replace, should they become destroyed, and it is common to have multiple plates of each size in case one becomes damaged, so that the day's work can continue. Each system has its advantages and disadvantages (**Box 4**), with the best system chosen to match the needs of the practice.[3,7]

Image quality depends a great deal on the software used to process the image. Software allows for the manipulation and enhancement of the image and integration with veterinary software. Images are viewed on a computer screen which allows for image enhancement, magnification, and sharing with the clients. Images can easily be emailed to a specialist for interpretation or consultation.

There are many systems available to veterinarians with differences in image quality, software capabilities, software user-friendliness, vendor support, and training. Each practice should assess their needs, caseload, and compare systems with an experienced vendor and consult with a Diplomate of the American Veterinary Dental College (www.avdc.org) or European Veterinary Dental College (www.evdc.org) in your region.

Cone-beam computed tomography (CBCT) has become an essential imaging modality for dental and oral surgical referral practices. It provides increased detail of dentoalveolar and maxillofacial hard tissues and a higher diagnostic yield than dental radiography.[15]

## COMPUTER

Computer stations are needed for access to the hospital software and for interface with dental X-ray.[3] Laptop computers may be located on an adjacent counter or swing

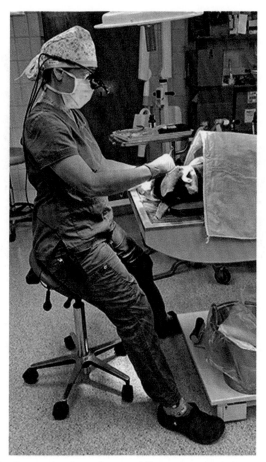

**Fig. 8.** Photograph of a veterinarian using a saddle stool promoting a neutral spine position for improved ergonomics.

arm/shelf. Wall-mounted workstations (ie, www.ergotron.com) are available with articulating arms for the display, keyboard, and mouse, or as compact units with a keyboard that folds to within 3.5″ of the wall in the storage position. The monitor can be placed in the operatory within direct view of the DVM.[4] This allows the assessment of the dental radiographs for diagnosis and treatment planning as well as postoperative evaluation. The authors use patient workflow software (ie, SmartFlow) that uses a large TV to display each patient's status and integrates with dental charting and anesthetic monitoring on tablets (**Fig. 10**).

## DENTAL DELIVERY SYSTEM

Dental delivery systems (**Fig. 11**) are powered by pressurized air from a compressor connected to the unit.[4] There are 2 basic styles of dental delivery systems: external compressor systems and built-in compressor systems. With external compressor systems, the compressor can be placed in a basement or a closet. This eliminates room noise and allows multiple dental delivery units to be run off one compressor. Careful

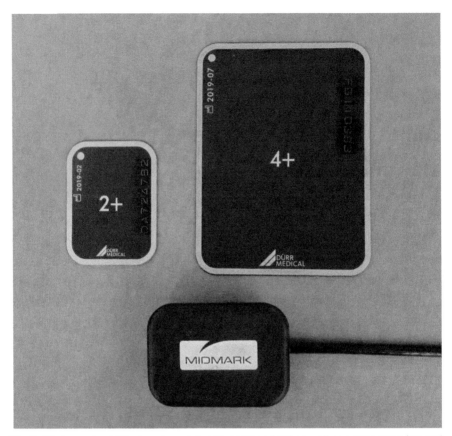

**Fig. 9.** Photograph of CR phosphor plates (sizes #2 and #4) as well as a DR sensor (#2 size). (*Courtesy of* IM3. Inc- The Veterinary Dental Company and Midmark Animal Health [Versailles, Ohio]: with permission.)

placement of air and suction lines is an important consideration with this style of the delivery system.

The main advantage to the built-in compressor systems is their mobility. These units plug into an electric outlet and can be repositioned for operator preference. These systems have refillable water bottles as the water source for the handpieces and powered scaler, eliminating a water line running from the plumbing source to the unit.

Dental delivery units have a high-speed handpiece (to remove alveolar bone, section multi-rooted teeth, smooth sharp boney surfaces), a low-speed handpiece (to polish teeth), and an air–water syringe (to rinse the mouth before, during, and after procedures).[8] Depending on the design or manufacturer, the unit may be equipped with suction, a fiberoptic light source, an integrated power scaler, and dual water reservoirs. Moreover, practitioners should consider units equipped with 2 high-speed handpieces which will enhance workflow by eliminating the need for removing one bur to replace it with another.

High-speed handpieces and ultrasonic scalers can be illuminated by fiber optics or LED lighting integrated into their handpieces to provide detailed illumination to the operative field.[16] Also, high- and low-speed handpieces are available with a swivel design for better ergonomics, reducing, hand, and wrist fatigue (**Fig. 12**). The authors

**Box 4**
**Disadvantages of digital systems**

- Digital radiography (DR or direct system)
  - The DR sensor has a small landscape/size when compared with a CR plate. In larger patients, it will often take 2 images to attain diagnostic views of a canine or molar tooth.
  - The thickness of the sensor can be difficult to place inside the mouth of very small patients for certain views, and compromises must be made.
  - The sensors are expensive and can take many days to replace should the patient's plane of anesthesia get light enough that they bite down on them and damage them.
  - The sensor can also be damaged by dropping it onto the hard surface of the floor.
  - One could consider a back-up system to prevent this unfortunate downtime.

- Computed radiography (CR or indirect system)
  - Phosphor plates require disposable plastic sleeves for protection.
  - A scanner requires countertop space.
  - Image acquisition time is slower than with DR.
  - CR systems are more cumbersome than DR systems to operate because the phosphor plate must be removed from its protective sleeve and placed into a scanner to obtain the image. The operator must either walk away from the patient to process the plate or hand it to another person for it to be processed. With practice however, radiographs can be taken with plates in succession without waiting for the previous image to appear on the screen, thus speeding up the process.
  - Phosphor plates wear and tear over time, need to be handled carefully, and with clean hands, and eventually need to be replaced.

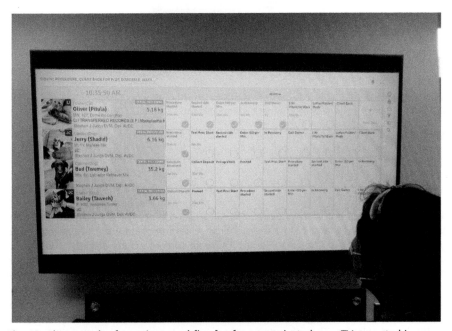

**Fig. 10.** Photograph of a patient workflow] software projected on a TV mounted in a central location of the hospital.

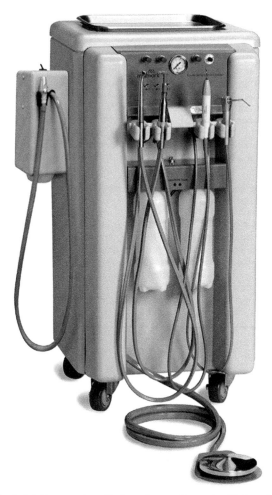

**Fig. 11.** Mobile dental delivery system that can be configured with 1 or 2 high-speed hand-pieces and suction. (*Courtesy of* Midmark Animal Health [Versailles, Ohio]: with permission.)

recommend that practices have more than 1 back-up handpiece, perform daily cleaning and maintenance/conditioning, or learning how to perform turbine replacement for high-speed handpieces.

## POWERED SCALER

Ultrasonic scalers are preferred over sonic scalers for the removal of plaque and calculus deposits above and below the gumline. Ultrasonic scalers are available in 2 types: magnetostrictive and piezoelectric.[16] These scalers vibrate at a high frequency with water-cooled tips to efficiently remove calculus as well as produce a "cavitation effect" that disrupts biofilm and destroys bacteria.

Choosing between a magnetostrictive and a piezoelectric unit is operator preference, as each handpiece and tip function somewhat differently. Magnetostrictive tip motion is elliptical, creating a rolling motion in which all sides of the tip are active on the tooth and calculus. These handpieces require more water coolant and are heavier. Piezoelectric tip motion is linear in which only the sides of the tip are used to shave off

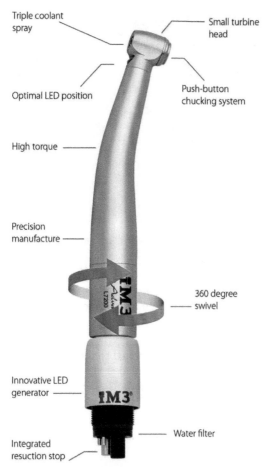

Triple coolant spray

Small turbine head

Optimal LED position

Push-button chucking system

High torque

Precision manufacture

360 degree swivel

Innovative LED generator

Water filter

Integrated resuction stop

**Fig. 12.** High-speed handpiece with integrated LED light and 360° swivel on coupling for improved ergonomics. (*Courtesy of* IM3. Inc- The Veterinary Dental Company.)

calculus. These handpieces are wider, lightweight, have less handpiece vibration, and can be considered more ergonomic. Regardless of the unit selected, the authors recommend that the practice selects one type of ultrasonic unit for multi-table operatory designs (either magnetostrictive or piezoelectric), as each type is technique sensitive, and staff only have to learn to use 1 type.

Ultrasonic scalers are available with LED lighting (**Fig. 13**) to illuminate the working area and come with a variety of tip inserts. These tips range from a thick tip to be used on large accumulations of supragingival calculus to longer thin tips designed for scaling subgingivally. A guide is used by placing the tips over a corresponding image to visualize wear and to determine if it is time for the replacement.

## ANESTHESIA FOR THE DENTAL PATIENT

Anesthesia with intubation is necessary to perform a proper cleaning of the tooth structures.[1,2] The dental operatory should be equipped similarly to the surgical operatory (**Box 5**). Hospitals should use individualized patient plans, procedure-specific anesthetic protocols, dental nerve blocks, IV fluid therapy, thermal support, and

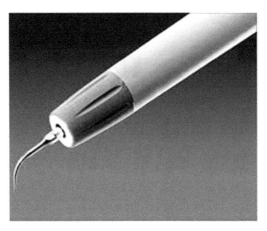

**Fig. 13.** LED Piezo ultrasonic scaler for improved illumination of the working area. (*Courtesy of* IM3. Inc- The Veterinary Dental Company.)

patient monitoring to provide patient safety and rapid recovery. Moreover, patients should be closely observed until they are alert, normothermic, and ambulatory.[17-19]

### Anesthetic machine

Depending on the size and layout of the dental space the anesthetic machine maybe rolling or mounted. Rolling anesthetic machines may connect with medical gas via a wall or ceiling outlet. Oxygen generators mount under the rolling anesthetic machines. Oxygen concentrators are cost-effective, relatively quiet, and extract oxygen from the

---

**Box 5**
**Dental anesthesia equipment**

- IV catheters
- Fluids and IV pump
- Endotracheal tubes
- Laryngoscope
- Anesthetic machine
  - Rolling or mounted
- Rebreathing tubes
- Rebreathing bags
- Nonrebreathing circuit with manometer
- Safety pop-off valve relief
- Oxygen
  - Medical gas, tank, or generator
- Monitoring (blood pressure, ECG, pulse oximeter, ETCO2, and body temperature)
- Thermal support
  - Water and hot air blanket
  - Towels and fleece

air to supply up to 4 L/min of medical grade oxygen to the machine.[20] There are FDA approved and UL tested concentrators available in the veterinary market that have a small footprint (18 x 18″) and an E tank as a backup supply.

Mounted anesthetic machines are available that attach (flush) to the wall, attach to the wall with an articulating arm (12–28″), or maybe mounted to an articulated swing arm from a dental table or wet lift table.

### Rebreathing and non-rebreathing setup

Anesthetic gases are delivered from the machine to the patient by rebreathing or non-rebreathing systems. Rebreathing systems are used in patients over 5 kg and allow lower flow rates and lower amounts of inhalants. These circuits come in 2 sizes (pediatric and adult) and various lengths (40″, 60″, and 72″). The patient's weight dictates the size of the circuit. The length of the circuit can be dictated by the location of the machine (mobile or wall-mounted) with the goal to select the minimum length to reduce dead space. Nonrebreathing circuits are commonly used in veterinary medicine, specifically for cats and small dogs less than 3 to 5 kg.[17–19,21] Two essential safety features to have on every anesthetic machine are an in-circuit manometer and a safety pop-off valve.[18,19] A manometer allows safe delivery of manual and mechanical breaths, visual indication of rise in airway pressure, and leak checking of the seal of the endotracheal tube cuff within the trachea. Safety pop-off valves prevent excessively high airway pressure and thereby prevent barotrauma. Both should be installed on every anesthesia machine.[18,19] Because the non-rebreather circuit bypasses these on the anesthesia machine, a Bain Block should be installed either on the circuit or on the anesthesia machine (**Fig. 14**).

### Checklist

Preanesthesia and procedure checklists are invaluable to ensure the procedure day goes smoothly and safely. Similar lists can be made for the end of anesthesia, end of procedure, and end of day to ensure the room is ready for the next patient and for the following day. An anesthetic safety checklist is published by the Association of Veterinary Anesthetists and can be adopted for your hospital's use (https://www.thinkanesthesia.education/sites/default/files/2019-04/AVA%20Anesthesia%20Safety%20Checklist.pdf)

### Anesthesia monitoring

There is no substitute for well-trained anesthesia monitoring personnel. Monitoring the patient should ideally not be done by the clinician performing the procedure.[22] An anesthetist should be present and on constant watch from induction of anesthesia until the patient has recovered and ambulatory. Hands-on monitoring of the patient's mucus membranes, capillary refill time, jaw tone, eye position, and pulse quality cannot be multi-tasked. The use and knowledge of a multi-parameter monitor with ECG, pulse oximetry, capnography, blood pressure, and body temperature are the responsibility of one trained person dedicated to monitoring the patient.[19,22] Although many complications occur throughout anesthesia, 47% of all dog and 60% of cat anesthetic-related deaths occur during the postoperative period, and most of those within the first 3 hours following anesthesia.[23–25]

### Thermal support

Hypothermia, core body temperature less than 98°F, can result in an array of adverse physiologic effects including delayed drug metabolism, cardiovascular dysfunction, impaired perfusion, respiratory compromise, and cerebral depression. It also

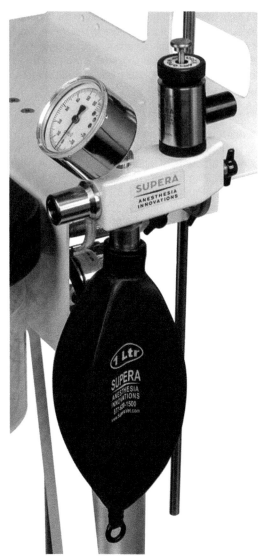

**Fig. 14.** Bain nonrebreathing circuit with a safety pop of valve. (*Courtesy of* Supera Anesthesia Innovations [Estacada, Oregon]: with permission.)

decreases clotting ability and increases the incidence of wound infection.[26] Hypothermia during anesthesia can decrease the MAC requirements of inhalant anesthetics which can result in detrimental effects on cardiac output (bradycardia). Compounding things further, hypothermia can make patients less responsive to anticholinergics when treating bradycardia during anesthesia. Delayed drug metabolism and cerebral depression can result in prolonged recovery.[27]

Maintaining normothermia or heat preservation is a goal in every dental patient, and patients should have continuous body temperature measurement. The most effective methods for patient warming are the use of warm air circulating systems and circulating warm water blankets.[18] When used simultaneously, the patient can be kept normothermic during even very lengthy dental procedures. Supplemental methods of slowing heat loss that may be helpful include warm IV fluids, use of a fluid line warmer, and insulation on the patient's feet (bubble wrap, baby socks, and so forth). The authors "sandwich" the patient in the following manner: a towel or yoga mat on the dental table, then a water circulating blanket, then fleece blanket, then patient, then forced air blanket wrapped, and then another fleece blanket. Only the patient's head is exposed, and a small folded towel is used as a head rest. This small towel can be separated from the blankets that are around the patient. This way the head towel can be replaced frequently when it gets wet and the separation between it, and the blankets under the patient are kept dry. Do not use supplemental heat sources that are not designed specifically for anesthetized patients, as they can cause severe thermal injury.

## INSTRUMENTATION

Instrumentation of a dentistry service depends on the level of care the clinician, staff, and hospital offer. Many practices design separate dental packs for examination and dental cleaning, periodontal surgery, tooth extraction, rabbit and rodent dentistry, or specialized packs for more advanced procedures. The AAHA Dental Care Guidelines recommend the instrumentation listed in **Box 6**. Dental instrumentation, their design, and intended use are beyond the scope of this article, but information is available in several references[8,16,28–31].

---

**Box 6**
**Instruments to include in a dental surgical pack**

- Retraction aid (eg, speculum, University of Minnesota retractor)
- Tartar forceps
- Scalers
- Curettes
- Probe/explorer
- Periosteal elevators
- Assortment of burs
  - Cross-cut fissure bur (701, 701L)
  - #1/4, #1/2, #1, #2, #4 carbide round burs (surgical length [S] when available)
  - Medium grit diamond burs (round, football, or cylindrical)
- Scalpel handle
- Dental luxator or elevator sets
- Extraction forceps
- Root tip pick and root tip forceps
- Miller curette or similar
- Thumb forceps (1 x 2 teeth)
- Hemostats
- Scissors (Iris, LaGrange, or Dean)
- Needle holders
- Sharpening materials

---

## SUMMARY

Excellent dental care for companion animals begins in the examination room with an oral examination and pet-owner education to deliver a preliminary diagnosis with a written treatment plan. Every veterinary facility should have a dedicated space for a dental operatory that is uniquely equipped to provide general anesthesia and dental/oral surgical services. Preplanning of the dental space depends on equipment selection, table design, and utility/supply line placement within the hospital. The environment should be an efficient, organized, and safe workspace for both patients and staff. The operating space should be a room of its own. The authors' goals are to expand the understanding and highlight the necessity of proper design and equipment for a dedicated veterinary dental operatory. We encourage the use of the 2013/2019 AAHA Dental Care Guidelines as well as AAFP and AAHA Anesthetic Guidelines when designing and equipping this space.

## DISCLOSURE

The authors have nothing to disclose.

## REFERENCES

1. Holmstrom SE, Bellows J, Juriga S, et al. 2013 AAHA dental care guidelines for dogs and cats. J Am Anim Hosp Assoc 2013;49:75–82.
2. Bellows J, Berg ML, Dennis S, et al. 2019 AAHA dental care guidelines for dogs and cats. J Am Anim Hosp Assoc 2019;55:49–69.
3. Adney J, Evers K, Freytag J, et al. Animal hospital design strategies for better care. Am Anim Hosp Assoc 2021. Available at: https://www.aaha.org/globalassets/04-practice-resources/hospitaldesignstrategies_web.pdf. Accessed February 2021.
4. McReynolds T. A practical guide to veterinary hospital design. Am Anim Hosp Assoc 2018. Available at. https://www.aaha.org/publications/newstat/articles/2018-10/a-practical-guide-to-veterinary-hospital-design/. Accessed February 2021.
5. Gladysz P. Considerations for adding a dedicated veterinary dental space. DVM 360 2020;115(7):12–3. Available at: https://cdn.sanity.io/files/0vv8moc6/dvm360/6ee2536e58047a4f6373abc24644cec32dc10db1.pdf.
6. Dianat I, Sedghi A, Bagherzade J, et al. Objective and subjective assessments of lighting in a hospital setting: implications for health, safety and performance. Ergonomics 2013;56:1535–45.
7. Niemiec B. Oral radiographic imaging. In: Lobprise HB, Dodd JR, editors. Wigg's veterinary dentistry. 2nd edition. Hoboken, NJ: Wiley & Sons, Inc.; 2019. p. 41–61.
8. Eubanks D. Equipping the dental operatory. J Vet Dent 2013;30:52–4.
9. American Dental Association Council on Scientific Affairs, US Food & Drug Administration. Dental Radiographic Examinations: Recommendations for patient selection and limiting radiation exposure. 2012. Available at: https://www.ada.org/~/media/ADA/Member%20Center/FIles/Dental_Radiographic_Examinations_2012.pdf. Accessed April 20, 2019.
10. Brame JL. Seating, positioning, and lighting keep your body injury-free with these cornerstones of ergonomics. Dimens Dent Hyg 2008;6(9):36–7.
11. Gladysz P. Add bite to your dental business. Today's Veterinary Business. 2019. Available at: https://todaysveterinarybusiness.com/add-bite-to-your-dental-business/. Accessed March 2021.

12. Szczygieł E, Zielonka K, Mętel S, et al. Musculoskeletal and pulmonary effects of sitting position - a systematic review. Ann Agric Environ Med 2017;24:8–12.
13. Pirvu C, Patrascu I, Pirvu D, et al. The dentist's operating posture – ergonomic aspects. J Med Life 2014;7:177–82.
14. D. Beevis, I.M. Slade Applied Ergonomics Volume 34, Issue 5, September 2003(5); 413-418
15. Döring S, Arzi B, Hatcher DC, et al. Evaluation of the diagnostic yield of dental radiography and cone-beam computed tomography for the identification of dental disorders in small to medium-sized brachycephalic dogs. Am J Vet Res 2018;79:62–72.
16. Bellows J. Small animal dental equipment, materials and techniques. Ames, IA: Blackwell; 2004.
17. Bednarski R, Grimm K, Harvey R, et al. AAHA anesthesia guidelines for dogs and cats. J Am Anim Hosp Assoc 2011;47:377–85.
18. Grubb T, Sager J, Gaynor JS, et al. 2020 AAHA anesthesia and monitoring guidelines for dogs and cats. J Am Anim Hosp Assoc 2020;56:59–82.
19. Robertson S, Gogolski S, Pascoe P, et al. AAFP feline anesthesia guidelines. J Feline Med Surg 2018;20:602–34.
20. Burn J, Caulkett NA, Gunn M, et al. Evaluation of a portable oxygen concentrator to provide fresh gas flow to dogs undergoing anesthesia. Can Vet J 2016;57: 614–8.
21. Warne LN, Bauquier SH, Pengelly J, et al. Standards of care anesthesia guidelines for dogs and cats. Aust Vet J 2018;96:413–27.
22. Stepaniuk K, Brock N. Anesthesia monitoring in the dental and oral surgery patient. J Vet Dent 2008;25:143–9.
23. Brodbelt DC, Pfeiffer DU, Young LE, et al. Risk factors for anesthetic-related death in cats: results from the confidential enquiry into peri- operative small animal fatalities (CEPSAF). Br J Anaesth 2007;99:617–23.
24. Matthews NS, Mohn TJ, Yang M, et al. Factors associated with anesthetic-related death in dogs and cats in primary care veterinary hospitals. J Am Vet Med Assoc 2017;250:655–66.
25. Brodbelt DC, Pfeiffer DU, Young LE, et al. Results of the confidential enquiry into perioperative small animal fatalities regarding risk factors for anesthetic-related death in dogs. J Am Vet Med Assoc 2008;233:1096–104.
26. Haskins S. Monitoring anesthetized patients. In: Tranquilli WJ, Thurmon JC, Grim KG, editors. Lumb and Jones' veterinary anesthesia and Analgesia. 4th edition. Ames, IA: Blackwell; 2007. p. 86–105.
27. Pottie RG, Dart CM, Perkins NR, et al. Effect of hypothermia on recovery from general anesthesia in the dog. Aust Vet J 2007;85:158–62.
28. Holmstrom SE, Frost-Fitch P, Eisner ER. Veterinary dental techniques for the small animal practitioner. 3rd edition. Philadelphia, PA: WBSaunders; 2004.
29. Charlier C. Oral surgery extractions. In: Lobprise HB, Dodd JR, editors. Wigg's veterinary dentistry. 2nd edition. Hoboken, NJ: Wiley & Sons, Inc.; 2019. p. 229–45.
30. Dental instrumentation and maintenance (Proceedings). *DVM 360.* 2008. Available at: https://www.dvm360.com/view/dental-instrumentation-and-maintenance-proceedings. Accessed April 3, 2021.
31. Theuns P, Niemiec BA. Periodontal hand instruments. J Vet Dent 2012;29:130–3.

# Communication, Veterinary–Client–Patient Relationship, and Teledentistry

Brenda L. Mulherin, DVM[a],*, Kristin M. Bannon, DVM[b]

## KEYWORDS

- Communication • Relationship-centered • Referral expectations
- Veterinary–client–patient relationship (VCPR) • Telemedicine • Teledentistry

## KEY POINTS

- Owners who have a strong relationship with their veterinarian are more likely to follow their recommendations.
- A relationship-centered model of communication builds on the mutual understanding between the veterinarian and the client for overall satisfaction between parties.
- Referring a case to a specialist should be considered an extension of the care the referring veterinarian is already providing.
- State and federal regulations governing what a valid veterinarian–client–patient relationship entails should be consulted before offering care.
- The use of e-mail, text messaging, video conferencing, and directly contacting a client or colleague is providing telemedicine.
- Teledentistry can be an income-generating source for specialists as well as a resource for general practitioners.

## INTRODUCTION

"Good communication is the bridge between confusion and clarity."[1] This famous expression epitomizes the importance of communication within the medical field. The process of communication, whether verbal, nonverbal, written, or visual, is critical in conveying an accurate picture to those that surround us within the field of veterinary dentistry. Whether giving treatment options to the owner of a cat with a suspected neoplasm, writing a laboratory prescription for a prosthodontic crown for a working dog, or demonstrating the proper way to brush the teeth on a newly adopted pet,

[a] American Veterinary Dental College, Department of Veterinary Clinical Sciences, College of Veterinary Medicine, Iowa State University Lloyd Veterinary Medical Center, 1809 South Riverside Drive, Ames, IA 50011-3619, USA; [b] Fellow Academy of Veterinary Dentistry, Diplomate American Veterinary Dental College, Practical Veterinary Dentistry, 5 Camino Karsten, Algodones, NM 87001, USA
* Corresponding author.
E-mail address: bmulher@iastate.edu

Vet Clin Small Anim 52 (2022) 25–47
https://doi.org/10.1016/j.cvsm.2021.08.002
vetsmall.theclinics.com

communication is and always will be an important component to the success or failure of a business. Society looks to veterinary professionals to provide the highest standard of care possible to their 4-legged friends. Unfortunately, even with providing high-quality care, poor communication can diminish any efforts made to improve the quality of life for the patient. To provide optimal care for the veterinary patient, the clinician needs to understand and master the importance of communication between all of those involved in the treatment process.

## TYPES OF COMMUNICATION

There are 4 main types of communication: verbal, nonverbal, written, and visual (**Box 1**). Veterinarians and health care providers commonly use all 4 forms of communication daily. Whether it is directly speaking to a client, nodding in agreement, preparing discharge instructions, or showing an owner a lesion within the oral cavity, all forms of communication are used. Many pet owners surveyed within the United States have a growing human–animal bond and consider their companion animals a member of their family.[2] Being a veterinarian is like being a pediatrician. As a veterinarian, we communicate with the "parent" or client, who must describe the clinical signs and behavior that is, occurring in the "child" or animal. The veterinarian relies on the owner's description and combines it with the clinical examination findings to determine the next course of action in diagnosing a patient.[3] The communication that occurs between the veterinarian and the client sets the stage for the patient to receive the care it needs.

Communication skills are a strong component to building a relationship between an owner and their veterinarian.[2] A clinician's ability to communicate with the owners and educate them about their pets' needs is of utmost importance.[2] Studies have shown that 69% of owners who have a strong relationship with their veterinarian will more likely follow their recommendations.[2] The relationship formed between the veterinarian and the client will enhance the ability to gather information, form a complete picture of the condition of the pet and allow for improved clinical evaluation and treatment of the pet.

## VERBAL

Veterinarians use many strategies to gather, interpret, and covey information. There are 3 main models of verbal communication: Directive style, consumerism model, and relationship-centered model (**Box 2**). Frequently, veterinarians use a directive model of communication to consult with clients.[4] The directive model allows for minimal client input and dominates the consultation with the clinician's agenda with minimal input from the client.[4,5] It has been described as a more "paternalistic role" regarding client interactions. The paternalistic relationship between the clinician and

| Box 1 Types of communication | |
|---|---|
| **Types of Communication** | |
| Verbal | Speaking with a client |
| Nonverbal | Gesturing, nodding, changes in body language |
| Written | Medical literature, handouts, discharge instructions |
| Visual | Photographs, radiographs, models |

| Box 2 | |
|---|---|
| **Models of communication** | |
| Directive Model | Clinician takes on paternalistic role regarding client interactions. Clinician sets the agenda for the appointment. |
| Consumerism Model | Client sets the agenda for the appointment. Clinician plays the role of a consultant and provides options for treatment based on client's demands. |
| Relationship-Centered Model | Balance between Directive Model and Consumerism Model. Model builds on mutual understanding between the veterinarian and the client. |

the owner is demonstrated by the clinician setting the agenda for the appointment.[5] There is an assumption by the clinician that the owner maintains the same thoughts and values as the clinician. With this model, a caretaker or guardian role is assumed by the clinician. This style of communication has been criticized for minimizing the client's opinion and perspective regarding the care of their pet.[5]

The consumerism model is another communication style that has been used in medical conversations. This style is described as the client setting the agenda of the appointment.[5] The clinician plays the role of a consultant and provides information and options for treatment, based on the client's demands. The consumerism style is focused on client control, with clinician input limited to responses to the questions asked by the client. This style of communication has also been criticized for limiting the role of the clinician or expert in the field.[5]

The third style of communication, the relationship-centered model, is a balance between the first 2 styles.[5] The relationship-centered model builds on a mutual understanding and agreement of the veterinarian and the client. It allows the veterinarian to take on a role of an advisor or counselor. This relationship-centered style allows for collaboration between the client and the veterinarian for a mutual transfer of information.[5]

One study reported that many veterinarians (58%) use the directive or more paternalistic style of communication.[5] The remaining veterinarians in the study used a technique similar to the relationship-centered model (42%). These veterinarians incorporated lifestyle and social topics in the discussion and spent time establishing rapport with the client. This was perceived as building a relationship with the clients and encouraging them to ask questions and participate more in the visit.[5]

The same study found that male clinicians were more likely to use the directive style of communication and female clinicians were more likely to use other styles of communication.[5] Overall, it was found that using the directive approach may have decreased satisfaction for the veterinarian, the client and the eventual outcome of patient therapies and treatment. Although a directive approach may be taken in busy practices in an attempt to work more efficiently, it has actually been found that an appointment that uses this approach lasted on average 1.5 minutes longer than one using the relationship-centered approach.[5]

Adaptation and flexibility to adjust to the client, patient, and situation are essential to the success of communication. Adjusting to the client's preferences and adapting to the communication pattern the client puts forth can help establish rapport between the clinician and the client. This rapport builds a collaborative relationship, thus providing optimal care to the patient. A strong veterinary–client–patient relationship (VCPR) with clear and concise communication can increase client compliance. When communicating with clients, there are several questions the clinician needs to consider.

(1) What am I trying to communicate?
(2) Why am I trying to communicate?
(3) Who am I communicating with?
(4) How am I going to relay my information?
(5) Do I need to adapt my communication style to fit the client's needs?

Asking these questions, gathering needed information, conveying options, and discussing the findings in a clear and concise manner can help shape the consultation to give satisfaction to all participants. This will help the clinician build a stronger relationship with the client and encourage the client to comply with the recommendations offered by the medical expert. The relationship-centered approach to communication between the veterinarian and the client has been shown to facilitate this process. This exchange of information and communication will help the clinician build a stronger relationship with the client and encourage them to comply with the recommendations and treatment options offered.[3] Clients who respect their veterinarian and have trust in the information delivered are more likely to remain loyal. Increased client understanding allows for increased adherence to recommendations, which is a direct reward of building a veterinary–client relationship.[3] The ability of a veterinarian to develop communication skills and rapport with the client not only affects the relationship between the veterinarian and the client but also the health of the animal.[3] Providing clear communication and ensuring understanding of the information delivered will allow for better patient care. This may be in terms of choosing the proper form of medication (liquid or tablet), frequency delivered (once or twice daily), or follow-up care needed to improve the quality of life for the patient as well as the client.

## OPEN-ENDED QUESTIONS

Open-ended questions are used frequently to gather as much information as possible from a client. An open-ended question is one in which it is difficult for an owner to give a single-word answer. This type of question is often phased more as a statement, encouraging the client to give a response (**Box 3**).

The use of open-ended questions allows the client to describe their concerns and encourages them to build a relationship with the clinician. The use of open-ended questions helps to build a more relationship-centered model of communication. In a medical interview, using open-ended questions has shown to help gather more information from the client than the use of closed-ended questions.[6]

## CLOSED-ENDED QUESTIONS

A closed-ended question is one for which the client can respond with a single-word answer (**Box 4**). This type of questioning can be intimidating to some clients, as it can be perceived almost as accusatory. Although a clinician can be trying to ask all the right questions, phrasing them in the proper manner will encourage the client to

---

**Box 3**
**Examples of open-ended questions**

Examples of open-ended questions
(1) What brings you in today?
(2) Describe the behavior the dog is exhibiting.
(3) Tell me about the change in eating habits.
(4) What questions do you have?

---

**Box 4**
**Examples of closed-ended questions**

Examples of closed-ended questions
1) How are you today?
2) Has your cat shown any evidence of sneezing?
3) Is there anything else you would like to discuss?
4) Do you have any questions?

---

open a dialogue with their concerns. Open-ended questions are more likely to improve client satisfaction by allowing the client to provide additional information in contrast to a closed-ended question.[7] Using open-ended questions at the beginning of the appointment can establish a rapport and allow the client to tell their story and concerns. These can be followed by closed-ended questions to gain additional information that may be useful.[8] The consultation can then be concluded with open-ended questions to allow the client to verify understanding and make any final comments. This combination approach can help improve the satisfaction of both the client and clinician and help provide the most information possible for appropriate patient treatment and care.

## EMPATHY

To be successful in veterinary medicine, a practitioner needs to develop skills in empathy. Empathy is the ability to appreciate or sense what another individual is experiencing. It is a process by which one person puts themselves in the place of another attempting to comprehend how the other person may be feeling.[8] Veterinarians need to combine the empathy they feel toward the patient, the client, and their colleagues to be able to be successful in their practice.[9] Veterinarians who demonstrate skills in empathy have been shown to exhibit more professionalism, clinical competency, confidence, and have higher emotional intelligence and well-being. Demonstrating empathy to a client is a clinical skill that can help the clinician develop rapport with the client and establish trust. Trust builds on the veterinarian–client relationship and can contribute to increased client compliance and better outcomes for the patient.[9] If a doctor can learn to empathize with the client, the ability to connect and communicate is improved making it easier to form a trusting relationship.[8]

## NONVERBAL

Nonverbal communication is described as communication that is not controlled with speech.[10] This form of communication allows the clinician to listen to what the client is saying to help them gather information without interrupting. When clinicians take the time to stop and listen to the client's concerns regarding their animal, they hear and understand the verbal, nonverbal, and the paralinguistic cues the client may be giving.[10] Paralinguistic cues modify the meaning of the spoken word or elicit emotion. Examples of paralinguistic cues include the tone, pitch, volume, and rate of speed of spoken word. The clinician should support the client with reciprocal nonverbal cues encouraging the client in short exchanges, but not interrupting the client. Using terms such as "yes," "please continue," and "I see,"[10] can reassure the client that they are being heard. Developing the ability to identify nonverbal cues from the client can improve the veterinarian's ability to respond to the client's emotions.[3] Facial expressions, body tension, movements of the client, and the space created between the client, pet, and veterinarian are all nonverbal cues that can be identified by the veterinarian and used to help shape the relationship between those involved.[3]

Active listening and nonverbal communication are important components of an effective conversation that should not be underestimated. Clinicians should attempt to allow for silence in the examination room to allow the client the opportunity to describe their concerns. When nonverbal communication is used in a positive manner such as smiling, nodding, and positive comments, they are generally reciprocated.[11] When nonverbal communication from the veterinarian is aloof and distant, this is usually reciprocated in kind with a reserved, unfriendly, or unapproachable behavior from the client.[11]

## BODY LANGUAGE

The use of movement can help to encourage clients to continue to discuss their concerns. Nodding or tilting of the head, smiling, and eye contact can reassure clients and encourage them to continue.[10] A consultation can be improved by the effective use of body language. Body language can enhance communication by demonstrating empathy and understanding to the client. The usage of body language to establish rapport and empathy between a client and a patient is an important skill for the clinician to learn.[8] The human body can be used to express emotions and concerns as well as interpret those same feelings from both the doctor and the client perspectives. The ability of a doctor to interpret the client's body language may be just as important as listening and hearing what the client is saying verbally.[8] Using open body language will encourage more open dialogue between the client and the clinician. Open body language is when an individual positions the trunk of their body in an exposed position to allow for open and friendly interaction. Examples of open body language are uncrossed arms and legs and not having a barrier between the individuals exchanging information. Closed body language includes an individual sitting or standing with crossed legs, their arms crossed or folded, or placing a barrier between them, such as an examination table. An open body language interaction is more likely to result in a mutually agreed on understanding.[8]

## WRITTEN COMMUNICATION

The communication style used for clinician and client interactions can have direct consequences on the care the patient receives, the perceived satisfaction of the client as well as client compliance regarding treatment recommendations. Regardless of the type of communication used, clear communication needs to occur to ensure the patient receives proper care. This includes directions related to the administration of any dispensed medications (timing, dose, route, and so forth), discharge instructions (dietary or exercise restrictions, and so forth), and follow-up care (re-evaluations, suture removal appointments, discontinuing of restrictions, and so forth).[5]

Clients who do not fully comprehend what the veterinarian is recommending may pretend they understand and feign compliance rather than ask for clarification.[12] This may be because they are embarrassed to ask for clarification or because they thought they understood, but in reality, did not comprehend their role in the pet's care. Refraining from asking for clarification may also be a result of a breakdown in the relationship between the clinician and the client. If the veterinarian makes an incorrect assumption about a client's ability to understand diagnostic or therapeutic options, and thus implement instructions, patient care can be compromised.[12]

## DISCHARGE INSTRUCTIONS

Written instructions should be composed clearly and concisely. Clients receiving a clear recommendation were 7 times more likely to comply with the recommendations compared with a confusing recommendation.[13] Clients will also be more satisfied with their interaction, resulting in increased client adherence to instructions and more relationship-centered care for the patient. Veterinarians who make specific recommendations have a greater chance for client adherence.[13] A study in humans reported that less than half of surveyed patients were able to list their personal diagnosis, medication regimen, medication purpose, and major side effects the medication may cause.[14] Client compliance improves with knowledge and understanding of the medications and their use. After a patient is discharged, the client assumes the role of the health care provider for the patient that was released. Clients need to have a basic knowledge of the disease that was diagnosed, medications that were dispensed, major side effects of the medications, the dosing schedule, and what follow-up care is needed for the patient. Using clear and concise instructions that are verbally discussed with the client as well as having written instructions available for reference can help to improve client understanding, compliance, and follow through. Clearly writing instructions so that there is no question as to what the client can expect and what or when they need to care for their pet is key to improved client comfort and trust in the care that was given. These instructions should also be reinforced by the health care team demonstrating a unified front, enhancing client understanding and compliance and ultimately patient care and outcome.[14]

When dispensing medications, the name of the drug, milligram strength, number of pills/tablets/caplets/capsules, and so forth, route of administration, number to be administered, and dosing frequency should be included. The specific time the next dose should be administered is also beneficial to make sure the client knows exactly when the next dose of medication is due and other circumstances that need to be considered. For example, avoid: "Clavamox: Give 1 tablet orally twice daily."

Providing detailed written communication will help to avoid any ambiguity. Try to avoid the opportunity for the client to interpret the dosing schedule. For example, use: "Clavamox: 62.5 mg, #14 tablets; Give 1 tablet by mouth once every 12 hours for 7 days. The first dose of this medication should be given this evening at 6:00 PM, if Ramsey is eating."

Remember to include any major side effects of the medication and if the medication needs to be administered with or without food, refrigerated, or kept at room temperature. Having complete and detailed written instructions regarding patient medication will increase compliance, and thus improve patient care.

## REMINDER CARDS

Many veterinary software systems include programs to manage inventory, invoicing, prescription label creation, medical record creation, appointment scheduling as well as reminders for wellness and preventative care. Veterinarians frequently use the system to send either paper or electronic reminder cards to their clients for follow-up appointments, vaccination reminders, and recommended procedure reminders.[15] Clients generally respond 3 times less frequently to a reminder for a vaccination appointment compared with a reminder for any other recall. Clients were far more likely to respond to a reminder recall for a dental procedure, laboratory testing, or progress examinations. In fact, clients were twice as likely to respond to a recall reminder regarding a dental procedure than they were an annual vaccination reminder. Therefore, veterinarians may consider refraining from contacting clients for annual vaccinations and instead promote other veterinary services such as wellness and preventative screenings.[15] This study would support the use of reminders to clients for preventative care including a thorough oral examination and professional dental cleaning and not specifically just for vaccinations.

## MEDICAL LITERATURE

Medical literature should be prepared so that any pet owner can read and understand the information provided. Considerations for creating medical literature include the intended/expected outcome or objective of the material, as well as the readability or complexity of the material.[16] The readability of a document is its ability to be easily read and understood. Educational materials that are poorly written or written above the level that can be comprehended by a nonmedical audience can have negative consequences to pet health and client compliance.[17] The Internet is a common source of information related to health care for clients.[18] It is becoming expected of veterinarians to use online resources to communicate with clients as well as provide them with the education they are looking for regarding diseases that may affect their pets.

The National Assessment of Adult Literacy determined that 14% of Americans have below basic literacy skills. Literature should be easy to read and targeted to be written at a 6th to 8th-grade reading level.[16,19] When evaluating the top 10 client handouts that were downloaded from a veterinary trade journal, 9 out of the 10 were written at or above an 8th-grade reading level, which is well above the recommended 6th-grade reading level recommended by the American Medical Association. Literature also suggests that much of what is written online for clients regarding human health care fails to meet the National Institute of Health and American Medical Association guidelines, which should be written for the comprehension level of a 3rd to 7th grader.[18] Medical information can be very complex; therefore, it is imperative that any information given to owners is written in a manner that maximizes the readers' ability to comprehend the information. It has been found that over 73% of articles on a website intended as a source of health care information for patients were written for reading comprehension of over a 12th-grade level, well above suggested 7th grade levels.[18] When creating handouts or other medical literature, it needs to be understandable to the intended target audience, regardless of their age, background or reading comprehension level.[16]

There are online programs that evaluate a document for its readability. Using a program designed to evaluate the document for its readability can serve as a guide so that the message you want to give to the target audience is clearly understood.[16]

## VISUAL COMMUNICATION

The use of photographic, radiographic, and diagnostic images, videos and demonstrations are powerful tools to help improve client and referral communication. Techniques such as demonstrating medication administration can help increase client compliance.[20] Making medication administration as simple as possible will also be helpful to clients. For example, drawing up oral dosing syringes with an appropriate amount of pain medication and labeling the dispensing bag will help avoid any dosing errors by the client.

Photographs obtained before and after professional dental cleaning are very impactful visual tools to help demonstrate the care a pet received (**Fig. 1**). When performing a dental cleaning or treatment for a dental abnormality, it is important for the clients to understand the treatment their pet received, and why they received it. The lips of the patient cover the teeth. Most pet owners do not know or realize

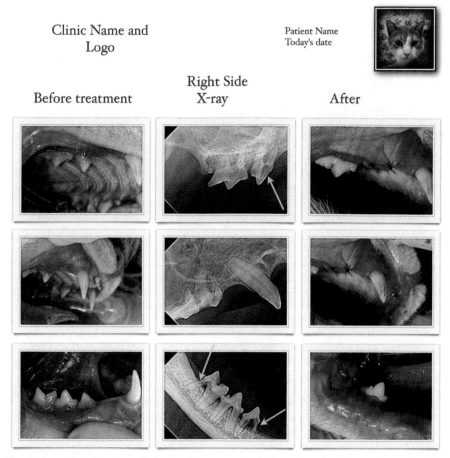

Clinic Name and
Logo

Patient Name
Today's date

Right Side
X-ray

Before treatment

After

**Fig. 1.** Example of patient discharge documents including clinical photographs and radiographs demonstrating pre and postcleaning, diagnostics, and treatment.

that a pathological condition exists in their pet's mouth. Ideally, the attending clinician or a staff member would review the before and after photographs and any relevant radiographs with the client before the presentation of their invoice. This will provide a better understanding of the treatment and give the client a higher perceived value to the care that was given. Using clinical or diagnostic images to show owners that a pathological condition exists below the gingival margin (ie, gumline) is also impactful. A dental cleaning just scratches the surface of what pathological conditions may be present. A cosmetic cleaning of the crown surface does not address pathology condition that lurks below the gingival margin. Clinical and diagnostic images are very important visual tools to help owners understand the importance of an anesthetized professional dental cleaning and oral evaluation including dental radiographs and periodontal probing (**Fig. 2**A, B).

## WEBSITES AND SOCIAL MEDIA

Providing easy access regarding what a clinic has to offer should be available to clients and other colleagues. Social media presence and having a website for the clinic

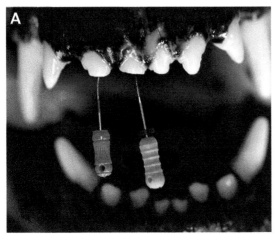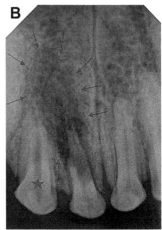

**Fig. 2.** (*A*) Usage of clinical images of a canine patient with pulp exposure of the right maxillary 1st and 2nd incisors (101, 102) that visually look normal. Endodontic pathfinders were used to demonstrate that pulp exposure existed within the pulp of these teeth. (*B*) Usage of an intraoral radiographic image of the right maxillary 1st and 2nd incisors (101, 102) using bisecting angle technique to demonstrate why endodontic therapy is not recommended for the treatment of the teeth with pulp exposure. The radiograph depicts significant resorption of the apical extent of the right maxillary 1st incisor (101) and associated periapical lucency (*arrows*) and evidence of significant root resorption. The radiograph also depicts the increased pulp canal width of the right maxillary 2nd incisor (102) (star) and the loss of periodontal ligament space associated with the resorption of the tooth root.

can inform clients of the services the clinic has to offer(**Box 5**). When developing a website for the clinic, keep it simple. The website should focus on the essential information and be user-friendly. Just as in the readability of medical literature, the website should be able to be navigated by a 6th–8th grader. It needs to be easily navigated if you want prospective clients to spend any time investigating what services and care the clinic has to offer. Whatever purpose the website has, the objective should be clear. Using clear, single words as hot buttons to identify information that clients

---

**Box 5**
**Essentials for an attractive website**

Keep it simple

Focus on essential information

Easily navigated

Clear objectives

Focus on the takeaway information

Clutter-free

Color to enhance

Videos and graphics to ADD not DISTRACT

Mobile device friendly

may find useful is important.[21] For example, having a button to click if the desired information is needed for an emergency should be obvious. Clicking the emergency hot button may provide the user with the phone number, directions to the hospital, and hours of operation listed clearly and concisely.

The website should focus on important information about the clinic and the services offered. Contact information, directions to the clinic, services, hours of operation, and types of patients seen would be just a few items the website may focus on. A website that is free of unnecessary information including overwhelming amounts of pictures and graphics can help to improve the website's readability. Too much of a good thing can be distracting to clients when an overwhelming amount of visual information to process is present. Using color to improve the attractiveness of the website with associated accent colors to highlight the important links or pages is recommended. The size and type of font that is used should be easy to read and large enough for viewers to see. Usually, a 16pt or 12pt font is the minimum size recommended for website creation.

The use of videos and images may be beneficial for engaging clients within the website.[21] Videos and pictures should enhance the website, not be used as a visual distraction. Websites also need to be easily viewed by a mobile device as this is how many clients will access the information.[21] Many web designers use a responsive design format. This type of formatting compresses images and shrinks the design automatically if viewed on a mobile device. There are online tools that help provide you with the information to ensure your clinic's website is mobile device friendly. Some of these tools may even provide you with a screenshot of how the website will appear on a mobile device, as well as recommendations for improving the mobile viewing experience.

## REFERRING VETERINARIANS' EXPECTATIONS WHEN REFERRING CASES

Many veterinarians who refer a case to a referral center or veterinary specialist feel that the specialist is an extension of the care the referring veterinarian is already providing.[22] Referring veterinarians and specialists can mutually benefit by having an open dialogue and establish a mechanism for communicating and sharing information. A survey of veterinarians who refer cases to veterinary specialists and referral centers have identified 5 areas that are important to the success of a relationship between the referring veterinarian and the specialist (**Box 6**).[22] These areas are as follows:

(1) Referring veterinarian–client relationship
(2) Referring veterinarian involvement during referral care
(3) Collegial referring veterinarian–specialist relationship

| Box 6<br>Considerations for making a referral a success |
| --- |
| Referring veterinarian–client relationship |
| Referring veterinarian involvement during referral care |
| Collégial referring veterinarian–specialist relationship |
| Communication between referring veterinarian and specialist |
| Boundaries of referral care |

(4) Communication between referring veterinarian and specialist
(5) Boundaries of referral care

## RELATIONSHIP BETWEEN THE REFERRING VETERINARIAN AND THE CLIENT

Focus groups have evaluated why veterinarians may refer a case to a specialist for care. Many veterinarians in one study described that they perceived referral as an extension of the care that they already provide to the patient.[22] They concluded that they want clients to be satisfied with the care received and that the client may judge the referring clinician based on the care they received at the referral hospital.[22] Many clients are more comfortable when the referring veterinarian is still involved with the care of their animal. Clients have developed a relationship with the referring veterinarian and trust them to know what is right for their animals. Many surveyed veterinarians have described that if they continue to be involved with the patients care, it demonstrates their continued interest in the case and the well-being of the patient.[22] This emphasizes that when a specialist is treating a patient, they are not only treating the client, but the referring veterinarian as well.

## INVOLVEMENT OF THE REFERRING VETERINARIAN WHILE IN THE CARE OF THE SPECIALIST

When a veterinarian refers a patient to a specialist, they typically want to remain involved with the case.[22] Communication regarding the diagnostics and treatment plan recommendations needs to be shared with the referring veterinarian to keep them apprised of the care the patient is receiving. Communication throughout the time the patient is at the specialty clinic will help to reduce repeat diagnostics the referring veterinarian has already performed. Veterinarians may be concerned with the perception that repeated diagnostics and workup could reflect poorly on the referring veterinarian as a sign the specialist did not trust their judgment and skill.[22] Referring veterinarians can improve the clinical outcome for the client and the patient by providing insight into the patient's history and their previous interactions with the client. They can offer input as to what the aftercare and follow-up could look like from a historical perspective from working with the client.[22]

## RELATIONSHIP BETWEEN THE REFERRING VETERINARIAN AND THE SPECIALIST

Communication based on respect, trust, and honesty will help improve any relationship. Referring veterinarians want to be heard by the specialist and would like the specialist to respect their opinions and the bond they have formed with the client who was referred.[22] They would also like specialists to be respectful of the referring veterinarian's time. The relationship that is, formed between the specialist and the referring veterinarian can impact the referring veterinarian's likelihood to refer additional cases as well as the specialist's likelihood to follow the trajectory of the plan of care for which the patient was referred.[22] More comfort and trust can be placed in a specialist for which the referring veterinarian has an existing relationship. They are more confident in the communication they will receive and the patient care that will be provided. When the referring veterinarian does not know or does not have a relationship with the specialist, there may be more uncertainty regarding the communication and the care the client and the patient could receive. When specialists are willing to support the referring veterinarian remotely by giving advice and talking through cases, this increases the familiarity with the specialist and begins to strengthen the bond between the 2 parties.[22]

## COMMUNICATION BETWEEN THE REFERRING VETERINARIAN AND THE SPECIALIST

Effective, concise, and prompt communication strengthens the relationship between a referring veterinarian and a specialist. Referring veterinarians want timely communication with the specialist to keep them apprised of the patient's condition. If the veterinarian is not knowledgeable regarding the patient's current condition and they encounter a client, it can reflect poorly on the veterinarian.[22] The specialist should initiate contact with the referring veterinarian to keep them apprised of the care the patient is receiving. Whether the communication is written, verbal, or both, it needs to be thorough, accurate, and contain any follow-up treatment or care the referring veterinarian may need to provide.[22] The discharge summary needs to be sent as soon as possible to keep the referring veterinarian apprised of any follow-up care that would be needed before the client arrives on their doorstep. If the follow-up care can be provided by the referring veterinarian, the client should be directed back to their primary care doctor. Frustration has been seen when the specialty hospital directs the client to return to their care for services that could be performed by the referring veterinarian.[22]

## SPECIALTY CARE BOUNDARIES

When a veterinarian refers a case to a specialist, they are acknowledging that they do not have the time, experience, staffing, or ability to provide the care that they feel a patient and client need. They recognize they may be losing the income that could be generated in providing the care. Specialists need to respect the referring veterinarian and set boundaries for providing services that could be performed by the primary veterinarian. Specialists who provide services and care beyond the reason for referral may find that referring veterinarians are reluctant to send them additional cases for fear of losing income the specialist generates beyond the reason for referral. Referring veterinarians' express displeasure with specialty clinics who actively try to convince clients to come to the specialty clinic for their primary care needs.[22]

## COMMUNICATION WITH THE PATHOLOGIST

One of the more common procedures performed in veterinary dentistry is a biopsy of an oral lesion. This may involve a mass in the maxillofacial region or an ulcerated area of the gingiva, alveolar, labial, buccal or sublingual mucosa, tongue, palatine tonsils, or palate. When obtaining a biopsy, it is important to take photographs of the area before the biopsy. It is also ideal to take another photograph of the area after the biopsy, or biopsies, have been collected. This is to show the exact location of the tissue submitted. Intraoral dental radiographs or 3D imaging such as a cone-beam CT or a traditional CT are extremely useful to the pathologist. These photographs and diagnostic images should be shared with the pathologist when a sample is submitted. Just as the veterinarian needs a complete history from the client and must perform a thorough physical examination before making a diagnosis, the pathologist needs detailed information to help make an accurate diagnosis. In many cases, especially in the oral cavity, the morphologic features of different diseases can appear very similar histologically.[23] Having a complete clinical and diagnostic picture will add additional information to assist the pathologist in distinguishing between morphologically similar diseases. This aids in identifying the primary diagnosis, as well as one or more likely differential diagnoses.

Working with a pathologist that has experience with oral and maxillofacial diseases will often facilitate a more accurate diagnosis. There are several diseases that are unique to the oral cavity. Odontogenic tumors are most notable due to their embryologic origin from the tooth germ.[24] The histologic characteristics of odonto-genic tumors are complex and there is a significant similarity among the various types of these tumors, which is an area of frustration for pathologists that do not routinely study these tissues. In these situations, the experience level of the pathologist and their interest in dental and oral pathological conditions may be key to identifying the unique diagnostic features that will allow for proper classification.[23]

## COMMUNICATION WITH THE DENTAL LABORATORY

There are situations in veterinary dentistry when a dental laboratory may be needed to fabricate a prosthodontic crown or an orthodontic appliance. It is very important that the clinician have a good working relationship with the dental laboratory. Communication between the clinician and the dental laboratory technician to discuss exactly what is needed from each party is imperative to obtain the desired result. Examples of this may include the dental laboratory requesting submission of specific impressions, or the clinician requesting a specific material for appliance fabrication. Many laboratories appreciate seeing photographs of the teeth so that the impressions submitted can be visualized to match the current condition of the oral cavity.

For a prosthodontic crown, some laboratories prefer to have high-quality impressions of the entire maxillary and mandibular dentition, as well as detailed impressions of the tooth that has been prepared for the crown. Other laboratories may not need or want the impressions of the entire mouth and would prefer to have only impressions of the tooth that has been prepared for the crown. If there is significant damage or loss of the crown that is being repaired, the laboratory may be requested to build the tooth up. Having an impression of the undamaged contralateral tooth can be extremely helpful. In most cases, photographs of the mouth are not necessary when creating and designing a prosthetic crown, but they can aid in providing additional information. It is important to communicate with the laboratory about the desired material to be used to fabricate the crown. If the crown is to be made from a tooth-colored material, such as zirconia, photographs can be very useful to match the color of the crown as closely as possible.

For an orthodontic appliance, high-quality impressions of both the upper and lower dental arches are best. A bite impression which demonstrates how the upper and lower jaws interdigitate allows the laboratory to fit the dental models together to create the needed appliance. Orthodontic cases often benefit from photographs of the oral cavity and how the teeth interdigitate. It is also important to ensure that the laboratory understands the goal of the orthodontic appliance for canine and feline patients. It is difficult to fabricate an appliance if they are unsure of the desired result and purpose of the appliance.

A dental laboratory that has experience working with veterinary patients is highly recommended. The occlusal forces between animals and humans are different. Humans have been found to have a maximum bite force of up to 511 N when measured at the level of the first molar teeth.[25] A study evaluating the bite forces of domestic canids showed ranges of 524 to 3417 N when measured at the second M tooth.[26] A dental laboratory that has experience and working knowledge of the occlusal forces in animals will produce a more functional and reliable outcome.

## THE VETERINARIAN–CLIENT–PATIENT RELATIONSHIP

The relationships between a veterinarian, the client, and the patient are important components to the care a pet receives and the overall health of the animal. According to the American Veterinary Medical Association (AVMA), there are 7 established requirements of a veterinarian–client–patient relationship (VCPR) (**Box 7**).[27]

(1) The licensed veterinarian assumes medical responsibility for making decisions regarding the health of a patient and the need for treatment. The veterinarian has communicated with the client the appropriate course of treatment for the patient.
(2) The veterinarian has enough knowledge of the patient to be able to formulate a preliminary diagnosis of its condition.
(3) The client agrees with the recommendations offered by the veterinarian.
(4) The veterinarian is available for continued care or has arranged for another competent veterinarian to provide care if unavailable. This individual has access to the medical records and can provide continued medical care for the patient.
(5) The licensed veterinarian oversees the treatment of the patient.
(6) The veterinarian has adequate knowledge of the patient by having performed a physical examination and has continued to provide care to the patient in accordance with state and federal regulations.
(7) The patient has an up-to-date medical record.

There are state and federal regulations that may have additional requirements governing the VCPR. Consulting state veterinary practice acts, state pharmacy laws, state licensure requirements, state and federal VCPR requirements are recommended to maintain standards in accordance with governing bodies regarding the relationship (**Box 8**).[28]

## TELEMEDICINE AND TELEDENTISTRY

As veterinarians, we provide telemedicine daily without even realizing it. Telemedicine services frequently involve the exchange of digital information and acquisition of medical information between a client and a clinician.[29] The use of e-mail, text messaging, video conferencing and directly contacting a client or colleague over a networking system can be considered telemedicine. A telemedicine device requires information to be

---

**Box 7**
**The veterinary–client–patient relationship (VCPR)**

(1) The licensed veterinarian assumes medical responsibility for making decisions regarding the health of a patient and the need for treatment. The veterinarian has communicated with the client the appropriate course of treatment for the patient.

(2) The veterinarian has enough knowledge of the patient to be able to formulate a preliminary diagnosis of their condition.

(3) The client agrees with the recommendations offered by the veterinarian.

(4) The veterinarian is available for continued care or has arranged for another competent veterinarian to provide care if they are unavailable. This individual has access to the medical records and can provide continued medical care for the patient.

(5) The licensed veterinarian oversees the treatment of the patient.

(6) The veterinarian has adequate knowledge of the patient by having performed a physical examination and has continued to provide care to the patient in accordance with state and federal regulations.

(7) The patient has an up-to-date medical record.

---

**Box 8**
**American Veterinary Medical Association Veterinary–Client–Patient Relationship Guidelines for Individual States**

https://www.avma.org/sites/default/files/2020-II/VCPR-State-Chart-NOV-2020.pdf

---

transferred from the device over some type of network. Telemedicine occurs any time a veterinarian answers a phone call from a client in which they have provided treatment recommendations. An exchange of information occurs, and advice is given. The addition of technology to provide more information including visual and audio conferencing can assist in providing a better picture of the patient's overall condition and progress, therefore, improving patient care. Mobile devices with software and hardware applications are frequent modes of telemedicine.[29]

There are state and federal regulations that need to be consulted before offering telemedicine services. The AVMA has guidelines related to the VCPR as well as regulations regarding telemedicine. As telemedicine and teledentistry are fairly new in the sense of an organized structure, it is important that the clinicians familiarize themselves with what is appropriate and what the regulations are for each individual state (and country).

Telemedicine services are very beneficial in allowing the distance between a client/patient and veterinarian to become obsolete. The AVMA does not support the use of telemedicine for consultation purposes when a valid VCPR has not been established.[30,31] The only exception to this is in the case of an emergency. When a veterinarian offers telemedicine services to a client who lives in another state, the AVMA advises that the veterinarian be licensed in the state the patient resides.[31] The importance of being licensed in both states is to protect the veterinarian if legal issues arise in the care of the patient. If veterinarians are not licensed in the state whereby the patient resides, they are not legally authorized to treat the patient via telemedicine services. If the veterinarian is licensed in both states, both the veterinarian and the patient are legally protected.[31]

For the veterinarian who is consulting with a specialist, the attending veterinarian must maintain a valid VCPR with the patient and a license to practice in the state for which the veterinarian practices as well as the state the patient resides.[31] As a specialist, the AVMA does not require the specialist to have the same criteria as the attending veterinarian. This is because the specialist is working through the attending veterinarian to treat the patient. However, a specialist who begins the direct treatment of a patient outside the care of the original attending veterinarian needs to establish a valid VCPR as well as licensure within the patient's state.[31] When maintaining ongoing treatment of a patient, having the client bring the patient to the state for which the veterinarian is providing the service is the most legally seamless way in which treatment can be provided. Telemedicine services that are provided to a patient living in another state can be difficult if the veterinarian does not maintain a license in the state for which the patient resides. This can result in issues prescribing medication within a state for which the veterinarian does not have a valid license to practice veterinary medicine.

*Telehealth* is defined as the use of some form of telecommunication or technology to provide services including delivering information, medical care, and education on a virtual platform.[32] Telehealth is the all-encompassing term of using technology to acquire knowledge and deliver information and education to individuals remotely. The AVMA divides telehealth into 2 categories, those individuals who have an existing

VCPR and those that do not. For those individuals that do not maintain a valid VCPR, telehealth information provided should be based on general topics of advice or education.[32] For individuals who maintain a current valid VCPR, advice, and education can be delivered with specific information regarding a patient or condition under the care of the veterinarian. There may be some legal implications questioning if a valid VCPR can be established remotely through telemedicine consultation. The AVMA stands firm that an in-person visit and examination are needed before a valid VCPR can be established.[33]

*Telemedicine* is the exchange of information regarding a specific patient from one location to another.[32] This could include photos of a patient's postoperative incision following a procedure. Many owners view the addition of telemedicine to a traditional VCPR as a positive complement to the care their pet is already receiving.[34] *Teletriage* is used for remote assessment of a patient to guide the client in the urgency for referral to a veterinarian for care.[32] The patient's condition is assessed electronically based on an owner's response to questions as well as any additional information the owner feels would be helpful in the assessment of the patient, such as photos and videos.[32] *Teleconsulting* is described as a referring veterinarian consulting a specialist to gain advice regarding the care for a specific condition.[32]

*Teleadvice* is the delivery of education or information that is, not related to a specific patient's condition.[32] It is general advice that is, given as a guideline for all patient care. It is not intended to diagnose or treat a condition. Daily, veterinarians and their clinic staff provide generalized information relating to non–patient-specific advice to the public, over the phone, email, or through updating the clinic's social media presence or website. Many times, the information is provided at no charge to the client. Teleadvice services can be offered by all members of a veterinary practice, as long as they are delivering information within the scope of what is allowed through their state and federal regulations. Structured delivery of teleadvice within a clinic can provide an opportunity for the veterinarian and their staff members to be compensated for utilizing their education to convey information and advice to existing clients and the potential for new clients.[32] Adding a teleadvice service can offer an additional revenue stream to the practice if the fee structure system is organized.

*Telemonitoring, mHealth, or mobile health* is a mode of health communication in which a monitoring device is used to transmit information to augment the care of an animal under the care of a veterinarian. Others are designed for clients to gathering information without input from a veterinarian.[32]

## TELEHEALTH PROTOCOLS

According to the AVMA guidelines for the use of telehealth in a veterinary practice,[32] the telehealth protocol should concentrate on the following 3 goals:

(1) Improve the level of patient care.
(2) Increase access to veterinary medical care to underserved populations.
(3) Improve the utilization of all veterinary health care team members.

*Teledentistry* is that part of telemedicine that combines the use of telecommunication and dentistry knowledge, as it exchanges clinical information, photographic or radiographic images remotely.[35] Teledentistry occurs when a client, whether the owner or a referring veterinarian, contacts an individual who has greater knowledge and expertise in the field of dentistry.[36] The interaction can be asynchronous when the specialist reviews information previously collected (such as radiographs) or synchronous when the patient may be on the table and the specialist can see what is happening, as it is occurring live stream via video conferencing. The goal of teledentistry in humans is to use technology and telecommunications for the improvement of oral care through consultations, education, and public awareness of dental issues. In human dentistry, teledentistry has been shown to have great potential to increase access to dental care for those located in underserved locations or those who have limited access to care.[36] Many veterinary dental specialists are already using teledentistry as means to advise general practitioners in diagnostic or treatment options that may be available for a patient. Barriers to the use of teledentistry can be related to the different regulatory boards used to govern its use.[36] Acquiring reimbursement for the services can be difficult due to inconsistent or absent clinic policies as to when a fee should be collected for teledentistry services.[36]

Technology can enable fast access to the patient history, diagnostic images, and documents related to patient care and transmit the information to a specialist for evaluation. Photographs, videos, and other information regarding the patient can be sent easily from a client to their veterinarian. These examples are a form of telemedicine that can relate to teledentistry if the information is related to a perceived oral issue. Although this information can be helpful to provide information regarding the patient's condition, it is not without shortcomings. Radiographic and clinical images are in a 2-dimensional view of a 3-dimensional object.[37] This can affect the accuracy of a diagnosis as well as not providing the clinical information needed to present treatment options to the client. Other limitations include the clinic, practitioner, or client's ability to capture diagnostic images or photographs.[37] The ability to acquire radiographic images is a skill that takes time and cannot be reliably produced at every veterinary clinic. Patients, like children, cannot be relied on to cooperate for the client to take a conscious diagnostic image of an area they are concerned with. Teledentistry limits the practitioner from performing full evaluations of the patient as well as limits the information that can be gathered during the consultation.[36] For the veterinary client, teledentistry is much less useful, as the information the client can provide is not as useful as what the veterinarian can acquire with a conscious or better yet anesthetized oral examination.

Clinics and consultants that are able to provide telemedicine and teledentistry services have discovered that this can generate an increased revenue stream. One teledentistry service that can be easily offered includes teleradiology services. This is whereby boarded veterinary dentists interpret diagnostic images such as radiographic, conventional computed tomography (CT), and cone-beam CT images submitted by referring veterinarians for interpretation and advice for a fee. This service can be used on a first opinion or second opinion basis. General practitioners may need assistance in the rapid interpretation of radiographic images while a patient is under anesthesia for a procedure. Services offered to help interpret images quickly can help the practitioner make educated decisions with assistance from an expert who is only a phone call or e-mail away. This is of benefit to the practitioner, the client, and most importantly the patient. Many teleradiology services offer different levels of service including stat readings, end-of-day readings, and no rush readings. There may be different pricing tiers for the different levels of treatment. Practitioners can pass the cost of these readings off to the client, with a convenience fee for service to help support the software and technology that may be needed to facilitate the submission of images.

## CONFIDENTIALITY AND SECURITY OF TELEMEDICINE SERVICES

Veterinary patients are not protected by the Health Insurance Portability and Accountability Act (HIPAA) regulations that protect medical privacy in human patients. However, like people, the information found in a patient's medical record, whether a companion animal or livestock patient, is protected by law. The confidentiality of the medical information of a veterinary patient is at the purview of the state for which the patient and the veterinarian reside. In some states, information that is found within the medical record such as treatments, medications, and diagnoses is considered privileged and confidential.[38] In many states this information must be kept confidential and not released except by the consent of the owner or by a court order (**Box 9**).

Telehealth services offered for veterinary patients are not without the risk of patient information becoming public. Data transmissions directly sent from a patient through a mobile app or a medical device may be shared with third-party advertisers if appropriate security measures are not used.[29] This shared information and data can give manufacturers and advertisers information concerning the patient's medical condition and target them for unsolicited information on products related to the information that was collected.[29] For example, a patient who has a device implanted for glucose monitoring may receive information on needles, syringes, or diabetic diets that may be used to help control or treat the condition. This can lead to decreased trust of the veterinarian that patient, or in the case of veterinary medicine, the client's information transmitted through a telemedicine service or device is secure. Collection of client and patient data resulting in unsolicited information from advertisers regarding products or therapeutic options can be considered intrusive to clients. Unsolicited information may upset clients as they may consider the information and data transmitted to the telehealth services no longer confidential. Thereby, questioning what other information provided to telehealth services is also not confidential and protected (eg, phone number, address, financial information, etc). For human patients, enforcement of HIPAA regulations is at the discretion of the Office for Civil Rights (OCR) at the Department of Health and Human Services. As of January 2021, due to the COVID-19 pandemic, the OCR is authorized to use its discretion to impose penalties for being incompliant with regulatory requirements concerning telehealth services.[39] At the time of this article, there is no regulatory body enforcing the regulations of telemedicine for veterinary patients.

Although telemedicine and telehealth services provide a significant convenience to the client, patient, and veterinarian, they are not without risk. Privacy concerns regarding a lack of control in relation to the use of the information collected are warranted. Disclosure of client information, patient information, diagnoses, treatment options, care, and financial information can be inadvertently shared through telehealth services.

When a veterinarian communicates electronically with a client, confidentiality can be breached during the collection and transfer of information. To avoid unauthorized access from unwanted individuals, encryption of the information is important. Encryption of data is whereby a mathematical series locks the data and ensures that a person who attempts to gain access to the encrypted information, will be unable to do so without having the key to the encryption.[29] If a person accesses the information without the encryption key, the information is useless, as it does not make any sense and is just a mathematical code. An individual who has the encryption key can retrieve the data and the information is meaningful and able to interpret. Information can also

---

**Box 9**
**American Veterinary Medical Association Confidentiality of Veterinary Patient Record Guidelines by State**

https://www.avma.org/advocacy/state-local-issues/confidentiality-veterinary-patient-records be controlled by restricting access to individuals by use of an authentication system based on the individual's role within the clinic.[29]

## COMMUNICATION AND MENTAL HEALTH

Veterinarian job satisfaction has been linked to relationships veterinarians have built with their clients.[11] Good communication helps to build self-esteem and the well-being of the veterinary clinician. Veterinarians who learn to develop self-care habits to improve their own well-being will be able to continue to provide compassionate care to their clients and patients. The implications of developing communication skills and self-care habits to help improve job satisfaction can be vital to a profession that struggles with mental health issues and depression.[11]

## EDUCATION AND COMMUNICATION

Many veterinarians seek additional education on how to better communicate with their clients. Communication is best learned using small groups, role-playing, and a discussion setting rather than a didactic lecture format.[5] Training can be conducted in the form of simulated consultations whereby actors play the role of a pet owner and through online training.[40]

Many veterinary schools are adding communication education into the veterinary curriculum. According to the Association of American Veterinary Medical Colleges Council on Education (COE) requirements regarding the curriculum, Standard 7.9.e states that universities must provide opportunities for students to learn how to acquire information from clients.[41] This includes opportunities to gather a complete history and read medical records. The COE also requires that students learn to retrieve information and develop skills to effectively communicate with clients and colleagues.[41]

Teaching effective communication to veterinary students has been suggested as an integral part of the curriculum for a successful veterinary practitioner.[3] Teaching communication skills to veterinary students can help shape their career as a practitioner. Developing skills to deliver bad news to clients can assist in decreasing the stress associated with having this type of conversation in practice.[3] Veterinary students who master communication skills used every day in practice will be able to deliver information regarding appropriate diagnostic and treatment options to clients as well as convey information that is, necessary to specialists to provide optimal care for their client and the patient.

A study of veterinary practitioners in the United States and the United Kingdom found that 98% of veterinarians feel that communication skills were as important, if not more important than clinical knowledge.[40] In this study, it was also found that 41% of veterinarians had received formal training in veterinary school regarding improving skills in communication. When surveyed, many veterinarians would like to have additional training regarding improving their communication skills.[40]

## SUMMARY

As John Powell, English Motion Picture Composer and Conductor stated, "Communication works for those who work at it."[42] Veterinary medicine is a profession of constant change and constant learning. Learning new therapies, medications, and diagnostics are just a part of the future. Good communication skills can be inherent within the individual, but also can be improved on by taking opportunities to refine the delivery. Every day gives the opportunity to demonstrate communication skills.

Veterinary practitioners who take advantage of opportunities to refine the skills they possess will build relationships with their clients and colleagues that can lead to an overall better experience for each person that they communicate with.

## DISCLOSURE

The authors have nothing to disclose.

## REFERENCES

1. Turner N. Nat Turner quotations. Available at: https://www.quotetab.com/quotes/by-nat-turner. Accessed February 5, 2021.
2. Lue T, Pantenburg D, Crawford P. Impact of the owner-pet and client-veterinarian bond on the care that pets receive. J Am Vet Med Assoc 2008;232:531–40.
3. Pun J. An integrated review of the role of communication in veterinary clinical practice. BMC Vet Res 2020;16:1–14.
4. Bard A, Main D, Haase A, et al. The future of veterinary communication: partnership or persuasion? A qualitative investigation of veterinary communication in the pursuit of client behaviour change. PLoS ONE 2017;12:1–17.
5. Shaw J, Bonnett B, Adams C, et al. Veterinarian-client-patient communication patterns used during clinical appointments in companion animal practice. J Am Vet Med Assoc 2006;228:714–21.
6. Takemura Y, Sakurai Y, Yokoya S, et al. Open-ended questions: are they really beneficial for gathering medical information from patients? Exp Med 2005;206:151–4.
7. Marcinowicz L, Chlabicz S, Grebowski R. Open-ended questions in surveys of patients' satisfaction with family doctors. J Health Serv Res Policy 2007;12(2):86–90.
8. Lindsley I, Wood S, Micallef C, et al. The concept of body language in the medical consultation. Psychiatr Danub 2015;27:41–7.
9. Stackhouse N, Chamberlain J, Bouwer A, et al. Development and validation of a novel measure for the direct assessment of empathy in veterinary students. J Vet Med Educ 2020;47:452–64.
10. Kacperek L. Non-verbal communication: the importance of listening. Br J Nurs 1997;6:275–9.
11. Shaw J, Adams C, Bonnett B, et al. Veterinarian satisfaction with companion animal visits. J Am Vet Med Assoc 2012;240:832–41.
12. Milani M. The Art of Private Veterinary Practice; Communication: Too compliant client communication. Can Vet J 2018;59:1123–4.
13. Kanji N, Coe J, Adams C, et al. Effect of veterinarian-client-patient interactions on client adherence to dentistry and surgery recommendations in companion-animal practice. J Am Vet Med Assoc 2012;240:427–36.
14. Makaryus A, Friedman E. Patients' understanding of their treatment plans and diagnosis at discharge. Mayo Clin Proc 2005;80:991–4.
15. Adams V, Waldner C, Campbell J. Analysis of a practice management computer software program for owner compliance with recall reminders. Can Vet J 2006;47:234–40.
16. King R, Baum N. How to write easy-to-read healthcare materials for blogs and websites that result in new patients. J Med Pract Manage 2018;33:392–4.
17. Royal K, Cheats K, Kedrowicz A. Readability evaluations of veterinary client handouts and implications for patient care. Top Companion Anim Med 2018;33:58–61.

18. Hansberry D, Agarwal N, Baker S. Health literacy and online educational resources: an opportunity to educate patients. AJR Am J Roentgenol 2015;204: 111–6.

19. Badarudeen S, Sabharwal S. Assessing readability of patient education materials: current role in orthopaedics. Clin Orthop Relat Res 2010;468:2572–80.

20. Glick A, Farkas J, Nicholson J, et al. Parental management of discharge instructions: a systematic review. Pediatrics 2017;140(2):1–16.

21. Shannon. How to create an engaging website design. In: AddThis Academy. Available at: https://www.addthis.com/academy/how-to-create-engaging-website-design/. Accessed March 15, 2021.

22. Best C, Coe J, Hewson J, et al. Referring equine veterinarians' expectations of equine veterinary specialists and referral centers. J Am Vet Med Assoc 2018; 253:479–89.

23. Murphy BG, Bell CM, Soukup JW. Veterinary oral and maxillofacial pathology. Hoboken NJ: Wiley Blackwell; 2020.

24. Verstraete FJM, Lommer MJ, Arzi B. Oral and maxillofacial surgery in dogs and cats. 2nd edition. St. Louis, MO: Elsevier; 2020.

25. Sidorowicz L, Szymanska J. The relationship between facial skeleton morphology and bite force in people with a normal relation of the bases of jaws and skull. Folia Morphol 2015;74:508–12.

26. Ellis JL, Thomason JJ, Kebreab E, et al. Calibration of estimated biting forces in domestic canids: comparison of post-mortem and in vivo measurements. J Anat 2008;212:769–80.

27. American Veterinary Medical Association. The veterinarian-client-patient relationship (VCPR). Available at: https://www.avma.org/resources-tools/pet-owners/petcare/veterinarian-client-patient-relationship-vcpr. Accessed March 12, 2021.

28. American Veterinary Medical Association. VCPR state laws. 2020. Available at: https://www.avma.org/sites/default/files/2020-11/VCPR-State-Chart-NOV-2020.pdf. Accessed March 15, 2021.

29. Hall J, McGraw D. For telehealth to succeed, privacy and security risks must be identified and addressed. Health Aff 2014;33:216–21.

30. American Veterinary Medical Association. Telemedicine. Available at: https://www.avma.org/resources-tools/avma-policies/telemedicine. Accessed March 12, 2021.

31. American Veterinary Medical Association. Telehealth and the VCPR: exploring the legal landscape of virtual care. Available at: https://www.avma.org/resources-tools/practice-management/telehealth-telemedicine-veterinary-practice/telehealth-and-vcpr. Accessed March 12, 2021.

32. American Veterinary Medical Association. AVMA guidelines for the use of telehealth in veterinary practice: Implementing connected care. Available at. http://avma.org/telehealth. Accessed March 11, 2021.

33. Watson K, Wells J, Sharma M, et al. A survey of knowledge and use of telehealth among veterinarians. BMC Vet Res 2019;15(1):474.

34. Roca R, McCarthy R. Impact of telemedicine on the traditional veterinarian-client-patient relationship. Top Comp Anim Med 2019;37:1–4.

35. Jampani N, Nutalapati R, Donatula B, et al. Applications of teledentistry: a literature review and update. J Int Soc Prev Community Dent 2011;1(2):37–44.

36. Daniel S, Kumar S. Teledentistry: a key component in access to care. J Evid Based Dent Pract 2014;I 4S:201–8.

37. Khan S, Omar H. Teledentistry in practice: literature review. Telemed J e-health 2013;19(7):565–7.

38. State Policy Analyst, AVMA Division of State Advocacy. Confidentiality of Veterinary Patient Records. Available at: https://www.avma.org/advocacy/state-local-issues/confidentiality-veterinary-patient-records. Accessed March 11, 2021.
39. Office for Civil Rights (OCR). Notification of enforcement discretion for telehealth remote communications during the Covid-19 nationwide public health emergency. In U.S. Department of Health and Human Services, Health Information Privacy. 2021. Available at: https://www.hhs.gov/hipaa/for-professionals/special-topics/emergency-preparedness/notification-enforcement-discretion-telehealth/index.html. Accessed March 12, 2021.
40. McDermott M, Tischler V, Cobb M, et al. Veterinarian-client communication skills: current state, relevance, and opportunities for improvement. J Vet Med Educ 2015;42:305–14.
41. American Veterinary Medical Association. COE accreditation policies and procedures: requirements: 7.9 Standard 9, Curriculum. Available at. https://www.avma.org/education/accreditation/colleges/coe-accreditation-policies-and-procedures-requirements. Accessed March 11, 2021.
42. Powell J. Meaning In. Available at: https://meaningin.com/quotes/john-powell/9809-communication-works-for-those-who-work-at-it–. Accessed March 15, 2021.

# Role of the Veterinary Technicians and Hygienists in Veterinary Dentistry and Oral Surgery

Check for updates

Mary L. Berg, BS, LATG, RVT, VTS (Dentistry)[a],[*],
Jeanette M. Eliason, CVT, RDH, VTS (Dentistry)[b]

## KEYWORDS

• Veterinary technician • Dental hygienist • Home care • Prevention • Examination

## KEY POINTS

- Describe the role of a veterinary technician, registered dental hygienist, and veterinary assistant in veterinary dentistry.
- Review conscious and unconscious examination.
- Review instrumentation in periodontal health.
- Review machine maintenance.
- Discuss oral home care and the role of the veterinary technician/nurse, registered dental hygienist, and veterinary assistant.

## INTRODUCTION: A TEAM EFFORT

Companion animals have become an essential part of our lives, and many people consider the pet a part of their family. This bond is important to the veterinary team, as it has made clients more interested in dental care for their pets. Communication must remain open between all parties and the entire veterinary team to project the same message to the client. All members of the veterinary team must be excited and motivated. The veterinarian and their team must educate the client about the need for dentistry and demonstrate the importance of good oral hygiene to the pet's overall health. Clients need to hear the same message several times to ensure they retain and understand the importance. About 25% of your clients accepts whatever you say immediately; another 60% takes a little time to accept your

---

[a] Beyond the Crown Veterinary Education; [b] The University of Pennslyvania - School of Veterinary Medicine, 91 Cobalt Ridge Drive North, Levittown, PA 19057, USA
* Corresponding author. Beyond the Crown Veterinary Education, 1002 East 850th Road, Lawrence, KS 66047.
E-mail address: mlberg@btcveted.com

Vet Clin Small Anim 52 (2022) 49–66
https://doi.org/10.1016/j.cvsm.2021.09.007

recommendations, and the remaining 15% may not accept your suggestions.[1] As veterinary professionals, we need to concentrate on the 60% to ensure they understand the need for dental care. The entire team plays a role in the success of a dental program in veterinary hospitals. This article concentrates on the role of veterinary technicians/nurses and dental hygienists (registered dental hygienist [RDH]), but each member of the team is essential.

## RECEPTIONISTS

The receptionist is the first and last person the client sees in the practice and is the bridge between the client and the rest of the veterinary team. These individuals must be friendly and confident and provide the client with accurate information. Receptionists demonstrate their interest in the client and pet through body language and words. A receptionist that projects a positive attitude regarding dentistry and home care is essential for success. The acceptance of dentistry within a practice can be significantly affected if the receptionist is not entirely on board. This interaction may begin with a telephone conversation. All practices have phone shoppers who are seeking the best deal on a dental procedure.

## VETERINARY ASSISTANTS

The veterinary assistant plays an important role in dentistry within the practice. The assistant's role can be divided into 3 areas: preoperative, intraoperative, and postoperative patient care.

Preoperatively, the veterinary assistant should ensure that the dental suite is cleaned, fully stocked, organized, set up, and ready for each patient. The assistant should inform the veterinary technician or practice manager when an instrument needs sharpening or replaced. In addition, attention should be paid to when ultrasonic tips or dental burs require replacement, and when any supplies need to be ordered. The assistant should organize and pack the dental kits to optimize use for the veterinarian.

Intraoperatively, the veterinary assistant supports the technician/nurse and dental hygienist (RDH) in dental procedures by recording findings on the dental chart, positioning the patient if needed, and assisting with preoperative and postoperative dental photographs and radiographs. Four-handed dentistry in which 2 people work together to perform an oral examination, record findings on the dental chart, and assist with the dental software during radiographic processing can decrease the total procedure time.[2] The assistant can also transcribe findings into the practice management software, upload photographs and radiographs, and prepare the discharge paperwork.

Postoperatively, the veterinary care assistant should ensure that the pet is cleaned and ready for discharge before release. The pet should be dry and have its hair brushed and any remnants of blood removed before being presented to the owner. Taking a few extra minutes to perform these tasks can ensure the pet owner feels that this was a pleasant and vital procedure. The assistant should also perform maintenance on the dental equipment, such as cleaning and autoclaving the instruments, assessing the instruments' sharpness, and performing routine maintenance on the dental unit by releasing the compressor's pressure, wiping all surfaces, lubricating the handpieces, and preparing the operatory for the next patient.

## CREDENTIALED VETERINARY TECHNICIANS/NURSES

Credentialed veterinary technicians/nurses are essential members of the dental team as pet advocates and client educators. They are often eager to be empowered, and dentistry is one of the veterinary practice areas where technicians/nurses can be fully used. It is important to remember that a credentialed technician/nurse can do everything but diagnose, perform surgery, prescribe drugs, and give a prognosis. Empowering a technician/nurse to become the go-to dental person of the practice allows for professional growth and pride in their chosen profession. It increases the dental revenue for the practice. This person would be the source for all dental things and would be responsible for the entire staff's training so that everyone understands the importance of good oral health.

Each practice should have a veterinary technician/nurse whose main emphasis and training are in dentistry.[1] The veterinarian is the only one who can diagnose disease; however, credentialed veterinary technicians/nurses with training in dentistry can assist the veterinarian by gathering an accurate history and recognizing abnormalities that are brought to the attention of the veterinarian (**Table 1**). The technician/nurse's responsibilities include the following:

- Patient intake
- History gathering
- Oral examination
- Dental charting
- Dental radiography
- Professional dental cleaning
- Assisting in dental/oral procedures
- Delivering postoperative instructions
- Home care discussion
- Client education
- Follow-up visits
- Medical record keeping
- Instrument/equipment maintenance

## CREDENTIALED REGISTERED DENTAL HYGIENIST

The credentialed RDH can play an essential role alongside the veterinary community regarding education and treatment of periodontal health by following the laws provided under the state regulations for veterinary dentistry. Dental hygienists have advanced knowledge and clinical skills that enable them to perform oral health assessment and periodontal therapies.[3] They can perform the same duties as the veterinary assistant and veterinary technician/nurse as mentioned above but cannot provide anesthesia to patients unless fully trained and under the supervision of a licensed veterinarian.

The American Veterinary Dental College (AVDC) provided a mission statement pertaining to the safety of veterinary patients when dental care is being provided by nonveterinary dental team members stating: "The AVDC recognizes that dentists, registered dental hygienists and other dental health care providers in good standing may perform those procedures for which they have been qualified under the direct supervision of the veterinarian. The supervising veterinarian will be responsible for the welfare of the patient and any treatment performed on the patient."

## HISTORY GATHERING

The veterinarian uses education and observation in dentistry, comparing abnormal findings with normal findings to determine a treatment plan.[4] The veterinary technician/nurse and RDH can help the veterinarian by gathering the relevant dental

**Table 1**
**Role of the veterinary technicians and hygienists in veterinary dentistry and oral surgery**

| | |
|---|---|
| History gathering | Gathering medical health history and relevant dental information to aid in development of a treatment plan by the veterinarian |
| Patient intake | Educate, review, and complete all consent forms with the owner before admission after the veterinarian has evaluated and discussed with owners |
| Operating room setup | Important role completed before the anesthetic procedure. Operatory is prepared; check all parts of the anesthetic machine, monitoring devices, and dental equipment. Failure to do so results in lagged anesthetic procedures and decreased optimal patient care |
| Conscious and unconscious examination | Technician/nurse or dental hygienist can conduct both examinations, but all finding must be reported and evaluated by the veterinarian. Physical examination is completed on conscious examination. Extraoral and intraoral evaluations are to be completed on both conscious and unconscious examination. During extraoral examination, one must include the neck and ears for evaluation, as some findings can be related to oral disease |
| Dental charting | Comprehensive periodontal evaluation, including missing teeth, probe depths, gingivitis, gingival recession, mobility, furcation involvement, plaque, calculus evaluation, tooth defects, and lesions/growths. All finding must be reported to veterinarian for determination of treatment |
| Dental radiography | Evaluation of the tooth pertaining to structural, pathologic, and periodontal findings completed before or after dental charting and oral examination. Advanced practices veterinary technicians/nurses/dental hygienists, in addition, can assist with imaging modalities, such as CT, CBCT, and MRI |
| Local anesthetic administration | Administration completed by properly trained clinical veterinary technicians/nurses and dental hygienists. Aids in decreasing inhalation anesthesia and intraoperative/postoperative pain management |
| | *(continued on next page)* |

| Table 1 (continued) | |
|---|---|
| Professional dental cleaning | Measure taken for prevention and progression of oral disease with the usage of power scalers (eg, magnetostrictive, piezoelectric, or sonic) and hand instruments (eg, sickle scaler, curette) |
| Scaling and root planning | Aid in periodontal therapy removing biofilm, plaque, and calculus subgingival from tooth surface to improve or sustain periodontal health |
| Assisting in dental/oral procedures | Conducting 4-handed dentistry is the optimal means of practicing to provide sufficient patient care |
| Obtaining dental impressions and stone model preparation | Obtain and prepare dental impression and stone models. Provides the clinician the ability to study and measure architecture of the oral cavity and fabrication of prosthetics and provides documentation |
| Client education | Vital role to gain compliance. Home care instructions must include postoperative medications, dietary restrictions or recommendations, an explanation of the procedure performed and aftercare needs, and long-term home oral hygiene recommendations |
| Follow-up visits | Follow-up postoperative care aids in discussion of home care and allows time for demonstration of recommendations |
| Medical record keeping | Aid in monitoring oral health to assess oral disease and treatment warranted. It is important to provide thorough record keeping, including patient pictures, radiographs, and dental charting |
| Instrument/equipment maintenance | Daily, monthly, biannual, yearly maintenance of instruments plays a vital role during surgical procedures. It allows conduction of proper oral care with the use of full functioning machines and a decrease biofilm in waterlines. Check manufacturer recommendations when purchased to provide optimal care |

information and obtaining an accurate overall health history to develop the treatment plan. Doing so allows the doctor to enter the examination room with an understanding of the pet's oral condition and overall health and work with the technician/nurse/hygienist and client to prepare the best treatment options for the pet.

The patient's history is valuable information that can assist the veterinarian in determining the treatment plan.[1] Having a complete history of previous oral examination findings and dental procedures performed helps the veterinarian to understand the present oral condition and predict a procedure's outcome. For example, an 8-year-old Yorkshire terrier who has not had any previous oral examinations and/or treatments is likely to have severe oral disease. In contrast, a similar patient with annual dental assessments and cleanings may only have mild disease.

Some clients are educated and recognize a problem with their pet's oral cavity; however, most seem to be unaware that their pet may have a dental concern.[1,4,5] A pet owner may see signs of excessive salivation, inappetence, swelling, difficulty swallowing, or indications of oral discomfort.[4,5] When a client suspects the pet has a problem with the oral cavity, it is necessary to interview the client to gather the needed information and perform an oral examination. This information and the complete history, including past oral examinations and treatments, current diet, chewing habits, and home care performed, are pieces of the puzzle that must be put together.[5] The most common symptom noticed by owners is malodor; however, many owners (and veterinary professionals) think that halitosis may be normal in pets ("puppy breath").

Most commonly, the owner may not be aware that there is a problem with their pet's mouth. Thus, any dental issues may only be discovered during the oral portion of the physical examination. Finding a dental concern during an examination is the perfect time for the veterinary technician/nurse or dental hygienist to educate the client on oral disease and its importance to overall health (**Fig. 1**).

Just as the veterinary technician/nurse or dental hygienist interviews the client regarding the pet's lifestyle to allow the veterinarian to determine the appropriate vaccine protocol and flea/tick prevention, questions should be asked about the pet's oral health. The client should be encouraged to volunteer information, if possible, but some questions need to be asked. Open-ended questions are the best way to gather information. If a client is not aware of any problems with their pet's oral cavity, questions that could be asked are as follows:

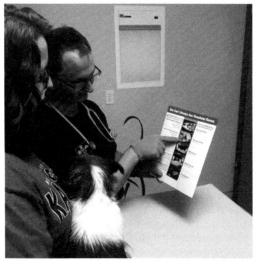

**Fig. 1.** A veterinary technician/nurse showing the client an area of concern in the pet's oral cavity.

- "Has Bea had any previous dental work?" Let the owner volunteer information for you. If the client responds with "Yes, Bea did have two teeth extracted at my previous veterinarian," you can now ask more direct questions about when the extraction procedure was performed, and so on.
- "What is the pet's favorite chew toy?" Some pets are very orally fixated, whereas others may not be chewers. Some toys, such as tennis balls, ice cubes, cow hooves, pig ears, and hard nylon bones, can cause tooth fracture.[1] A client may not realize the harm that could come from what they thought was a great toy, allowing for an opportunity to educate your clients about possible harm.

If the client is aware of a dental problem, ask them when they first noticed a problem. Many owners think that bad breath is expected and are not aware that periodontal disease is likely responsible for the malodor.[6] The following questions could be asked in situations whereby the owner is concerned about a problem:

- "Has Gypsy had any problems eating? Does she tend to drop food or chew on one side of the mouth? Has she stopped eating altogether, or will she only eat soft food?"
- "Does Frank seem to salivate excessively?"
- "Does Lisa appear to have problems drinking or swallowing?"
- "Has there been a change in Cooper's habits or behavior?"
- "Does Susi rub her face on the carpet or paw at her face?" Face rubbing can be a sign of oral pain or inflammation.

## ORAL EXAMINATION IN THE CONSCIOUS PATIENT

The veterinarian must perform the general health examination. The entire animal should be examined from nose to tail. A thorough examination should include the eyes, ears, skin, heart, lung, and abdomen. One should also check for internal parasites. Before anesthesia, routine blood tests (complete blood count and biochemical serum profile) are performed, and a urinalysis should be added as needed.

In a well-managed practice (ie, with effectively used staff), the veterinary technician/nurse or dental hygienist can perform the initial oral examinations on both the conscious and the anesthetized patient and report the findings to the veterinarian. The conscious examination is limited to smell, visual, and tactile examination. The examination should include the symmetry of the head. Do both sides appear to be uniform, or does 1 side look different?[4] Is there swelling in any area of the head? If swelling appears below the eye, look for a fractured maxillary fourth premolar tooth. Do the jaws appear symmetric? If 1 side of the jaw is swollen or not symmetric, rule out tooth pathologic condition, jaw fractures, or oral masses.

A detailed oral examination should be performed before anesthesia if possible. Check for occlusion, tooth fractures, gingival recession, inflammation, and mobile teeth. Count the teeth to determine if there are supernumerary teeth present or if teeth are missing. Inflammation in the oral cavity can contribute to the swelling of the lymph nodes. The temporomandibular joint should also be palpated for indications of discomfort. An oral examination may sometimes be a difficult task, as not all patients are willing to allow a good look into their mouth, especially if they are head shy or a young puppy.

Although it is most important to evaluate the periodontal tissues under general anesthesia when the various indexes (for plaque, calculus, pocket depth, furcation involvement, and tooth mobility) can be evaluated, it is essential to observe the gingiva to determine a preliminary degree of periodontal inflammation. Healthy gingiva is pink and has a stippled appearance with defined margins, whereas red, swollen gums indicate inflammation. Gingival recession and enlargement are crucial elements of periodontal disease and should be noted. A complete examination can only be performed under general anesthesia. However, the conscious patient's examination already yields vital information that can help to determine the need for additional diagnostic tools and create an initial treatment plan and cost estimate.

## COST ESTIMATE (DIAGNOSTIC AND TREATMENT PLAN)

Diagnostic and treatment procedures cannot be done without the owner's permission. The client needs to understand the presence of pathologic condition and the need for therapy. The technician/nurse and dental hygienist play a vital role in providing this education to the client. The diagnostic and treatment plan should be itemized and as accurate as possible. The technician/nurse or dental hygienist should go through this plan with the client, explaining each item's need and value. For example, preanesthetic blood work may find systemic problems that can increase the patient's anesthetic risk and affect the anesthesia protocol. Also, dental radiographs are necessary to determine if there is pathologic condition that is not visible to the naked eye.

Explaining the diagnostic and treatment plan line by line helps the client understand the need for and importance of the different procedures. Clients see and understand the pathologic condition more easily in pictures, models, or videos than in their pet's oral cavity. The treatment plan should also address the patient's anesthetic risk level and explain the precautions necessary for a positive outcome. It is good to provide a cost estimate to the client before any diagnostic and treatment procedures are undertaken. This practice prevents distress over unexpected expenses and helps the clients understand that the procedure is vital to their pet's health. Providing an estimate in advance can also help the client make arrangements for payments.

An exact diagnostic and treatment plan cannot be determined in the examination room on a conscious patient, but a close "estimate" can be created from the oral examination. The veterinary technician/nurse or dental hygienist should explain that this is only an estimate and that a more accurate range of anticipated costs can be prepared once a complete oral examination and dental radiography are performed with the animal under anesthesia. Providing a cost estimate that is higher than anticipated can have a twofold benefit. First, it provides an allowance if the oral pathologic condition is more advanced than thought on the initial examination. Second, the client can be pleasantly surprised to have a lower cost for the procedure. If the client wants a more precise estimate before the procedure, prepare a "worst-case scenario" and explain this to the client.

The veterinary technician/nurse and dental hygienist should recognize the owner's commitment and ability to perform home care.[1] This knowledge is of importance, as it can serve the veterinarian to decide whether diseased teeth should be extracted or whether the pet should be referred to a dental specialist for a tooth-salvaging procedure.

## ORAL EXAMINATION IN THE ANESTHETIZED PATIENT

Before the anesthetic procedure, the veterinary technician/nurse or dental hygienist should ensure that the operatory room is prepared and check all parts of the anesthetic machine and monitoring devices. As stated earlier, a thorough oral examination can only be completed under general anesthesia. The veterinarian and technician/nurse should work together to determine the patient's best anesthetic protocol. The technician/nurse prepares and administers the drugs for sedation, provides preoxygenation, and then induces anesthesia with the veterinary assistant or dental hygienist's assistance or another technician/nurse. If a licensed technician/nurse is not available, the veterinarian should induce anesthesia. The technician/nurse must ensure the patient is correctly connected to monitors and that heating devices have been appropriately placed. The patient should be at a surgical plane of anesthesia before beginning the oral examination.

One of the most common reasons clients are hesitant to have dental procedures performed is their fear of anesthesia. It is essential to explain that each patient is thoroughly evaluated, and the best anesthetic protocol is used for their particular needs. It is also reassuring for the client to know that a dedicated anesthetist closely monitors the patients during the entire procedure, ensures they are kept warm to prevent hypothermia, and keeps detailed records of the anesthesia event.

The veterinary technician/nurse or dental hygienist should perform a thorough oral examination on each tooth in the oral cavity while the veterinary assistant records the findings on a dental chart. Each tooth must be evaluated for gingivitis, periodontal pockets, gingival recession, mobility, and furcation involvement (on multirooted teeth). Extra or missing teeth are noted on the chart, and any other abnormalities that may be found. This chart and the dental radiographs are presented to the veterinarian to assess potential problem areas and develop a more detailed treatment plan.

The veterinary technician/nurse or dental hygienist also takes the dental radiographs (**Fig. 2**). It is highly recommended that full-mouth radiographs be taken on

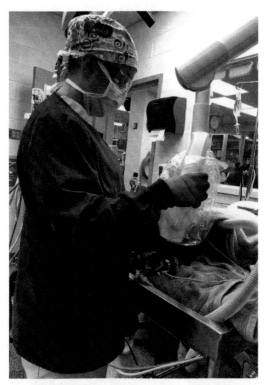

**Fig. 2.** Taking diagnostic dental radiographs is an essential skill that the veterinary technician/nurse and dental hygienist should master.

each pet every year. Training must be provided to successfully take diagnostic radiographic views in a timely manner and recognize abnormalities found on the radiographs. In more advanced practices, the technician/nurse should assist with other imaging modalities, such as computed tomography (CT), cone-beam CT (CBCT), and MRI. A dental hygienist may be able to help with CBCT, but assisting with CT and MRI often is state regulated and requires extensive training.

The veterinary technician/nurse or dental hygienist should complete the professional dental cleaning procedure. They must know how to properly and safely use each instrument involved and continually evaluate and train the staff on the proper techniques of scaling and polishing. The entire tooth must be cleaned below (subgingival) and above (supragingival) the gingival margin (gumline). The removal of plaque and calculus is vital to the success of the treatment. This can be completed by hand instrumentation and or by use of a power scaler. If dental deposits are not removed, bacteria can continue the inflammatory process, leading to the destruction of the periodontium, resulting in gingival recession, alveolar bone loss, and eventual tooth loss.

Calculus removal forceps can be used for quick removal of large deposits. This instrument has a long-curved tip (with a rubber insert) and a short tip. The former is placed over the crown of the tooth, and the latter is placed over/under the large calculus deposit. Closing the forceps will dislodge gross chunks of calculus. It is important to use caution and not grip and lacerate the gingival tissue while using the forceps. Regular extraction forceps should ideally not be used, as they can fracture the tooth when engaged against a cusp of the crown.

Power scalers are broken down into 2 types, ultrasonic and sonic, and are helpful to remove the biofilm/plaque and calculus deposits. The instrument is held the same as manual instruments using the modified pen grasp (but in a "light" modified pen grasp; **Fig. 3**). This allows the operator to roll the instrument between the thumb and pointer finger to properly adapt the scaler tip on the tooth surface. Once the modified pen grasp is established using a "light featherlike" pressure, the side of the tip is held at a 0° to 15° angle toward the tooth surface. It is important to keep the tip always moving (and not in a "stop-and-go" movement). Heavy pressure must not be applied, as this will cause damage to the tooth and decrease efficiency of the tip. Another rule of

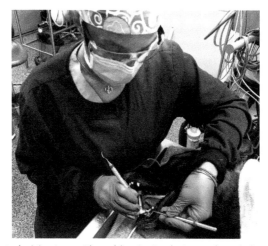

**Fig. 3.** Veterinary technician/nurse/dental hygienist during a dental cleaning.

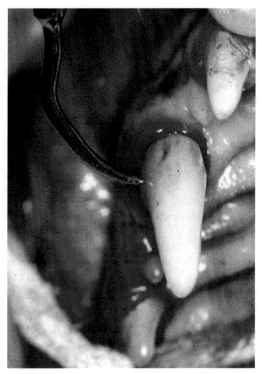

**Fig. 4.** Holding the scaler tip at a 90° angle to the tooth will cause structural and thermal damage.

thumb is to never hold the tip of the power scaler at a 90° angle to the tooth surface, as this will cause structural damage to the enamel and thermal injury to the pulp of the tooth (**Fig. 4**).

Tip selection for powered instrumentation has grown over the years, and numerous designs are offered for proper application of periodontal care. Tips vary in length, shape, diameter, and function, and it is important to have a general understanding for clinical application. In general, the universal tips are much wider and used for gross heavy debridement of debris. Thinner tips are used for deep periodontal pockets and furcation areas. Power and water settings must be set appropriately during use of either of these tips to not damage the tip of the instrument or cause damage to the tooth.

Hand scaling is a skill that takes time to learn. It is important to understand the anatomy of the instrument so that it can be used appropriately.[7] Hand scaling is best performed after power scaling and aids in the removal of residual plaque and calculus. A sickle scaler is used for supragingival debris only, as it has a triangular tip that will lacerate the gingival tissue if placed subgingivally. A curette is used for removal of subgingival plaque and calculus. It has rounded tip end, which will not traumatize the gingival tissue when adapted properly below the gumline. The operator must adapt, angulate, and activate these hand instruments appropriately to not cause trauma to the tooth, such as "gouging" the root surface. The first third of the tip is always applied to the tooth surface. Depending on the type of hand instrument selected and location of the tooth applied, the angulation can vary. For subgingival scaling, the face of the blade of the curette is held toward the tooth. Once the blade has reached the base of the tooth, the instrument is angled for the cutting edge to be placed below the dental deposit and pulled in an upward (coronal) direction. This procedure is repeated until all plaque and calculus are removed.

The fine tip of a dental explorer should be used to check the tooth surface for any remaining calculus. Air drying makes the calculus appear chalky white. The crown can be inspected for any residual plaque by applying a disclosing solution and gentle rinsing with water. This technique must be used with care, as it may cause staining of the hair around the patient's mouth.

Polishing with a slightly abrasive paste can remove any missed plaque and smooths out the minute scratches on the tooth surface. The cup on a prophy angle attached to a low-speed handpiece moves at approximately 3000 to 8000 rpm. A higher speed or staying on a tooth for longer than approximately 10 seconds can lead to overheating and result in thermal pulp damage. Disposable prophy angles are relatively inexpensive and are discarded after each use. There are many commercially available prophy pastes on the market, ranging in grit and hardness from flour and fine to extra coarse. Flour or fine grit pastes are recommended to ensure the enamel is as smooth as possible. Prophy paste can also be made by mixing flour pumice with water or glycerin.

Irrigation of the mouth following scaling and polishing is vital. All pieces of dislodged calculus and prophy paste must be removed from the mouth to avoid aspiration upon recovery. The gingival sulcus should be gently irrigated to remove debris. A final rinse with chlorhexidine gluconate (0.12%) provides additional control of bacteria because of its substantiveness (ability to adhere to oral tissues and release agents over an extended period).

The veterinary technician/nurse and dental hygienist should be training and prepared to assist the veterinarian in any additional dental procedures that may need to be performed, including retracting tissue, handing instruments, and blotting blood away for a cleaner work area. An experienced technician/nurse or dental hygienist would anticipate the next steps of the procedure and be prepared to assist when needed. Oral examination findings and procedures performed should correctly be recorded into the patient's dental and medical record. Extractions are considered oral surgery and therefore should not be performed by technicians/nurses or dental hygienists. Position statements of the AVDC, Academy of Veterinary Dental Technicians (AVDT), and American Veterinary Medical Association regarding task of veterinary technician/nurse, RDH, and veterinary assistant can be seen in **Boxes 1–3**.[8–10]

Postoperatively, the veterinary technician/nurse should postoxygenate, ensure that the oral cavity is clean, extubate and monitor the patient, and provide a comfortable recovery area. When the patient is fully recovered, the move from the recovery area to the hospital ward is supervised. The technician/nurse or dental hygienist should work with the veterinarian to determine appropriate dietary recommendations and postoperative pain management for the patient.

## HOME CARE INSTRUCTIONS

A client who understands the importance of oral care may be willing to perform home care. This ensures that their pet's mouth heals and remains healthy. The veterinary technician/nurse and dental hygienist should work with the client to develop an understanding of why home care is essential. Demonstrating how to administer it is critical to gaining compliance (**Fig. 5**). Home care instructions must include postoperative medications, dietary restrictions or recommendations, an explanation of the

---

**Box 1**
**Position statements for *Veterinary Clinics of North America: Small Animal Practice***

Extraction of teeth
- The AVDC considers the extraction of teeth to be included in the practice of veterinary dentistry. Decision making is the responsibility of the veterinarian, with the consent of the pet owner, when electing to extract teeth. Only veterinarians shall determine which teeth are to be extracted and perform extraction procedures.

Dental tasks performed by veterinary technicians
- The AVDC considers it appropriate for a veterinarian to delegate maintenance dental care and certain dental tasks to a veterinary technician. Tasks appropriately performed by a technician include dental prophylaxis and certain procedures that do not result in altering the shape, structure, or positional location of teeth in the dental arch. The veterinarian may direct an appropriately trained technician to perform these tasks providing that the veterinarian is physically present and supervising the treatment.

Veterinary technician dental training
- The AVDC supports the advanced training of veterinary technicians to perform additional ancillary dental services: taking impressions, making models, charting veterinary dental pathologic condition, taking and developing dental radiographs, performing nonsurgical subgingival root scaling and debridement, providing that they do not alter the structure of the tooth.

Tasks that may be performed by veterinary assistants (not registered, certified, or licensed)
- The AVDC supports the appropriate training of veterinary assistants to perform the following dental services: supragingival scaling and polishing, taking and developing dental radiographs, making impressions and making models.

Tasks that may be performed by dentists, RDHs, and other dental health care providers
- The AVDC recognizes that dentists, RDHs, and other dental health care providers in good standing may perform those procedures for which they have been qualified under the direct supervision of the veterinarian. The supervising veterinarian will be responsible for the welfare of the patient and any treatment performed on the patient. The AVDC understands that individual states have regulations that govern the practice of veterinary medicine. This position statement is intended to be a model for veterinary dental practice and does not replace existing law.

American Veterinary Dental College Position Statement (avdc.org) revised 2006/accessed 9/20/2021

---

procedure performed and aftercare needs, and long-term home oral hygiene recommendations.

Follow-up visits can often be scheduled with the veterinary technician/nurse or dental hygienist. A postoperative follow-up visit within 1 to 2 weeks allows evaluation of proper healing. The need for continued home oral hygiene can be reinforced, and any questions or concerns by the client can be answered. Tooth brushing and other home care techniques can be evaluated and discussed with the client during these visits. Some practices use a color-coding system for the follow-up examinations. A red code means the patient needs to have a follow-up visit every 3 months; orange means the patient needs to have a follow-up visit every 6 months, and green means the patient needs to have a follow-up visit every year. Patients can be upgraded or downgraded from 1 code to another, depending on the recheck results.

Handouts can be individualized for the patient by showing the client the importance of oral health.[4] They should include a simplified dental chart for making notations, such as pocket depth, furcation exposure, or missing/extracted teeth. The treatment performed should be included on this handout. A copy of the dental radiographs can

---

**Box 2**
**Academy of Veterinary Dental Technicians position statement**

AVDT extraction position statement
  The AVDT does not condone, endorse, nor recommend that veterinary technicians, credentialed or not, perform dental extractions on any species, especially cats, dogs, and horses. Extraction of teeth is oral surgery and should be performed by a licensed veterinarian, per the American Veterinary Medical Association. Several states allow for veterinary technicians to perform extractions, but the wording is often vague, some stating simple extractions only, others simply listing extractions as a task that can be performed by a credentialed veterinary technician.
  The duties of a veterinary technician during a dental procedure include charting, performing dental cleaning (subgingival and supragingival) and polishing, intraoral radiographs, performing nerve blocks, assisting with the dental procedures, and oral surgery. Diagnosing dental disease, prescribing treatment options and medications, and performing oral surgery are duties for the veterinarian. The veterinary technician may and should assist the veterinarian with these duties, thereby ensuring the patient receives the most thorough and efficient dental care.
  A veterinary technician specialist in dentistry is a credentialed technician with a special interest in dentistry and oral surgery. They have extensive knowledge and training in these areas (endodontics, exodontics, orthodontics, prosthodontics, and periodontics); however, they are not taught nor licensed to perform oral surgery. They may instruct veterinarians on proper extraction techniques under the direct supervision of a licensed veterinarian.
  Always refer to your state's veterinary practice act for the duties that you may perform legally.

AVDT Extraction Position Statement 2021 accessed 9/21/2021.

---

demonstrate the value of diagnostic imaging to the owner. The veterinary technician/ nurse or dental hygienist can create other handouts on common dental problems, home care options, and treatments. Handouts can be sent to clients after the procedure or problem has been discussed with them in the examination room.

---

**Box 3**
**Veterinary Dentistry/American Veterinary Medical Association (avma.org)**

In regards to equine dentistry, oral medicine, and oral surgery, "procedures which are invasive of the tissues to the oral cavity including, but not limited to, removal of sharp enamel points, treatment of malocclusions of premolars, molars, and incisors, odontoplasty, the extraction of first premolars and deciduous premolars and incisors, extraction of damaged or diseased teeth, treatment of diseased teeth via restorations and endodontic procedures, periodontal and orthodontic treatments, dental radiography and endoscopy of the oral cavity are veterinary dental procedures and should be performed by a licensed veterinarian." [1]

[1] Excerpt from AAEP Position on Equine Dentistry (2019) www.aaep.org, used with permission.

Concluding statements
  Veterinary dentistry, oral medicine, and oral surgery are, therefore, to be performed by licensed veterinarians in accordance with their state veterinary practice act. Appropriately trained veterinary health care workers may be allowed to perform certain nonsurgical oral and dental procedures only under the direct supervision of a licensed veterinarian in accordance with state regulations.
  As with other areas of veterinary practice, veterinary dentistry, oral medicine, and oral surgery require a veterinarian-client-patient relationship to protect the health, safety, and welfare of animals.

Veterinary Dentistry/American Veterinary Medical Association (avma.org) Accessed 9/20/2021.

---

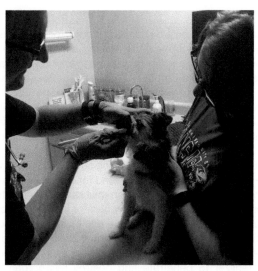

**Fig. 5.** Veterinary technician/nurse/dental hygienist demonstrating home care to a client.

The veterinary technician/nurse and dental hygienist should also consider themselves public educators. Education helps more pets receive proper oral care. Offering it shows that the veterinary practice embraces dentistry and its importance to the well-being of the patients. There are many options to get the word out about the importance of oral health, including social media posts with trivia questions, essential information, and interesting cases (with client permission). Consider your audience when posting cases and leave out the blood and gore, even though this can be a valuable tool to raise pet parent awareness of dental conditions.

Be creative, as there are many opportunities to educate the public about the importance of pets' oral health. A few ideas are as follows:

- Hold an open house and tours of the dental suite for clients, visitors, and youth groups.
- Provide informational brochures in the examination rooms.
- Post a video on your website, explaining the day of a dental procedure at your practice.
- Create a "smile book" with photographs before and after treatment and a pictorial step-by-step dental cleaning procedure.
- Write an article for a local newspaper.
- Visit an elementary school with a dog that loves to have its teeth brushed.
- Give an informational talk at a youth group meeting, such as 4-H or Scouts.
- Provide a booth at Mutt Strut or other dog-related events.

## EQUIPMENT MAINTENANCE

Maintenance of dental equipment needs to be done daily, monthly, and yearly and includes routine and emergency repair of larger items, such as the dental unit and radiograph generator, and inspection and sharpening of all instruments needed, such as for dental cleaning and surgical procedures.[11] If maintenance is not done routinely, the life expectancy of tools and instruments will shorten, and potential failure during surgical procedures can occur.

## Daily Maintenance

Water lines of dental machines must be flushed through for 2 minutes before use. This includes the powered instrument units, high-speed handpiece lines, and 3-way air-water syringe. A biofilm of microorganisms grows inside the dental unit lines when not in use, and flushing the lines before use will help decrease these colonies being introduced into the patient's oral cavity. The lines must also be flushed for 20 to 30 seconds between patients before the start of the next case. When flushing the waterlines, the technician/nurse or dental hygienist should make sure all handpieces are working, and an appropriate psi of 35 to 45 according to manufacturer instructions is maintained.

Instruments should be inspected when opening surgical packs to verify they are not broken, that all are accounted for that are needed for the procedure, and that all have been sharpened. Instrument sharpening is a special skill that needs to be mastered by the dental team. Dull instruments can lead to operator fatigue, musculoskeletal disorders, and insufficient removal of biofilm/plaque and calculus.[11] Following completion of procedures, instruments should be rinsed immediately to remove all bioburden, including inside the latches. This process is important, as if not removed, it will inhibit chemicals in the sterilizer to penetrate and destroy microorganisms. Dental units should be decompressed and wiped down with appropriate hospital grade disinfectant except for high-speed handpieces. High-speed handpieces should be cleaned with 70% isopropyl, as the disinfectant can damage the turbine.

## Weekly and Monthly Maintenance

Ultrasonic tips should be evaluated to make sure they have adequate length. Manufacturers provide wear guides. The instrument tip should be placed over the corresponding image. A tip loss of 2 mm indicates that 50% of effectiveness has been lost, and thus, the instrument will no longer sufficiently remove calculus or disrupt the biofilm. It is also important to make sure the magnetostrictive inserts are not bent or broken, as this can cause overheat production or insufficient tip movement to remove debris from the tooth surface.

Oil and oilless dental units are to be drained weekly to release the buildup condensation from the tanks. If machines are not drained on a routine basis, the condensation will accumulate, causing overheating of the unit. For compressors that require oil, the technician/nurse or dental hygienist should verify that oil is filled to an appropriate level, as this is another factor causing overheating of the unit.

Water filters associated with ultrasonic units and dental units should also be replaced. Water treatment of the dental unit should occur according to recommendations of the manufacturer. Some practices use a dilution of bleach, chlorhexidine, or iM3 straw.

## Yearly

Instruments that no longer have sufficient original blade required for surgery should be replaced. Oil and filters on all dental units should be replaced as recommended by the manufacturer. Water lines should receive a shock water treatment annually in addition to the monthly water treatment. Note that waterlines can be tested quarterly to insure proper control of microorganisms. Bacterial counts should be less than 500 colony-forming units. Waterlines can be tested in-house or sent out to specific laboratories.

## VETERINARIANS

The veterinarian is the team leader and must have a strong belief in the importance of dentistry. As the team leader, the veterinarian should set proficiency goals, schedule dental training meetings, work together with the team to develop a highly professional and efficient working group, and understand the importance of providing the best quality care possible. Veterinarians are the only team members that are allowed to diagnose disease. The veterinarian evaluates the data provided by the veterinary technician/nurse or dental hygienist and areas of concern. The combination of oral examination and dental radiography findings helps to establish a diagnosis and create a treatment plan. Veterinarians should perform all complex treatments and surgical procedures, including dental extractions. Veterinarians should be comfortable with the procedures they perform and know the limitations of their training. If the necessary treatment is outside of their training scope, they should refer the patient to a veterinary dental specialist for advanced procedures.

## PET PARENTS

The pet parents (ie, clients) also play a significant role in the veterinary practice. As a customer, they make the decisions on who cares for their beloved pet. They should feel comfortable with and work closely with the veterinary team to determine the best options for their pet's oral health. They are the home care provider for oral care and must have buy-in to the best home care options. Not all home care options work for everyone, so the team must work together to develop a customized oral hygiene program.

## SUMMARY

The success of a veterinary practice's dental program depends on all team members working together to accomplish common goals. With a well-educated and trained team wherein each member plays a vital and essential role, there is no limit to the success of the practice. Clients value the services provided by veterinary technicians/nurses and dental hygienists and will stay with a veterinary practice because of the stellar performance by the entire team.

## DISCLOSURE

Both the author and coauthor are not responsible for any liability, negligence, or otherwise and injury resulting in staff practicing outside their jurisdiction and guidelines according to state/countries pertaining to veterinary medicine. This article only contains an overview of information relating to roles of veterinary technicians/nurses and registered hygienists. Instrument care is the responsibility of the veterinary staff to follow manufacturer guidelines and use this information as a guide. The author and coauthor do not take responsibility of damage to or failure of dental materials.

## REFERENCES

1. Bellows J. Philosophy and teamwork. In: The practice of veterinary dentistry: a team effort. Ames, IA: Iowa State Press; 1999.
2. Lobprise HB, Wiggs RB. Oral examination and recognition of pathology. In: The veterinarian's companion for common dental procedures. Lakewood, CO: AAHA Press; 2000.
3. Reiter RM, Gracis M. Perioperative considerations in dentistry and oral surgery. In: BSAVA manual of canine and feline dentistry and oral surgery. 4th edition. Gloucester, UK: BSAVA; 2018. p. 338–70.
4. Berg ML. Building your dental practice through education. In: Companion animal dentistry for veterinary technicians. Minneapolis, MN: Bluedoor Publishing; 2020.

5. Niemiec BA. Oral examination. In: A color handbook small animal dental, oral & maxillofacial disease. London, UK: Manson Publishing; 2010.
6. Perrone J. The examination room and the dental patient. In: Small animal dental procedures for veterinary technicians and nurses. Hoboken, NJ: Wiley Blackwell; 2021.
7. Wilkins EM. Instrumentations and principles for instrumentation. In: Clinical practice of the dental hygienist. 12th edition. Philadelphia, PA: Wolters Kluwer; 2017. p. 664–84.
8. Position statement: veterinary dental healthcare providers. American Veterinary Dental College Website. 2006. Available at: http://avdc.org/about/#pos-stmts. Accessed September 20, 2021.
9. Position statement: veterinary dentistry. American Veterinary Medical Association. Available at: http://avma.org/resources-tools/avma-policies/veterinary-dentistry. Accessed September 20, 2021.
10. Position statement: AVDT extraction position statement. Academy of Veterinary Dental Technicians. 2021. Available at: http://Avdt.us/about-1. Accessed September 21, 2021.
11. Daniel SJ, Harfst SA, Wilder RS. Instrument design and principles of instrumentation. Instrument sharpening. In: Mosby's dental hygiene concepts, cases, and competencies. 2nd edition. St. Louise, Missouri: Mosby Elsevier; 2008. p. 188–201. Ch. 10 Instrument Sharpening.

# Diagnostic Imaging of Oral and Maxillofacial Anatomy and Pathology

Lenin A. Villamizar-Martinez, DVM, MS, PhD, Dipl. AVDC[a],*,
Anson J. Tsugawa, VMD, Dipl. AVDC[b]

## KEYWORDS

- Intraoral radiography • Dental digital imaging equipment • Image postprocessing
- Dental radiograph interpretation • CT CBCT maxillofacial skeleton
- CBCT high spatial resolution • Multiplanar reconstruction maxillofacial trauma
- 3D printing OMFS • MRI TMJ articular disc • Orbital ultrasound retrobulbar disease

## KEY POINTS

- The accurate and efficient interpretation of dental radiographs is built on a strong knowledge base of dental and maxillofacial anatomy-pathology and the application of a step-by-step approach to image analysis.
- Dental radiographic findings should be documented in report format and included as part of the veterinary medical record.
- Multidetector/multislice computed tomography (MDCT/MSCT) and cone-beam computed tomography (CBCT) are the current gold standard imaging modalities for the assessment of the maxillofacial skeleton in dogs and cats.
- Tridimensional (3D) reformatted images and printed models provide enhanced the visualization of the complex in the presurgical treatment phase of complex maxillofacial trauma cases than the evaluation of two-dimensional cross-sectional images.
- Magnetic resonance imaging (MRI) is primarily useful for the evaluation of the soft tissue components of the maxillofacial region and specifically of the temporomandibular joint (TMJ) articular disc.
- Diagnostic ultrasound in veterinary dentistry and maxillofacial surgery is used infrequently for sample collection (culture, cytology, and biopsy) and for the initial screening of the retrobulbar space.

[a] North Carolina State University College of Veterinary Medicine, Department of Clinical Sciences, 1060 William Moore Dr, Raleigh, NC 27607, USA; [b] Dog and Cat Dentist, Inc, 9599 Jefferson Boulevard, Culver City, CA 90232, USA
* Corresponding author.
E-mail address: lavillam@ncsu.edu

Vet Clin Small Anim 52 (2022) 67–105
https://doi.org/10.1016/j.cvsm.2021.08.003
0195-5616/22/Published by Elsevier Inc.

vetsmall.theclinics.com

## INTRODUCTION

This chapter will serve as a review, but not as a buying guide, of the imaging hardware readily available to the veterinary practitioner for evaluating the oral and maxillofacial region of the dog and cat. We also introduce a methodical, step-by-step approach to the interpretation of these different imaging modalities that encourage best practices and we hope that it will improve the practitioner's radiographic interpretation efficiency. The core foundation of dental imaging interpretation is built on a strong knowledge base of normal dental and orofacial anatomy and through flashcard recognition of common disease conditions "Aunt Minnie." This chapter is not intended as a replacement for entire textbooks and atlases dedicated to the subject matter. It rather should serve as a roadmap for the selection of the appropriate imaging modality for the evaluation of a patient's presenting symptoms by highlighting exemplar disease conditions. We begin this review with a discussion on traditional intraoral digital dental radiography, as it is the most universally available of the imaging techniques and widely accepted as the current minimum diagnostic standard, and also touch on the few indications whereby extraoral dental radiography (ie, extraoral use of intraoral sensors/plates and skull radiography) still serves a purpose. There will be in-depth coverage of the more advanced imaging technologies (multidetector computed tomography [MDCT], cone-beam computed tomography [CBCT]) as they represent, at the time of publication, the highest standard of imaging technology available to both the specialty and general veterinary profession. This will be followed by a brief discussion on magnetic resonance imaging (MRI) and diagnostic ultrasound which have limited applications in veterinary dentistry and oromaxillofacial surgery.

## INTRAORAL DENTAL RADIOGRAPHY

Similar in importance as the electrocardiogram and echocardiogram are to the complete cardiac examination, intraoral dental radiography is a mainstay complement to the complete oral examination and remains an essential component of a thorough oral health assessment.

### Equipment

The standard digital dental radiography setup includes an X-ray generator to produce photons (dental radiographic machine); these are available in a variety of configurations, either fixed (wall-mounted), mounted on a mobile stand with wheels or handheld/portable. The analog image produced by the dental radiographic machine is either captured directly by a solid-state digital intraoral sensor that is typically tethered by a cable of varying length and with a male USB-A connector at the other end, or indirectly, using reusable photostimulable phosphor (PSP) plates that stores a latent image which must be processed through a scanner and converted into a digital image using digital imaging software installed on a computer. Although indirect imaging has the disadvantages of the additional processing step, ease of collecting scratches and defects on the plate with usability of up to only 200 times before needing to be retired, it does offer several advantages over direct sensors, and these include: Familiar form factor to regular film (flexible), availability of all sizes of traditional dental films, and wider exposure range/latitude which translates to more forgiveness in exposure technique.[1] Due to the larger pixel size inherent to PSP plates they do, however, typically produce an image of lesser quality than direct digital sensors. Bite force damage to the sensor or plate may prove fatal to either hardware, but will be much more significant cost-wise with the sensor. Therefore, great lengths should be taken to avoid damage to the internal components of the sensor from excessively applied pressure onto the plastic housing of the sensor from the bite forces of teeth. Damage to the cord can be prevented by avoiding kinking of the cape and unnecessary tugging of the insertion point of the cable to the sensor and through the use of a short (1 m) USB extension cord attached to the sensor instead of sustaining wear to the actual USB end of the sensor from the daily plugging and unplugging of the sensor from the USB port of the computer. As this is not an exhaustive review of hardware care tips and tricks, as with any expensive medical device, please refer to the original equipment manufacturer's care and use instructions to maximize the image quality and longevity of the equipment.

### Technique and interpretation/image analysis

Dental radiographic images are obtained with the intraoral sensor or PSP plate positioned either intraorally, using a paralleling or bisecting-angle technique for most views, or extraorally, for the specific extraoral near parallel technique view in the cat (**Fig. 1**B). The number of views in the full-mouth radiographic series will vary, depending on species, size of the dog, and whether the clinician prefers to obtain multiple separate bitewing images using a smaller size sensor (eg, size 2) for the entire series, or use a variety of plate sizes (up to a size 4 occlusal plate; is a size that is not available in sensor form) to capture the entire tooth crown, root, and surrounding structures in a single view (periapical view). No method is necessarily incorrect, as long as the whole tooth and surrounding periapical region (at least 2 mm surrounding the root apices) is included as part of the complete survey.

The approach to dental radiographic interpretation begins with proper organization, and this can only occur through the acquisition of images into a labially mounted template (**Fig. 2**), which is universally recognized as the preferred mounting method. Each image is reviewed twice from top to bottom and in the same sequential order each and every time, whether this means starting with the review of images from the top left corner of the template with the left maxillary teeth, progressing horizontally along the top of the template with a review of the right maxillary teeth, and then down to the review of the mandibular teeth from the bottom right to left sides of the template,

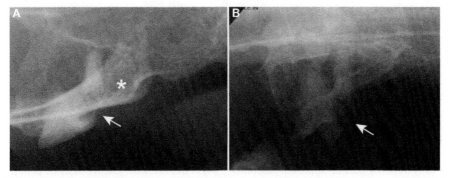

**Fig. 1.** Intraoral bisecting-angle and extraoral near-parallel technique views of the right maxilla in a cat. Intraoral view *(A)*. Note the crown and roots of the fourth premolar tooth and its tooth resorption lesion *(white arrow)* being obscured by the superimposed zygomatic arch *(asterisk)*. Extraoral near-parallel view *(B)*. The zygomatic arch is shifted dorsally in the image and away from the teeth and area of interest, and the tooth resorption lesion at the fourth premolar tooth is now in clear view *(white arrow)*.

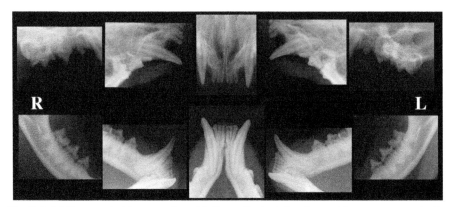

**Fig. 2.** Labially-mounted images of a cat full-mouth dental radiographic survey presented in a template using XDR Imaging Software (Cyber Medical Imaging, Inc). The radiographic views are mounted in anatomic order, from the perspective of the clinician viewing into the closed mouth of the patient with lips and cheeks retracted; the right-side teeth are positioned on the left side of the template (clinician's left), and the left-side teeth are on the right side of the template (clinician's right). The maxillary teeth are arranged with their crowns pointing down and reside on the top of the template, and images of mandibular teeth with their crowns pointing up are located along the bottom of the template.

in a clockwise fashion, or counterclockwise in direction. Viewing images in a deliberate order, if nothing else, encourages the careful evaluation of the entire radiographic survey, rather than allowing the eyes to focus on only what is abnormal. Systematic means step-by-step and methodical, and every clinician and establishment should adopt their own standard operating protocol that works for them (**Fig. 3**).

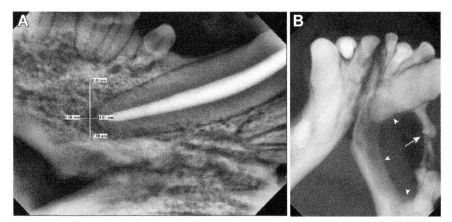

**Fig. 3.** The recommended approach to analyzing dental radiographs has been modified for brevity from the classical approach described.[40] (A) In this first example, we describe periapical pathosis at the right mandibular canine tooth of a dog that received standard root canal treatment as a 4.51 mm × 7.08 mm diameter ill-defined periapical radiolucency consistent with a periapical abscess. (B) The second example shows a well-defined ovoid-shaped unilocular radiolucency (*arrowheads*) consistent with a dentigerous cyst associated with an embedded left mandibular first premolar tooth (*white arrow*) that has expanded and resulted in a significant bodily displacement of adjacent teeth.

### Image postprocessing

One of the distinct advantages that digital dental imaging has over traditional dental film is the ability to manipulate (*image postprocessing*) the appearance of an image using computer software to improve its readability/diagnostic value. There is a myriad of digital postprocessing tools available to the practitioner, some are proprietary and highly complex mathematical algorithms, and others are common tools shared by virtually all software applications, akin to stock photo editor applications that most users are familiar with from their smartphones or tablets, without needing to have the skill set of a graphic designer. These include basic image enhancement tools that adjust sharpness, brightness, and contrast, and image analysis tools that provide magnification and digital rulers that are useful for measuring the size of lesions (**Figs. 4**C and **5**A). Although some image manipulation may enhance quality and improve an image's spatial resolution, excessive manipulation may introduce artifacts, pseudopathology (overshoot artifact), and actually degrades image quality.[2] Many dental radiography software systems produce an initial image that is, heavily filtered (sharpened) and digitally processed using unsharp masking/USM; this is undesirable, as the software force feeds the clinician a clarified image rather than providing an unbiased noncompressed RAW format image (see **Fig. 4**A). Some programs take this further by default saving the initial image in its postprocessed state (**Fig. 4**B).

### Dental radiographic reporting

Formal dental radiographic reporting is usually required only at training institutions, but if adopted into general use, may serve to optimize the information gained from the radiographic review process and facilitate the integration of clinical data with diagnostic data into the medical record. The basic requirements of the dental radiographic report, in addition to patient signalment and the date, when the images were obtained, should always begin with a brief clinical history, indication(s) or intended purpose/objective for the survey, description of the survey contents (eg, number of images), whether there are any comparison/prior studies available for review, and an assessment of the diagnostic quality and documentation of any identified technical errors of the images to be reviewed. Much like the patient physical examination in the objective section of the medical record, the body of the radiology report should include a description of the observed findings, and as suggested here, divided into the following categories: Anatomic/developmental, periodontal status, endodontal status, and

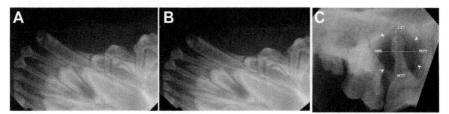

**Fig. 4.** RAW format image of the left rostral mandible in a 10-week-old dog obtained using a size 2 XDR Anatomic Sensor (Cyber Medical Imaging, Inc) and XDR Imaging Software (Cyber Medical Imaging, Inc.). Note the "soft" appearance of the RAW digital radiographic image *(A)*.[41] Same image as in *(A)* with unsharp mask (USM) filter applied for image sharpening *(B)*. A digital ruler tool is used to measure in millimeters and in 2 dimensions well-defined periapical radiolucency *(arrowheads)* at the distal root of the right maxillary fourth premolar tooth in a dog. Severe external inflammatory root resorption is present *(C)*.

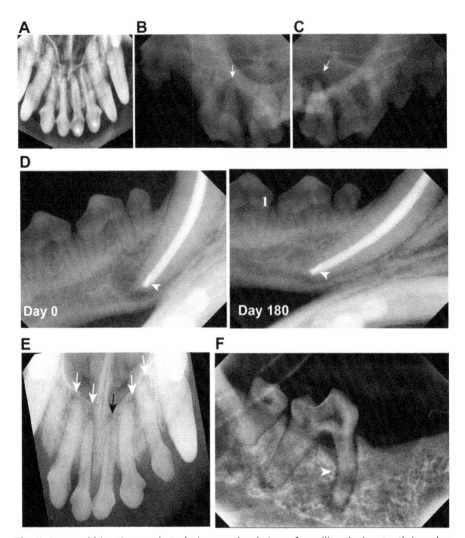

**Fig. 5.** Intraoral bisecting-angle technique occlusal view of maxillary incisor teeth in a dog. The comparatively wide pulp cavity and less thick appearance of dentinal walls of the left first and second incisor teeth are consistent with nonvitality of the pulp whereby there has been a cessation of secondary dentin production. A Caries-Endo postprocessing hard tissue filter (XDR Imaging Software, Cyber Medical Imaging) was used to increase local contrast of the grayscale of predominantly the hard tissues *(A)*. Ill-defined *(Image courtesy of* Anson Tsugawa) *(B)* and well-defined *(C)* periapical radiolucencies *(white arrows)* at the left maxillary fourth premolar tooth and right maxillary first molar tooth in 2 different dogs. Well-defined lucencies are often associated with chronic periapical periodontitis or periapical granulomas; whereas ill-defined lucencies are typically associated with acute periapical periodontitis or periapical abscessation. The reduction in the size of the periapical radiolucency at the right mandibular canine tooth 6 months following root canal therapy to almost near normal periodontal ligament space width is obvious despite the presence of a separated instrument file *(white arrow) (D)*. Artifactual chevron-shaped periapical radiolucencies may be seen at healthy canine, incisor, and mandibular carnassial teeth that mimic true periapical pathoses. The chevron lesion appears as a radiolucent apical extrapolation of the apices of the root, and the radiolucency does not "balloon-out" as one follows the

other. Followed by the clinician's overall impressions and suggestions for additional imaging tests, normal anatomy and specific treatment recommendations are not reported.

### Anatomic/developmental
The number of teeth is accounted for in this section. A basic chart that includes the tooth numbers and can be easily annotated may be useful for this purpose. Missing teeth, either congenitally missing or previously extracted (if immediately postoperative, this is referred to as a recently vacated tooth socket or sockets), persistent deciduous teeth (and whether the deciduous tooth has a permanent successor) (**Fig. 6**), anomalies of eruption (embedded/impacted teeth) or development (eg, craniomandibular osteopathy/CMO, periostitis ossificans), extra teeth (supernumerary), the size or shape of teeth (eg, fusion, gemination, concrescence, dilaceration, mandibular carnassial tooth malformation in the dog), are all described here (**Fig. 7**).

### Periodontal status (Figs. 8 and 9)
Evaluated here is the alveolar margin height in reference to the cementoenamel junction of the tooth, and if abnormal, greater than 1 to 3 mm, is documented, measured (in millimeters) or assessed as a percentage of root length. Also evaluated is the pattern of bone loss observed (horizontal or vertical), relative severity of bone loss (mild, moderate, severe), and overall extent (generalized, focal, multifocal) of disease throughout the mouth. Varying loss of opacity in the region of the tooth furcation (involvement or exposure) is recorded. The collection of periodontally related radiographic findings is correlated with a particular stage of periodontal disease.

### Endodontal status
The endodontic section focuses on the description of inflammatory pathoses of the periapical region. Inflammation destroys the regional bone resulting in the classic periapical radiolucency, and these lesions are measured (in millimeters and in 2 dimensions), characterized as well- or ill-defined, and any root resorption and/or pulp cavity changes (eg, failure of the pulp cavity to narrow in size/width from the cessation of secondary dentin production, indicating a loss of pulp vitality) are appropriately documented (**Fig. 5**). If a standard root canal treatment or other endodontic intervention has been performed on a tooth, radiographic documentation of each stage of the procedure, assessment of the quality of the procedure, and confirmation of any restoration (and/or prosthetic crown if applicable) are to be included in this section (**Fig. 10; Box 1**).

### Other
In this last section of the body of the report, we typically comment on tooth resorption (type/stage) (**Figs. 11** and **12**) and other diseases of the jaws such as traumatic

---

periodontal ligament space in an apical direction. In this maxillary occlusal view of a dog, classic chevron radiolucencies (*white arrows*) are observed at several maxillary incisor teeth; however, a true periapical radiolucency is present at the left maxillary first incisor tooth that also shows a wider pulp cavity and apical inflammatory root resorption *(E)*. In this view of the right mandibular second M tooth of a dog, there is evidence of severe periodontitis, vertical bone loss at the furcation, and a periapical radiolucency at both roots. Notice the union of the periapical lucency and vertical bone loss in the shape of an hour glass (*white arrow*) at the mid-root of the mesial root consistent with a true combined perio-endo lesion *(F)*.

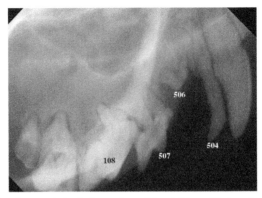

**Fig. 6.** Intraoral bisecting-angle technique view of the right maxilla in a dog with persistent deciduous right maxillary canine (504), second premolar (506), and third premolar (507) teeth. The permanent first premolar tooth is congenitally missing, and the deciduous second premolar and third premolar teeth lack permanent successors. In terms of their radiographic appearance, note that the deciduous teeth are less radiopaque, have longer, more slender, and divergent roots than their permanent counterparts. Also, take note of the morphologic similarities that deciduous teeth have to the permanent tooth located distal to it ("molarization"); in this view, the deciduous right maxillary third premolar tooth (507) has a similar appearance to that of the permanent right maxillary fourth premolar tooth (108). The periodontal ligament space in this younger patient is distinctly wider, and is a normal feature seen in developing dogs, and may decrease in width with age.

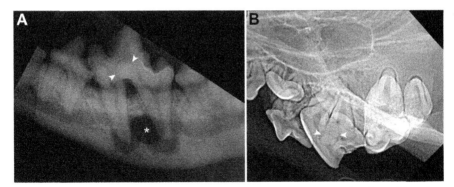

**Fig. 7.** Left mandibular carnassial-tooth malformation in the crown of a dog. This unique anomaly (radiopacity similar to dentin with a deviation of the pulp cavity; white *arrowheads*) neither originates from the enamel or dentin nor presents an invagination of the enamel. It had previously incorrectly been classified as dens invaginatus. Periapical pathosis and periodontitis are commonly reported clinical and radiographic features associated with this malformation.[42] Note the marked root convergence and the well-defined periapical radiolucencies that originate from both roots and have fused to create a single large radiolucency (*asterisk*) (A). A similar malformation may also be seen in the maxillary fourth premolar tooth (B). Image courtesy of G.G. Comet Riggs.

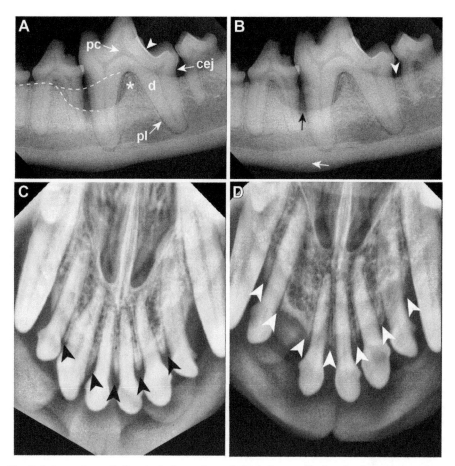

**Fig. 8.** Intraoral paralleling technique view of the left mandibular cheek teeth in a dog. Annotated salient periodontal anatomy and landmarks to be assessed during whole image analysis of a tooth: Enamel (*white arrow*head); dentin (*d*); cementum; cementoenamel junction (cej); pulp cavity (pc); periodontal ligament (pl) space; furcation bone (*asterisk*); alveolar margin (interrupted *lines*) *(A)*. In this same view, we note severe (greater than 50% of root length) combined horizontal and vertical pattern bone loss (*black arrow*) at the distal root of the fourth premolar tooth and mesial root of the first molar tooth with thickened but normal-appearing (as an indication of the chronicity of the periodontitis) ventral mandibular cortex (*white arrow*), moderate horizontal bone loss at the second M tooth (white *arrowhead*) *(B)*. More subtle signs of periodontal disease are appreciated in these serial maxillary occlusal views of the same dog over a 3-year time span. Wedge-shaped widening (black *arrowheads*) of the periodontal ligament space at several incisor teeth *(C)* is an early radiographic change seen with mild periodontal disease that progressed to horizontal pattern bone loss (white *arrowheads*) over the course of 3 years *(D)*.[43] Notice the absence of the right maxillary second incisor tooth (D). This tooth was extracted 3 years prior (C), as it was deemed non-vital, take note of its comparatively wider pulp cavity to other teeth in the same view.

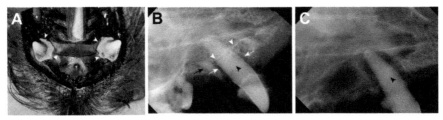

**Fig. 9.** In this anesthetized dog positioned in dorsal recumbency, note the heavy supragingival calculus accumulation along the palatal surface of both maxillary canine teeth (*arrowheads*), an appearance typically seen when deep periodontal pockets are present *(A)*. Intraoral bisecting-angle technique lateral view of the right maxillary canine tooth, showing severe combined horizontal–vertical pattern bone loss (*white arrows* indicate a vertical component of bone loss; the horizontal component of bone loss is outlined with black *arrowheads*). Although oronasal communication/fistula is predominantly a clinical diagnosis, dental radiographs can be complimentary. The white arrowheads delineate the radiopaque line that is, the nasal surface of the alveolar process of the maxilla, that is the separation between the oral and nasal cavities.[49] If oronasal communication had been present, the radiopaque line would be absent. The apical-most extent of bone loss at this tooth is, however, close to this radiopaque line, and therefore indicates near oronasal communication. There is a root remnant of the deciduous right maxillary canine tooth (*black arrow*) *(B)*. In this image from another dog, where there was clinically documented oronasal communication at the right maxillary canine tooth, we observe the absence of the radiopaque line (black *arrowheads*) *(C)*. Image courtesy of Jenna Winer.

injuries/jaw fractures, altered bone patterns from infections that have progressed into the bone marrow (**Fig. 13**) or oral neoplasia. The description of a tumor's radiographic pattern (permeative, moth-eaten, geographic) and its effect on the surrounding structures (eg, tooth displacement, root resorption) are described in this "catch-all" section (**Fig. 14**).[4]

## EXTRAORAL

Extraoral imaging, as it pertains to general veterinary dentistry, typically refers to an alternative view to the standard intraoral bisecting-angle technique view that is obtained to evaluate the maxillary premolar/molar region in the cat. This extraoral near-parallel view allows for improved visibility of the roots and their surrounding structures without the superposition of the zygomatic arch (**Fig. 1**). With respect to the practice of oral and maxillofacial surgery, this typically refers to the extraoral application of typically intraorally-positioned sensors or plates. Partial or whole skull views can be obtained from cats and smaller dogs in the initial screening of oral and maxillofacial trauma in the financially challenged case. A dorsoventral view may provide a suitable glimpse at the general positioning of the mandibular head of the condylar process within the mandibular fossa of the temporal bone, often to confirm its positioning postreduction of temporomandibular joint (TMJ) luxation (**Fig. 15**). As noted previously in reference to intraoral dental radiography, for the purposes of the radiologic assessment of oral tumors and jaw fractures, skull radiography (or orthopantomography in the human patient) is viewed as an outdated technique, and its shortcomings severely limit its use to initial screening/survey purposes only. It has largely been replaced by CT/CBCT for this purpose. But for the initial assessment and identification of common radiographic patterns involving the mandible (eg, periosteal reaction patterns, general

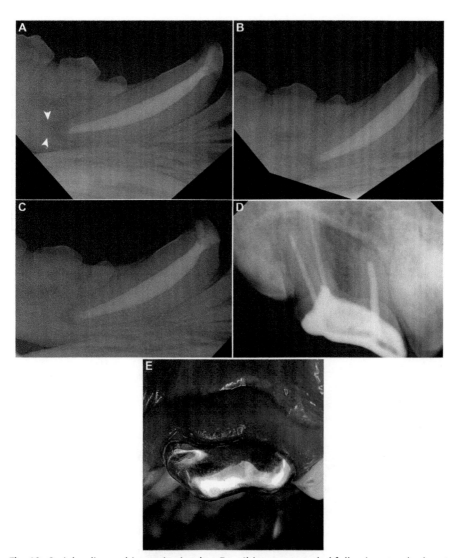

**Fig. 10.** Serial radiographic monitoring (see **Box 1**) is recommended following standard root canal therapy; this is especially important when a periapical radiolucency is documented on pretreatment radiographs; in this example of a right mandibular canine tooth, an ill-defined periapical radiolucency was present at the time of endodontic treatment *(arrowheads) (A)*. In this 3-month follow-up radiograph there is already a noticeable reduction in the size of the periapical radiolucency *(B)*, and at the 12-month follow-up, the periapical radiolucency has further reduced in size *(C)*. Images courtesy of Helena Kuntsi. A metal crown prosthesis was placed to protect endodontically treated maxillary carnassial teeth *(D)*.[47,48] For documentation purposes, dental radiographs should be obtained once the metal crown has been cemented *(E)*.

Box 1
**Recommendations for the radiographic assessment of standard root canal therapy in dogs[3]**

- Three-month follow-up, 1-year follow-up, and annually thereafter.

- The presence of pretreatment periapical radiolucency or root resorption may negatively impact the success rate of therapy; however, the quality of obturation (eg, presence of voids in the fill) may be of lesser importance.

- Treatment success: Normal periodontal ligament space; cessation of any preexisting root resorption.

- No evidence of failure: Same or decrease in size of preexisting periapical radiolucency and/or cessation of preexisting root resorption.

- Treatment failure: Development of periapical radiolucency and/or root resorption posttreatment; increasing size or progression of preexisting periapical radiolucency or root resorption.

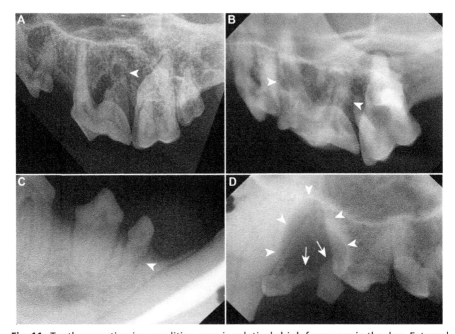

**Fig. 11.** Tooth resorption is a condition seen in relatively high frequency in the dog. External inflammatory root resorption (*arrowhead*) (*A*) and external replacement root resorption (*arrowheads*) (*B*) are the 2 most common types of resorption seen.[44] With external surface resorption, as seen in this example of the right mandibular first premolar tooth, there is a structural defect and defined periodontal ligament space along the mesial surface of the root (*arrowhead*) (*C*). External inflammatory root resorption is also a common feature seen with nonodontogenic oral malignancies and aggressive odontogenic tumors such as canine acanthomatous ameloblastoma.[45] This intraoral view of the left rostral maxilla is an example of unilocular cyst formation (*arrowheads*), tooth displacement, and resorption associated with oral malignancy (*arrows*); in this particular case, a histologically-confirmed papillary squamous cell carcinoma (*D*).

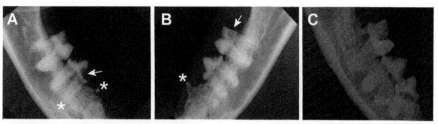

**Fig. 12.** Intraoral paralleling technique views of the mandibles of a cat obtained using a size 2 solid-state sensor. There is a type II (dentoalveolar ankylosis) tooth resorption lesion at the left mandibular third premolar tooth (*white asterisk*) and type I tooth resorption lesion at the left mandibular first molar tooth (*white arrow*) (*B*). With type I tooth resorption, the periodontal ligament space is preserved. There is a type II tooth resorption lesion at the right third premolar tooth (white *asterisk*) as well, demonstrating the typical symmetry seen with this disease, and a type III tooth resorption lesion at the right fourth premolar tooth, which has radiographic characteristics of both type I (*white arrow*) and type II resorption (*white asterisk*) (*A*). Although the size 2 sensor is of appropriate size for obtaining most of the intraoral views in the cat mouth, parallel positioning of the sensor intraorally for the mandibular premolar/molar view may be a tight fit, and the area of interest may not be shown in smaller sized or brachycephalic cats and dogs, whereby the use of a size 0 PSP plate may be preferable. Intraoral paralleling technique view of the right mandibular premolar/molar region in a Persian cat with a size 0 PSP plate (*C*).

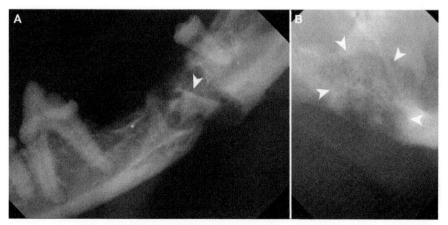

**Fig. 13.** Radiographic appearance of chronic osteomyelitis as suggested by the identification of a sequestrum "island" of nonvital/dead bone (*arrowhead*) in a nonunion left caudal mandibular fracture of a dog *(A)*, and in a less common location, the maxilla of a dog—the faintly visible sclerotic rim surrounding the region of permeative osteolysis (area of necrotic bone) is outlined with white arrowheads *(B)*.

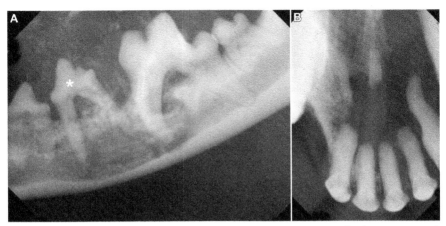

**Fig. 14.** Oral tumors, particularly benign tumors *(A)*, that are biologically slower in growth, through chronic exertion of pressure on the surrounding tissues, displace teeth and resorb roots, and in this example of a dog with histologically confirmed acanthomatous ameloblastoma, tumor tissue filling-up the periodontal ligament space has extruded teeth *(asterisk)*, than malignant *(B)* or biologically more aggressive, fast-growing tumors, as in this maxillary occlusal view example of a tubular subtype nasal adenocarcinoma in a dog, whereby the destructive impact on surrounding tissues has been much more rapid, and the regionally involved teeth, maxillary incisors, are seen as floating, and root resorption is less commonly seen.

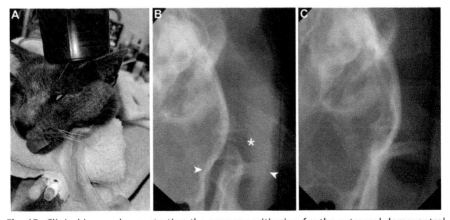

**Fig. 15.** Clinical image demonstrating the proper positioning for the extraoral dorsoventral view of the temporomandibular joint (TMJ) in a cat using a size 2 sensor *(A)*. The utility of this view is demonstrated here in this example of a left TMJ luxation in a cat. The condylar process *(arrowheads)* displaced rostrodorsally from the mandibular fossa *(asterisk)* of the temporal bone *(B)*. Postreduction image in the same cat *(C)*.

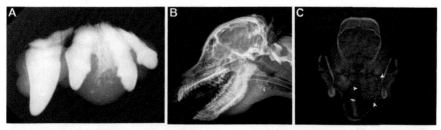

**Fig. 16.** Example of an extraoral view radiograph used for medicolegal documentation following a partial incisivectomy for the treatment of a peripheral odontogenic fibroma in a dog *(A)*. Skull radiograph of a 4-month-old female Corgi dog whereby skull radiographs, in combination with histopathology, were successfully used to diagnose craniomandibular osteopathy (CMO). The radiographic appearance of severe irregular bony proliferation along the ventral surface of the entire length of both mandibles is nearly pathognomonic for this disease but can be married with bone histopathology for confirmation *(B)*. CBCT 3D reconstruction of another dog with CMO. Note the caudal extension of the disease process *(arrowheads)* to involve this patient's right TMJ and tympanic bullae resulting in a significant restriction in mandibular range of motion. Image courtesy of Helena Kuntsi *(C)*.

direction of the fracture line in minimally comminuted mandibular fractures) or to image the excised portion of tissue following jaw resection surgery (**Fig. 16**A), skull radiographs may still hold some diagnostic-medical value.

There are still a few instances whereby the evaluation of a larger geographic region of the mandible is needed beyond the field of view that can be captured with the largest intraoral sensor or plate. Skull radiography is suitable from both an economics standpoint and to successfully screen for developmental diseases in the dog such as craniomandibular osteopathy/CMO (**Fig. 16**B) and periostitis ossificans (**Fig. 17**). The involvement of the TMJs and/or tympanic bullae in CMO, however, can only be formally evaluated by CT/CBCT (**Fig. 16**C).

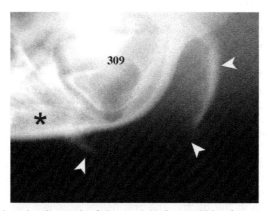

**Fig. 17.** Intraoral dental radiograph of the caudal left mandible of a young large breed dog with periostitis ossificans, a developmental condition that results in a firm mandibular swelling and a pathognomonic double-cortex radiographic appearance of the ventral surface of the mandible *(arrowheads)*.[46] (309) left mandibular first molar tooth, *(asterisk)* mandibular body. Image courtesy of Tony Woodward.

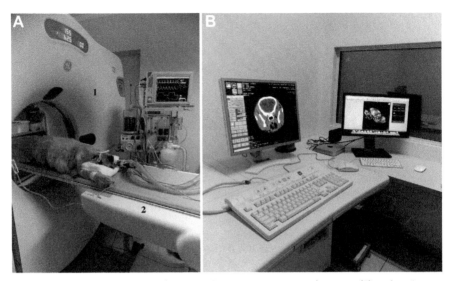

**Fig. 18.** CT scan parts. Gantry with its rotating X-ray generator, detectors (1) and patient table (2) *(A)*. Operator console whereby the reconstructed images can be manipulated using native software or on a different computer workstation using third-party DICOM software *(B)*. (Copyright Lenin A. Villamizar)

## COMPUTED TOMOGRAPHY

Computed tomography (CT) is a diagnostic imaging technique that uses X-rays and computer software to form cross-sectional images of the body without the overlap of anatomic structures. The basic components of a tomography unit are the gantry (X-ray tube and detectors), patient table, and control panel (**Fig. 18**).[5,6] CT scanners may be classified according to how the imaging data are acquired (axial or helical). With conventional axial CT scanners, which are discussed here for historical purposes, the X-ray tube within the gantry only emits X-rays when the gantry is rotating around the patient's body and when the table is stationary and not being advanced. Due to this incremental/sequential start–stop process, axial CT scans require longer study times to cover the entire area of interest. The patient table remains stationary during X-ray emission; which allows the operator to set the desired slice thickness and increment to the examination specifications (**Fig. 19**A).[7–9]

With helical (or spiral) CT, the more recent scan mode technology, there is continuous X-ray tube rotation around the patient combined with constant-speed advancement of the patient table through the gantry (see **Fig. 19**B). Helical scanners allow for the assessment of larger body areas in a shorter time frame, eliminate the blur/motion artifact associated with thoracic and abdominal movements and abdominal movement, however, this advantage may result in higher radiation exposure for the patient.

Image quality and resolution are associated with the number (and composition) of the X-ray detectors in the gantry. The first helical scanners had only one row of X-ray detectors and were referred to as single-slice scanners. The later incorporation of more rows of detectors gave rise to multi-slice (or multidetector) CT scanners (**Fig. 20**). The advanced CT scanners used in human medicine for the 3-dimensional

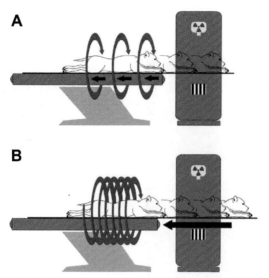

**Fig. 19.** Illustrations of axial *(A)* and helical *(B)* scanners. In axial scan tomography, axial thin sections of the anatomic field of interest are acquired at intervals and thickness previously established by the operator. In helical scanners, the patient table is displaced in a continuous pattern during the X-ray emission. (Copyright Lenin A. Villamizar)

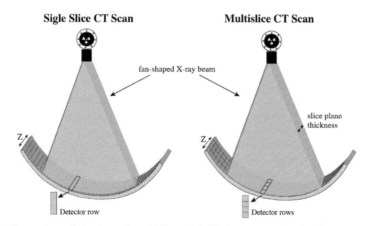

**Fig. 20.** Illustration of single and multislice CT helical scanners. Single slice scanners have only one detector row in the "Z" axis aligned at the gantry, whereas multislice scanners may have several rows of sensors aligned in the "Z" axis (eg, 4, 8, 16, or more detector rows). In multislice scanners, the multiple detector rows simultaneously collect the imaging data. In traditional CT scanners (axial or helical), the collimation of the fan-shaped X-ray beam corresponds to the slice plane thickness. (Copyright Lenin A. Villamizar)

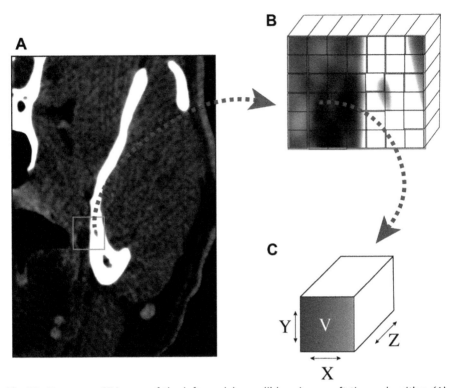

**Fig. 21.** Transverse CT image of the left caudal mandible using a soft tissue algorithm *(A)* and voxel illustrations *(B, C).* The reconstructed bi-dimensional CT images displayed on the screen are formed by a grayscale matrix of pixels, where high tissue density is depicted as white voxels. In contrast, low-density tissue is represented as black voxels *(B).* CT imaging voxels are nonisotropic *(C),* whereby the "Z" axis is larger than the "Y" and "X" axes. Voxel *(V).*

assessment of the heart and coronary artery disease screening may have more than 300 rows/slice count (256- to 320-slice) of detectors.[10,11]

The acquired CT data are reconstructed using complex mathematical processes to produce the CT image. In helical tomography, this process is known as interpolation. The reconstructed images are composed of a square matrix comprised of small units (pixels) which correspond to voxels of the CT image. A voxel is a 3D analog or volumetric unit of a pixel with a width (X-axis), height (Y-axis), and length (Z-axis). The Z-axis is also referred to as the slice thickness (**Fig. 21**).[6,9]

Generally, the voxels of a matrix in multislice scanners are isotropic, which means that one axis (Z-axis) is greater than the other 2 (X- and Y-axis). Although some multislice CT scanners can acquire the data with isotropic voxels (X = Y = Z), which translates into better spatial resolution, this feature has been associated with increased patient radiation dose and imaging acquisition time. The voxels are displayed in white, black, and on a wide scale of shades of gray. Each gray shade reflects the radiation coefficient attenuation of each tissue of the body. In other words, each tissue has a specific density associated with a specific gray shade.[6,12]

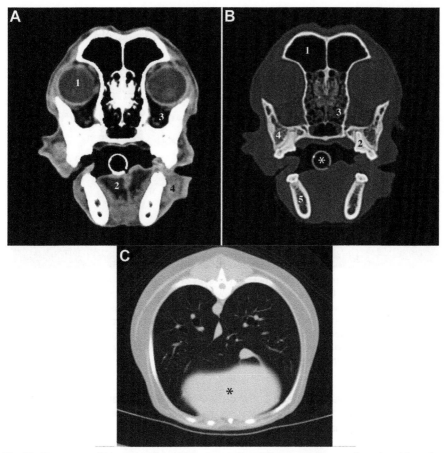

**Fig. 22.** Transverse CT images of an adult dog using different reconstruction algorithms for soft tissue *(A)*, bone *(B)*, and lung *(C)* tissues. *(A):* Eye *(1)*, lingual fat *(2)* and infraorbital region *(3)*. *(B):* Right frontal sinus *(1)*, left maxillary first molar tooth *(2)*, alveolar bone of right maxillary first molar tooth *(4)*, right mandibular body *(5)*, and endotracheal tube *(asterisk)*. *(C):* caudal lung lobes and liver *(asterisk)*.

The imaging data set can be manipulated using specialized viewer software to highlight different tissue types of the Hounsfield scale (eg, bone, soft, lung tissue windows). Windowing, or grayscale mapping, allows the clinician to evaluate changes in attenuation appearance in a particular anatomic area (**Figs. 22** and **23**). The raw data and reconstructed images can then be transferred from the PACS (Picture Archiving and Communication System) whereby they are stored to different computers or workstations as a DICOM file (Digital Imaging and Communications in Medicine). Any computer whereby the veterinary clinician can remotely access free or paid third-party DICOM viewer software to evaluate the images can serve as a workstation. Examples of free DICOM viewer software are: RadiAnt (Medixant, Poznań, Poland), OsiriX Lite (Pixmeo SARL, Bernex, Switzerland), and Horos (Nimble Co LLC d/b/a Purview, Annapolis, MD, USA).[12]

The tissue attenuation is measured with a linear radiodensity scale known as the Hounsfield scale in honor of Sir Godfrey Newbold Hounsfield, an electrical engineer

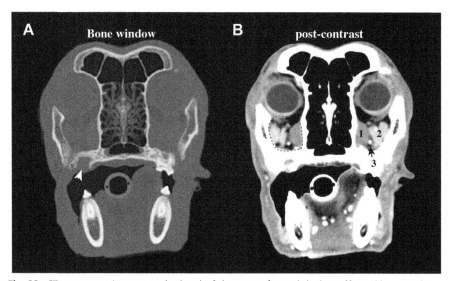

**Fig. 23.** CT transverse images at the level of the eyes of an adult dog affected by acanthomatous ameloblastoma. Bone tissue window showing a lytic lesion and missing right maxillary second M tooth *(arrowhead)* (A). The soft tissue window post-contrast image was displayed to rule out infraorbital invasion *(dashed line)*. The infraorbital structures are not affected and are easily identified in the post-contrast soft tissue window image *(B)*. Contralateral infraorbital structures for comparison: Medial pterygoid muscle *(1)*, zygomatic salivary gland *(2)*, and maxillary artery *(3)*.

who together with Allan MacLeod Cormack developed and introduced CT in 1972.[13] In the Hounsfield scale, the attenuation values are expressed as Hounsfield Units (HU). In this scale, the attenuation of water corresponds to 0 HU, air is −1000 HU, and bone is +1000 HU. Blood, muscles, and other soft tissue types reside above 0 HU, and fat has a lower value than water at −50 to −100 HU. Heavy metals are valued at +3000 HU.[6,12]

Although MRI is the recognized standard technique for soft tissue imaging, CT scan also provides detailed imaging information for soft tissue and blood vessels. Soft tissue and blood vessel visualization are improved by the administration of intravenous contrast agents.[14] Depending on the contrast phase for which the tomographic images are acquired (arterial, portal venous, nephrogenic, or excretion), the soft tissue attenuation and blood vessel appearance can change.[15]

CT scans of the head of veterinary patients are evaluated during the precontrast and post-contrast phases. The post-contrast phase corresponds to the arterial or late arterial phase that occurs 15 to 30 seconds after peripheral intravenous contrast agent administration. During these phases, the arteries and soft tissue structures (eg, masticatory muscles, salivary glands) of the head are impregnated by the contrast medium and appear as hyperattenuated on the scan.[16]

The contrast enhancement observed in the images is associated with vascular permeability and the concentration of iodine in the vascular system that reaches the target organs. Pathologic increases in the X-ray attenuation (ie, hyperattenuation) are associated with anomalous vascular permeability, blood vessel pattern, or neovascularization. On the other hand, hypoattenuation is associated with less vascularized (edematous) or devitalized (necrotic) tissue **(Fig. 24)**.[16,17]

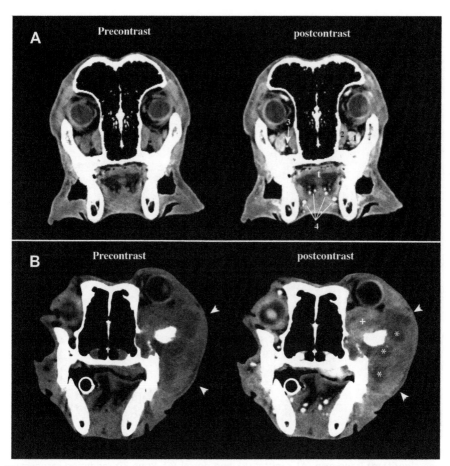

**Fig. 24.** CT transverse images at the level of the eyes of a normal dog. Note the contrast enhancement in the post-contrast image. Pre and post-contrast soft tissue window images. Left zygomatic salivary gland *(1)*, left medial pterygoid muscle *(2)*, left maxillary artery *(3)*, lingual and sublingual blood vessels *(4)*, and tongue *(t)* *(A)*. Pre and post-contrast soft tissue window images of a dog affected by a fibrosarcoma *(arrowheads)* *(B)*. Notice how the neoplastic process has a heterogeneous contrast enhancement pattern in the post-contrast phase. The hypoattenuating cavitary areas are associated with poor vascularization, suggesting edema or necrosis *(asterisks)*. A hyperattenuating area *(+)* in the infraorbital area suggests a denser soft tissue area. Areas of necrosis should be avoided, and tissue biopsies should be collected from more hyperattenuating areas. (Copyright Lenin A. Villamizar)

Multiplanar reconstruction (MPR) and 3D reconstruction are essential tools that allow the clinician to evaluate an anatomic area of interest from different perspectives. With MPR, the tomographic raw data can be simultaneously reconstructed into several planes, and for the head of veterinary patients, these planes are transverse, sagittal, and dorsal **(Figs. 25A–C)**. It is essential to follow the guidelines established in the veterinary literature when referencing the anatomic planes in veterinary patient CT images. For example, the expression "axial plane" is discouraged due to the possible confusion when referring to the imaging acquisition technique (ie, axial vs. helical).[12,18]

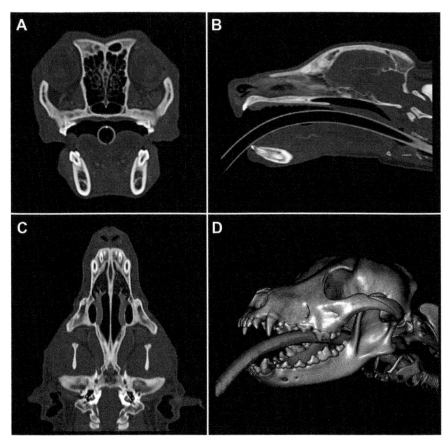

**Fig. 25.** Computed tomographic multiplanar reconstruction of an adult dog using a suitable bone algorithm. Transverse *(A)*, sagittal *(B)*, and dorsal *(C)*. Bone 3D rendering reconstruction of the same dog. (Copyright Lenin A. Villamizar)

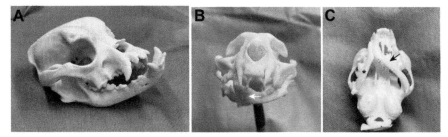

**Fig. 26.** 3D printed anatomic models. Note the relative mandibular prognathism of a class III malocclusion in an adult brachycephalic dog *(A)*. 3D printed model of a 7-month-old domestic shorthair cat affected by right temporomandibular ankylosis *(B, C)*. Note the deviation of the lower jaw to the right *(arrows)* and mandibular length asymmetry *(asterisk)*. *(Copyright Lenin A. Villamizar)*

The use of 3D volume rendering and 3D printing in maxillofacial surgery has increased in popularity in veterinary medicine due to their clinical benefit and educational application for veterinarians and animal owners (see **Figs. 25**D and **26**). 3D reconstruction and 3D printed models are used during the preoperative phase to plan various surgical procedures. In veterinary maxillofacial surgery, 3D applications for orthopedic, oncologic, and reconstructive surgery have been described.[19,20]

## CONE-BEAM COMPUTED TOMOGRAPHY

CBCT is an advanced diagnostic imaging technique that uses X-ray to display high-resolution (ie, due to its high spatial resolution) tomographic images of mineralized tissue structures. This technique has been widely used in humans to assess the head and appendicular skeleton.[21] The use of this diagnostic technique has dramatically increased in the last decade in veterinary dentistry and maxillofacial surgery. Several studies have demonstrated its value and superiority than other diagnostic imaging techniques for dentoalveolar, maxillofacial, and TMJ assessment in animals.[22–24]

CBCT units are a modification from traditional single and multislice CT scanners. In a CBCT system, the X-ray tube and a flat-panel detector (FPD) are mounted in a mobile C-arm gantry that rotates around the patient in a horizontal or vertical plane (**Fig. 27**). With CBCT, a single 360-degree gantry rotation acquires the necessary volumetric data to generate images; whereas traditional CT scans are reconstructed from the raw data acquired from multiple overlapping slices of the region of interest.[25,26] Unlike the flat fan-shaped X-ray beam of traditional CT scanners, the collimated X-rays in CBCT units form a pyramidal or cone-shaped beam. The cone-shaped

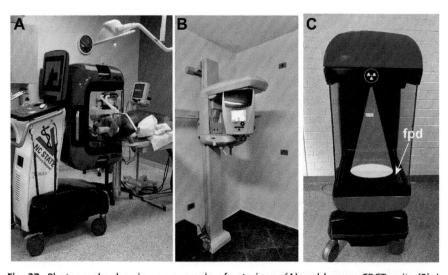

**Fig. 27.** Photographs showing an example of veterinary (A) and human CBCT units (B). In veterinary CBCT units, the patient is positioned on a table, whereas the gantry rotates in a vertical plane around the region of interest. In some human CBCT units, the patient stands, whereas the gantry rotates around the region of interest in a horizontal plane. CBCT gantry in a veterinary unit showing a graphic representation of the cone-shaped X-ray beam targeting the bi-dimensional flat-panel detector (fpd) (C). (Copyright Lenin A. Villamizar)

beam is projected through the region of interest, and the attenuated X-rays are captured in a bi-dimensional FPD (**Fig. 27**). The FPD transforms the attenuated X-ray photons into electrical information that is converted into raw data. Similar to traditional CT systems, the volumetric raw data from the CBCT are reconstructed into tomographic images using complex algorithmic processes.[26]

Compared with traditional CT scanners, CBCT systems expose the patient to lower radiation doses due to its pulsed X-ray emission and high-quality FPDs.[27] CBCT units use a low-power X-ray source that generates a collimated cone-shaped X-ray beam directed to a small field of view. In comparison, multislice scanners use higher-frequency power X-ray tubes that can produce high-quality diagnostic images of larger anatomic areas. Another factor associated with the lower radiation dose of CBCT scanners is that the X-ray beam is not overlapped as with multislice CT systems whereby several slices overlap over the patient's long axis to form the images. In CBCT systems, the imaging acquisition process occurs in a single 360-degree gantry rotation around the patient.[25,28]

In contrast to multislice CT scanners, whereby the images are generally formed of nonisometric voxels, the CBCT images are constructed with isometric voxels. As was previously explained in this chapter, isometric voxels result in better image spatial resolution. Current technology allows the reconstruction of high-quality images with submillimeter isometric voxels, making CBCT the ideal technique for dentoalveolar assessment.[29]

Even though CBCT scanners allow for the acquisition of high-definition images of mineralized tissue (eg, bone and dental hard tissues), current CBCT software does

---

**Box 2**
**CBCT[26,28,37]**

| Advantages* | Disadvantages* |
|---|---|
| • Lower radiation exposure (10 × less than multislice CT). | • Low contrast resolution than conventional CT scanners. Not indicated for soft tissue assessment. |
| • Shorter scan times. | |
| • Better spatial resolution and imaging accuracy than multislice CT scans. CBCT images are comprised of isotropic voxels. Ideal for evaluating maxillofacial and dentoalveolar structures. | • Image noise and movement artifacts. |
| | • Smaller field of view (FO). CBCT units are designed to scan small anatomic areas. Largest FO available in veterinary units is 24 × 14 cm. Larger head patients may require 2 scans for the full assessment of skull structures. |
| • Less expensive than multislice detector CT units. | |
| • Small footprint, requires less space than a conventional CT scanner. | • Tissue density measurement is not reliable, as CBCT does not use Hounsfield Units. |
| • Mobile CBCT units can be brought to the patient and allow scans to be performed in different rooms of a veterinary facility. CBCT units may be connected to a regular 110V electrical outlet. | |

*at the time of writing this chapter

| Box 3<br>CT and CBCT indications | | CT | CBCT |
|---|---|---|---|
| Soft tissue and bone inflammatory and infectious disorders | • Acute/chronic soft tissue swelling of the oral and maxillofacial structures<br>• Detection/localization of foreign bodies<br>• Masticatory muscle myositis<br>• Salivary gland pathology (eg, sialocele, sialadenitis, sialadenosis and necrotizing sialometaplasia)<br>• Osteomyelitis – osteonecrosis<br>• Odontogenic cysts | Yes<br>*IV-C | *Only for bone structures |
| Neoplastic disorders of soft tissue and/or bone involving the jaws, oral cavity proper, and salivary glands | • Malignant tumors (eg, melanoma, squamous cell carcinoma, fibrosarcoma, etc.)<br>• Benign tumors (eg, odontogenic origin)<br>• Lymph node staging<br>• Radiation therapy planning | Yes<br>*IV-C | *Only for bone structures |
| Maxillofacial trauma | • Fractures affecting the maxilla and mandible, palate, nasal passages, periorbital region, and zygomatic arch<br>• Dentoalveolar injuries | Yes<br>*IV-C optional | Yes |
| TMJ | • TMJ fracture, luxation, or subluxation<br>• Inability to open the mouth (intra or extraarticular ankylosis)<br>• Inability to close the mouth (open-mouth jaw locking)<br>• Degenerative diseases (eg, osteoarthritis, subchondral cysts, bone defects)<br>• Dysplasia<br>• Neoplasia (uncommon) | Yes<br>*IV-C optional | Yes<br>*Only for bone structures |
| Congenital or acquired disorders | • Primary/secondary cleft palate<br>• Skeletal malformation, anatomic malformation | Yes | Yes<br>*Only for bone structures |
| Endodontic disease | • Root fractures<br>• Root resorption – internal/external | No | Yes<br>+SR |

| | | | |
|---|---|---|---|
| | • Before endodontic therapy | | |
| | • Endodontic therapy follow-up | | |
| Periodontal disease | • Periapical disease<br>• Infrabony pocket assessment | Yes | Yes<br>+SR |
| | • Periodontic-endodontic infections | | |
| Complicated dental extractions | • Lingual/buccal alveolar bone loss<br>• Localization of fractured/ displaced root fragments in the nasal cavity | Yes | Yes<br>+SR |
| Dental implants | • Localization of tooth roots in relation to neurovascular structures – anatomic relationship<br>• Morphometric assessment of alveolar bone | Yes | Yes<br>+SR |

*IV-C, requires intravenous contrast agent; *IV-C optional, for evaluation of adjacent soft tissue structures; +SR, better spatial resolution.

not permit the reconstruction of soft tissue structures. The reduced soft-tissue contrast has been linked to the current FPD technology, cone-beam geometry, X-ray scatter, low radiation dose, and reconstruction algorithm.[30–32]

Another known limitation of CBCT systems is that they do not use HU, and therefore, tissue density measurements are not possible as with traditional CT scanners. Instead of HU, CBCT systems use gray values (GVs). Some studies have aimed to validate GVs as a density measurement of dentoalveolar structures. This, however, remains controversial, as GVs can vary and do not always correlate consistently with HU density values.[33–36] **Box 2** presents the advantages and disadvantages of CBCT systems.

## INDICATIONS FOR COMPUTED TOMOGRAPHY AND CONE-BEAM COMPUTED TOMOGRAPHY

Imaging of the dentoalveolar complex and maxillofacial structures may be initially performed through intraoral or skull radiography. However, due to the complexity of the regional anatomy and superimposition of bone and soft tissue structures, interpretation may be challenging. CT and CBCT allow the clinician to characterize a lesion's size and extent and facilitate the diagnosis of pathologic processes without the added burden of anatomic structure overlap.

CT and CBCT are considered the gold standard technique in veterinary patients to assess the bony structures of the head and TMJ. Disease conditions affecting soft tissue structures of the masticatory apparatus should be assessed by traditional CT instead of CBCT due to the lack of soft-tissue contrast provided by the latter. **Box 3** and **Figs. 28–35** present the main indications for tomographic examinations of the dentoalveolar and maxillofacial structures in dogs and cats.

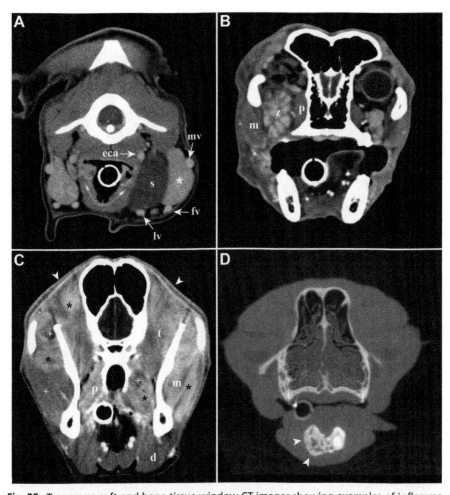

**Fig. 28.** Transverse soft and bone tissue window CT images showing examples of inflammatory disorders. CT post-contrast soft tissue image of an adult dog affected by a cervical sialocele (A). Note the soft tissue contrast difference between the left mandibular salivary gland (*asterisk*) and the hypoattenuating locular area filled by fluid (saliva) (S). The hyperattenuating regional blood vessels are easily identified due to the contrast enhancement: External carotid artery (eca), lingual vein (lv), facial vein (fv), and maxillary vein (mv). Postcontrast soft tissue image of an adult dog suffering from a zygomatic sialadenitis (B) (Copyright Lenin A. Villamizar). Note the zygomatic salivary gland (z) enlargement that produces partial obliteration of the right infraorbital space. Masseter muscle (m) and medial pterygoid muscle (p). CT post-contrast soft tissue image of an adult dog affected by masticatory muscle myositis (C) (Copyright Alexander M. Reiter). Note the bilateral temporalis muscle atrophy and the heterogenous contrast enhancement pattern affecting the masticatory muscles that close the mouth: Masseter (m), medial pterygoid (p), and temporalis (t). Hyperattenuating areas (*asterisks*) suggest areas of inflammation, whereas darker areas (hypoattenuating) (+) may suggest edema. The normally attenuating aspect of the digastricus muscle (D) suggests that it is not affected by the inflammatory process. Transverse CBCT bone tissue window image at the mandibular canine teeth level of an adult cat affected by osteomyelitis, showing moderate lytic and expansive process of the rostral aspect of the right mandible (*arrowheads*) (D).

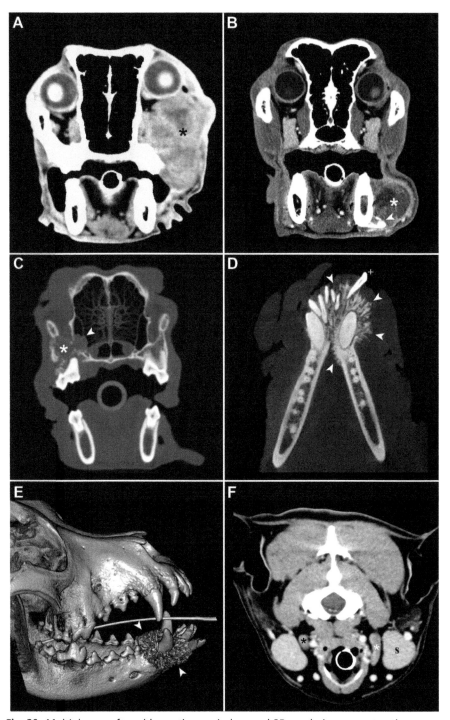

**Fig. 29.** Multiplanar soft and bone tissue window and 3D rendering reconstruction examples of patients affected by neoplastic processes. Post-Contrast transverse soft tissue

## MAGNETIC RESONANCE IMAGING

In the dog and cat, MRI is an infrequently used imaging modality for evaluating the soft tissues of the maxillofacial region, and examples of its uses include the assessment of salivary gland diseases, staging of oral tumors, metastatic lymph nodes screening, and early diagnosis of myopathies such as masticatory muscle myositis (**Fig. 36A**).[38,39] When used for imaging of the jaws, T1-and T2-weighted sequencing are most common. Long study acquisition times under general anesthesia, high cost, and differing needs of veterinary patients (ie, surgery of the TMJ is not commonly performed in dogs and cats), and the emergence of CBCT as the imaging method of choice for the examination of the osseous components of the TMJ are all reasons for the lack of popularity of MRI in veterinary dentistry and oral surgery. In the human side of the specialty, the use of MRI has seen a sharp decline, as the 1990s boom of surgical TMJ intervention has waned and the popularity of CBCT has increased. MRI studies, however, remain the reference method for evaluation of the soft tissue (articular disc) internal structures of the TMJ (**Fig. 36B**).

## ULTRASOUND

The use of diagnostic ultrasound in veterinary dentistry is extremely limited. However, with respect to oral and maxillofacial diseases, ultrasound does serve rare utility, especially in the identification/localization of cervical or intermandibular foreign bodies (eg, plant awn, penetrating injuries), diagnostically for the collection of fine-needle aspirates for cytology or culture, for obtaining biopsy samples from masses, lymph nodes or salivary glands, and also to conveniently evaluate less accessible orofacial regions such as the retrobulbar space before scheduling more definitive anesthetized imaging tests. Ocular ultrasound can be particularly helpful in the initial evaluation of the exophthalmic patient, allowing for the quick differentiation between a tissue- or fluid-filled retrobulbar swelling, and adjunctively in the diagnosis of masticatory muscle or extraocular myositis in dogs.

←————————————————————————————————————————

reconstruction at the level of the eyes of adult dogs affected by a maxillary malignant melanoma (A) and a mandibular fibrosarcoma (B). In (A), note the heterogeneous contrast enhancement, mass effect on the left eye, and obliteration of the infraorbital area (*asterisk*). The mandibular fibrosarcoma (B) appears as a lobulated soft tissue mass at the buccal aspect of the left mandible (*asterisk*). Note the bone proliferation (*arrowhead*) and soft tissue attenuation of the mandibular canal that suggests infiltration of the neoplastic process. CBCT bone tissue window transversal (C) and dorsal (D) reconstructions of different adult dogs affected by acanthomatous ameloblastomas. Note the predominant lytic pattern on the right maxilla at the level of the first molar tooth (*asterisk*) and the neoplastic infiltration of the maxillary recess (*arrowhead*) (C). In (D), note the predominant proliferative bone tissue pattern of the rostral region of the right mandible (*arrowheads*) with the displacement of the third incisor tooth (+). 3D volume rendering reconstruction (E) from the same dog displayed in (D). Note the bone proliferation of the rostral aspect of the right mandible extending up to the first premolar tooth (*arrowheads*). Transverse soft tissue post-contrast CT reconstruction at the level of the mandibular salivary glands of an adult dog affected by an oral malignant melanoma. The images are used for staging the neoplastic process. Note the enlargement of the left medial retropharyngeal lymph node (*asterisk*). Further cytology evaluation confirmed neoplastic cells.

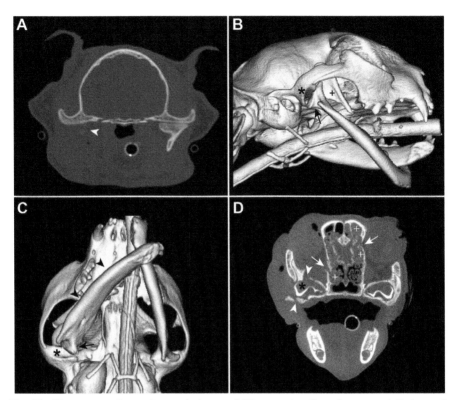

**Fig. 30.** CT transverse bone tissue window and 3D reconstructions from an adult domestic shorthaired cat with mandibular trauma. Note that the right condylar process is not located at the mandibular fossa (*arrowhead*) (*A*), luxation of the right TMJ (condylar process [*arrow*] and mandibular fossa [*asterisk*]), mandibular symphyseal separation, and mandibular deviation (*arrowheads*) (*B* and *C*), and fracture of the ramus of the mandible *(+)*. CBCT transverse bone reconstruction at the level of the eyes of a 3-month-old puppy. Several fractures affect the caudal maxilla (*arrowheads*) and medial aspect of the orbit *(arrows)*. Note that the maxillary fracture affects the alveolar bone of the unerupted permanent right maxillary first molar tooth. In this case, nasal opacification is associated with intranasal bleeding (+). (Copyright Alexander M. Reiter)

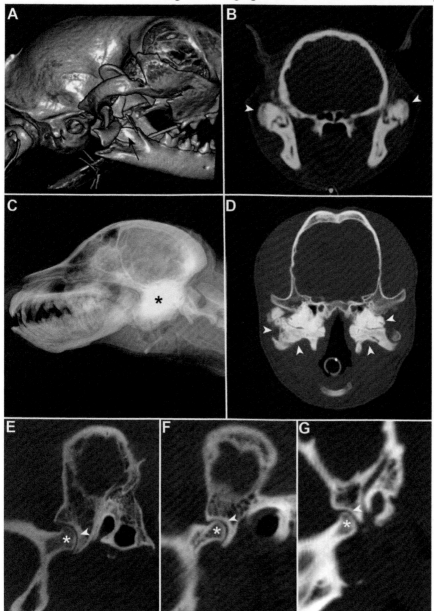

**Fig. 31.** CT and CBCT examples of veterinary patients with TMJ disorders. CBCT volume rendering reconstruction of an adult domestic shorthaired cat affected by a comminuted fracture at the condylar process (*arrow*) (*A*). CT scan transverse image of an adult cat affected by bilateral TMJ ankylosis (*B*). Note the bilateral bone proliferation at the level of both TMJs (*arrowheads*). Latero-lateral radiographic view and CT transverse reconstruction of a West Highland terrier suffering from craniomandibular osteopathy. Note the thickening of the ventral aspect of the mandibles and bone proliferation at the TMJ on the radiograph (*C*) and the same lesion observed in the CT image (*arrowheads*). CBCT images showing the normal conformation of the medial aspect of the TMJ in an adult German shepherd dog (*E*) and an adult domestic shorthaired cat (*F*). Note the dysplastic conformation in an adult Cocker spaniel (*G*). The mandibular fossa appears flattened, and the mandibular head of the condylar process does not show the round conformation observed in E and F. Mandibular head (*asterisk*), mandibular fossa (*arrowhead*).

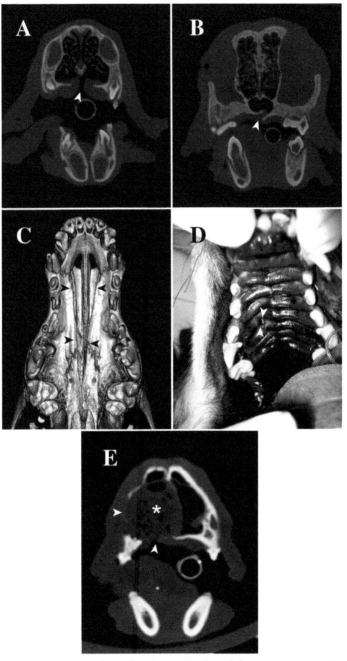

**Fig. 32.** CBCT and CT examples for cleft palate and palate defect assessment. CBCT transverse bone and 3D reconstructions of a 5-month-old Cocker spaniel affected by a secondary cleft palate (*arrowheads*) (*A–C*). Photography of a 1 cm palate defect in a 7-year-old mixed breed dog (*arrowheads*) (*D*). Note on the CT image the more extensive bone destruction of the right maxillary and palatine bones (*arrowheads*). Turbinate bones are not observed. Instead, a soft tissue attenuating material is present at the right nasal cavity (*asterisk*). Histopathology assessment was consistent with a chronic inflammatory process. (*Copyright Lenin A. Villamizar*)

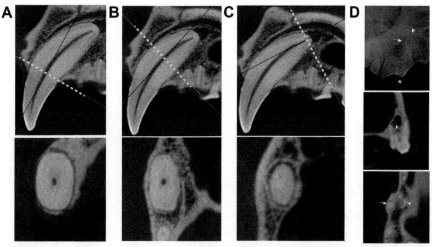

**Fig. 33.** CBCT examples of endodontic assessment. Sagittal reconstructions of a clinical healthy right maxillary canine tooth in a 4-year-old dog *(A–C)*. Dorsal reconstructions at different levels of the root *(dotted line A1-C1)*. Notice a well-defined periodontal ligament at the most coronal reconstruction (A1). At the middle aspect of the root, the periodontal ligament is not observed at the palatal surface of the root, suggesting dentoalveolar ankylosis *(arrowheads B1)*. Dorsal reconstruction of the root apex *(C1)*. Intraoral dental radiograph of the right maxillary fourth premolar tooth presenting an uncomplicated crown fracture *(asterisk)*. Note the normal appearance of the mesiobuccal root *(arrow)* and partial definition of the mesiopalatal root *(arrowhead) (D)*. Transverse *(D1)* and dorsal *(D2)* reconstructions of the same tooth. Note the tooth resorption at the buccal aspect of the mesiopalatal root *(arrowheads)* on *D1* and *D2*. Mesiobuccal *(white arrow)* and distal *(black arrow)* roots. (Copyright Lenin A. Villamizar)

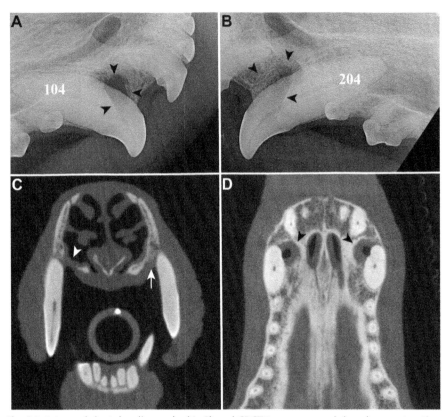

**Fig. 34.** Intraoral dental radiographs (*A*, *B*) and CBCT transverse and dorsal reconstructions (*C*, *D*) of a 5-year-old dog. Images show bilateral maxillary canine mesiopalatal bone defects as a consequence of bilateral linguoverted mandibular canine teeth. Intraoral radiographs show severe vertical bone loss (*arrowheads*) at the mesial aspect of 104 and 204 (*A*, *B*). CT images allow assessing the infrabony pockets in different planes (*C*, *D*). Note the oronasal communication at the palatal aspect of the right maxillary canine tooth (*arrowhead*). There is still bone separating the oral from the nasal cavity at the bottom of the left maxillary canine infrabony pocket (*arrow*) (*C*). These imaging findings can guide the veterinary practitioner in deciding when to perform periodontal procedures. Dorsal reconstruction showing the infrabony pockets at the maxillary canine teeth (*arrowheads*).

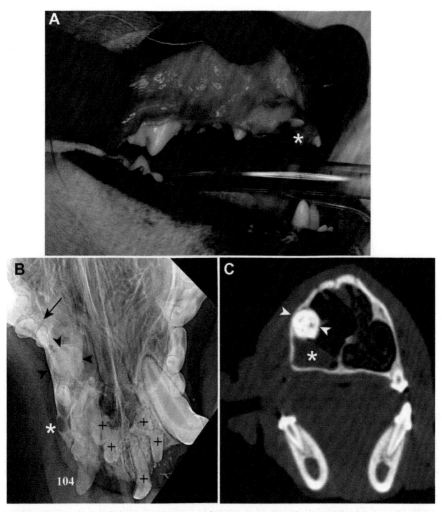

**Fig. 35.** Photograph of the lateral aspect of the oral cavity of 15-month-old dog showing a malformed and partially erupted right maxillary canine tooth (104) *(asterisk)* and several missing incisors and premolar teeth *(A)*. Intraoral radiograph showing the malformed 104, several malformed erupted and unerupted incisor teeth *(+)*, locular bone expansion at the buccal aspect of 104 *(asterisk)*, round dental radiopacity at the level of the missing right maxillary second premolar tooth *(arrowheads)*, and the unerupted and malformed maxillary third premolar tooth *(arrow)*. Transverse CBCT reconstruction at the level of the missing second maxillary tooth showing a hyperattenuating rounded structure located at the right nasal cavity *(arrowheads)* *(C)*. Note the soft tissue opacification at the nasal cavity suggestive of fluid accumulation.

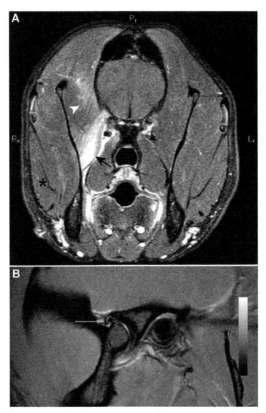

**Fig. 36.** T1-weighted postcontrast fat suppression (for improved identification of abnormal contrast enhancement) in a young dog with confirmed masticatory muscle myositis*(A)*. Note the intense contrast enhancement of the deep portion of the right temporalis muscle (*arrowhead*) and right medial pterygoid muscle (*arrow*). Image courtesy of Jeremy O'Neill. MRI may provide an earlier tentative diagnosis of inflammatory muscle diseases and enable an earlier start to treatment; whereas more definitive tests such as 2M-fiber antibody titers require a 1-week turnaround time, eventually delaying the start of treatment.[39] Open-mouth sagittal T1-weighted image of a normally positioned articular disc (green *arrow*) in a dog *(B)*. Image courtesy of Boaz Arzi.

## SUMMARY

Intraoral dental radiography remains an essential part of the comprehensive oral health assessment in the dog and cat. On a daily basis, the practicing veterinarian is likely to use the skill set of dental radiographic interpretation. Over the past decade, the veterinary imaging industry has seen tremendous growth in CBCT unit sales. Due to its excellent spatial resolution, CBCT has quickly become the gold standard for imaging of dentoalveolar tissues and the maxillofacial skeleton. CBCT units also have a small footprint, making it an easy addition to existing veterinary facilities, and are a lesser financial investment than traditional CT units that are significantly larger and more expensive. Multislice CT scanners and MRI units, although their usage is typically limited to larger multi-specialty veterinary facilities, shared regional facilities, or academic institutions, remain the reference standard for the assessment of maxillofacial tissues and for the evaluation of soft tissue diseases whereby improved contrast is needed. Although CT and CBCT provide cross-sectional images that already solve the superposition artifacts inherent with intraoral and skull radiography, they also provide additional diagnostic, pretreatment, and educational value when datasets are reconstructed using DICOM image processing software. These 3D-reconstructed images and 3D-printed models play an invaluable role in presurgical planning in maxillofacial trauma and patients with cancer. The utility of diagnostic ultrasound in veterinary maxillofacial imaging is limited; however, it can be helpful with diagnostic sample collection and for chairside screening of poorly accessible (intermandibular and retrobulbar) areas of the maxillofacial space.

## DISCLOSURE

The authors have nothing to disclose.

## REFERENCES

1. Bedard A, Davis TD, Angelopoulos C. Storage phosphor plates: how durable are they as a digital dental radiographic system? J Contemp Dent Pract 2004;5(2): 057–69.
2. Clark JL, Wadhwani CP, Abramovitch K, et al. Effect of image sharpening on radiographic image quality. J Prosthet Dent 2018;120:927–33.
3. Kuntsi-Vaattovaara H, Verstraete FJM, Kass PH. Results of root canal treatment in dogs: 127 cases (1995-2000). J Am Vet Med Assoc 2002;220:775–80.
4. Lee L. Inflammatory lesions of the jaws. In: White SC, Pharoah M, editors. Oral radiology principles and interpretation. 6th edition. St. Louis: Mosby (Elsevier); 2009. p. 325–42.
5. Assheuer J, Sager M. Priciples of imaging techniques. In: MRI and atlas of the dog. Blackwell Science; 1997. p. 449–61.
6. Tidwell A. Principles of computed tomography and magnetic resonance imaging. In: Thrall D, editor. Textbook of veterinary diagnostic radiology. 5th edition. Saunders, Elsevier; 2007. p. 50–6.
7. Farfallini D. Tomografia computarizada. In: Pellegrino F, Suraniti A, editors. El Libro de Neurologia para La práctica Clínica. Buenos Aires: Inter-Médica; 2003. p. 475–81.
8. Lell MM, Wildberger JE, Alkadhi H, et al. Evolution in computed tomography: the battle for speed and dose. Invest Radiol 2015;50:629–44.
9. Saunders J, Ohlerth S. CT physics and instrumentation - Mechanical design. In: Schwarz T, Sauders J, editors. Veterinary computed tomography. John Wiley & Sons, Ltd; 2011. p. 1–8.
10. Bardo D, Brown P. Cardiac multidetector computed tomography: basic physics of image acquisition and clinical applications. Curr Cardiol Rev 2008;4:231–43.
11. Nasis A, Mottram PM, Cameron JD, et al. Current and evolving clinical applications of multidetector cardiac CT in assessment of structural heart disease 1. Rev Comment Rev Radiol 2013;267:11–25.
12. Feeney DA, Fletcher TF, Hard R. Multiplanar imaging, basics of computed tomography. In: Atlas of correlative imaging anatomy of the normal dog. W.B Saunders Company; 1991. p. 344–52.
13. Farman AG, Scarfe W. Historical perspectives on CBCT. In: Scarfe WC, Angelopolous C, editors. Maxillofacial cone beam computed tomography. Principles, techniques and clinical applications. Springer International Publishing AG; 2018. p. 3–12.

14. Cavalcanti MG, Sales MA. Tomografia computadorizada. In: Cavalcanti MG, editor. Diagnóstico por imagem da face. Livraria Santos Editora; 2008. p. 3–43.
15. Groell R, Doerfler O, Schaffler GJ, et al. Contrast-enhanced helical CT of the head and neck. Am J Roentgenol 2001;176:1571–5.
16. Pollard R, Puchalski S. CT contrast media and applications. In: Schwarz T, Sauders J. Veterinary computed tomography. John Wiley & Sons Ltd; 57–66.
17. Bae KT. Intravenous contrast medium administration and scan timing at CT: considerations and approaches. Radiology 2010;256:32–61.
18. Saunders J, Schwarz T. Principles of CT image interpretation. In: Schwarz T, Saunders J, editors. Veterinary computed tomography. John Wiley & Sons, Ltd; 2011. p. 29–33.
19. Gyles C. 3D printing comes to veterinary medicine. Can Vet J 2019;60:1033–4.
20. Winer JN, Verstraete FJM, Cissell DD, et al. The application of 3-dimensional printing for preoperative planning in oral and maxillofacial surgery in dogs and cats. Vet Surg 2017;46:942–51.
21. Posadzy M, Desimpel J, Vanhoenacker F. Cone beam CT of the musculoskeletal system: clinical applications. Insights Imaging 2018;9:35–45.
22. Roza MR, Antonio Silva LF, Barriviera M, et al. Cone beam computed tomography and intraoral radiography for diagnosis of dental abnormalities in dogs and cats. J Vet Sci 2011;12:387–92.
23. Heney CM, Arzi B, Kass PH, et al. Diagnostic yield of dental radiography and cone-beam computed tomography for the identification of anatomic structures in cats. Front Vet Sci 2019;6:58.
24. Riggs GG, Arzi B, Cissell DD, et al. Clinical application of cone-beam computed tomography of the rabbit head: Part 1 - normal dentition. Front Vet Sci 2016;3:93.
25. Winter AA, Pollack AS, Frommer HH, et al. Cone beam volumetric tomography vs. medical CT scanners. N Y State Dent J 2005;71:28–33.
26. Jacobson MW. Technology and principles of cone beam computed tomography. In: Sarment D, editor. Cone beam computed tomography: oral and maxillofacial diagnosis and applications. John Wiley & Sons, Inc; 2013. p. 3–24.
27. Haridas H, Mohan A, Papisetti S, et al. Computed tomography: will the slices reveal the truth. J Int Soc Prev Community Dent 2016;6(8):S85–92.
28. Loubele M, Bogaerts R, Van Dijck E, et al. Comparison between effective radiation dose of CBCT and MSCT scanners for dentomaxillofacial applications. Eur J Radiol 2009;71:461–8.
29. Howerton WB, Mora MA. Use of conebeam computed tomography in dentistry. Gen Dent 2007;55:54–80.
30. Coscarelli CT, Oliva A, Cavalcanti M. Implantologia. In: Calvancanti M, editor. Diagnóstico por imagem da face. Editora Livraria Santos; 2008. p. 154–61.
31. Van Thielen B, Siguenza F, Hassan B. Cone beam computed tomography in veterinary dentistry. J Vet Dent 2012;29:27–34.
32. Pauwels R, Araki K, Siewerdsen JH, et al. Technical aspects of dental CBCT: state of the art. Dentomaxillofac Radiol 2015;44(1):20140224.
33. Patrick S, Praveen Birur N, Gurushanth K, et al. Comparison of gray values of cone-beam computed tomography with hounsfield units of multislice computed tomography: an in vitro study. Indian J Dent Res 2017;28:66–70.
34. Nasim A, Sasankoti Mohan R, Nagaraju K, et al. Application of cone beam computed tomography gray scale values in the diagnosis of cysts and tumors. J Indian Acad Oral Med Radiol 2018;30:4–9.
35. Mah P, Reeves TE, Mcdavid WD. Deriving Hounsfield units using grey levels in cone beam computed tomography. Dentomaxillofacial Radiol 2010;39:323–35.

36. Pauwels R, Jacobs R, Singer SR, et al. CBCT-based bone quality assessment: are Hounsfield units applicable? Dentomaxillofacial Radiol 2015;44:1–16.
37. Venkatesh E, Venkatesh Elluru S. Cone beam computed tomography: basics and applications in dentistry. J Istanbul Univ Fac Dent 2017;51:S102.
38. Cauduro A, Favole P, Asperio RM, et al. Use of MRI for the early diagnosis of masticatory muscle myositis. J Am Anim Hosp Assoc 2013;49:347–52.
39. Bishop TM, Glass EN, De Lahunta A, et al. Imaging diagnosis - Masticatory muscle myositis in a young dog. Vet Radiol Ultrasound 2008;49:270–2.
40. White SC, Pharoah M. Principles of radiographic interpretation. In: White S, Pharoah M, editors. Oral radiology principles and interpretation. 4th edition. Mosby, Inc; 2000. p. 256–70.
41. Yoon DC, Mol A, Benn DK, et al. Digital radiographic image processing and analysis. Dent Clin North Am 2018;62:341–59.
42. Ng KK, Rine S, Choi E, et al. Mandibular carnassial tooth malformations in 6 dogs—Micro-computed tomography and histology findings. Front Vet Sci 2019; 6:464.
43. Tsugawa AJ, Verstraete FJ. How to obtain and interpret periodontal radiographs in dogs. Clin Tech Small Anim Pract 2000;15:204–10.
44. Peralta S, Verstraete FJM, Kass PH. Radiographic evaluation of the types of tooth resorption in dogs. Am J Vet Res 2010;71:784–93.
45. Nemec A, Arzi B, Murphy B, et al. Prevalence and types of tooth resorption in dogs with oral tumors. Am J Vet Res 2012;73:1057–66.
46. Blazejewski SW, Lewis JR, Gracis M, et al. Mandibular periostitis ossificans in immature large breed dogs: 5 cases (1999-2006). J Vet Dent 2010;27:148–59.
47. Coffman CR, Visser L. Crown restoration of the endodontically treated tooth: literature review. J Vet Dent 2007;24(1):9–12.
48. Wingo K. Cementation of full coverage metal crowns in dogs. J Vet Dent 2018; 35(1):46–53.
49. Tsugawa A. Tooth extractions. In: Griffon D, Hamaide A, editors. Complications in small animal surgery. Wiley Blackwell; 2016. p. 249–62.

# Oral Microbiome in Dogs and Cats: Dysbiosis and the Utility of Antimicrobial Therapy in the Treatment of Periodontal Disease

Eric M. Davis, DVM[a],*, J. Scott Weese, DVM, DVSc[b]

KEYWORDS

- Canine oral microbiome • Feline oral microbiome • Periodontitis • Antibiotic therapy

KEY POINTS

- The oral microbiome of dogs and cats is composed of hundreds of different bacterial species, archaea, viruses, and microscopic eukaryotes that cover all mucosal and dental surfaces as a biofilm.
- Immune tolerance of the microbiome prevails in health without evoking an inflammatory response.
- If the equilibrium between the microbiome and host immune surveillance is disturbed, immune tolerance shifts to a proinflammatory response.
- Despite decades of research, specific bacteria have not been shown to initiate the transition from health to inflammation; however, the proportion of more virulent species is increased (dysbiosis) at sites of inflammation and tissue destruction.
- Systemic antimicrobial therapy neither prevents nor effectively resolves inflammation resulting from disrupted homeostasis between the microbiome and host.
- To date there is no evidence that adjunctive systemic antimicrobial treatment for days before, postoperatively, or as a substitute to surgical treatment of periodontitis is medically beneficial in canine or feline patients.

## INTRODUCTION

Advances in gene sequence technology and data analysis have enabled the detection and taxonomic identification of microorganisms in vivo based on their unique RNA or DNA sequences compared to standard culture techniques which can only detect those organisms that readily grow on artificial media in vitro.[1] Because the specific growth requirements of most of the microorganisms are as yet unknown, culture-

[a] Animal Dental Specialists of Upstate New York, 6867 East Genesee Street, Fayetteville, NY 13066, USA; [b] Ontario Veterinary College, University of Guelph, Guelph, ON, Canada
* Corresponding author.
E-mail address: emdavisdvm@gmail.com

Vet Clin Small Anim 52 (2022) 107–119
https://doi.org/10.1016/j.cvsm.2021.08.004
0195-5616/22/© 2021 Elsevier Inc. All rights reserved.

independent technology has been used to provide a more accurate assessment of the richness (total number of species) and diversity (relative abundance of each species) of microorganisms present in a defined location.[1-3] The *microbiota* refers to living microorganisms including bacteria, archaea, and microscopic eukaryotes (fungi and protozoa), but excludes viruses, virusoids, prions, and plasmids which are considered to be nonliving particles.[4,5] The *metagenome* refers to all DNA sequences of the microbiota in a particular environment.[4,5] The *microbiome* has been defined as the genes and genomes of all microbial inhabitants (including viruses) within a defined environment.[5] The microbiome consists of a polymicrobial community that has distinct properties and functions and which interacts with the host environment as part of a specific ecologic niche.[4,5] Microorganisms within a microbiome interact with each other as well as with the host. A microbiome is dynamic and may change over time as conditions within the defined environment become altered.[5]

The Human Microbiome Project (HMP) was a U. S. National Institutes of Health (NIH) initiative which sought to sample, categorize, and define the microbial constituents from healthy human volunteers.[6,7] As part of the HMP (2007–2019), 9 specific oral sites were sampled that provided the basis to establish the Human Oral Microbiome Database (HOMD).[8,9] The oral microbiome of dogs, and later of cats, was subsequently surveyed using gene sequencing technology and similar open-access curated databases were created.[10,11] In oral health, neither gingivitis nor periodontitis is present and the host and microbiome coexist symbiotically without evoking an inflammatory response. The circumstances that cause a shift from immune tolerance to a proinflammatory response remain unknown, and a unified, all-encompassing hypothesis to explain how and why periodontal disease develops has yet to be described (**Fig. 1**).[12] The purpose of this review is to clarify the current understanding of the role played by the oral microbiome in dogs and cats, describe how the microbiome changes in periodontal disease, and offer guidance on the utility of systemic antimicrobial agents in the treatment of periodontitis in companion animals.

## CULTURE-INDEPENDENT TECHNOLOGY

All microorganisms contain ribosomal subunit genes that can be used for phylogenetic discrimination.[13] The16S rRNA gene in prokaryotes (bacteria and archaea) and the 18S rRNA gene in microscopic eukaryotes (protozoa and fungi) contain both conserved regions and uniquely variable regions that together can permit taxonomic identification.[14,15] Although the healthy oral cavity is occupied by a wide range of microbial inhabitants, the inventory of bacterial species is most complete because the 16S rRNA gene has been used for more than 20 years as a marker gene in oral microbiome studies.[16,17] PCR (polymerase chain reaction) primers are used to amplify the 16S rRNA gene, and the hypervariable regions can then be sequenced.[17] Next-generation sequencing (NGS), also called high-throughput, or massively parallel sequencing, refers to the automated, simultaneous reading of thousands of marker gene sequences in a sample.[18-21] Technical improvements have recently allowed the entire 16S rRNA gene to be sequenced rapidly, for lower cost, and with greater accuracy.[18-21] Sequencing the entire 16S rRNA gene instead of selected variable regions have made it possible to differentiate closely related bacterial species and to detect sequence variations in a genome to identify subtypes or strains.[19-21] A strain of a species is a small but consistent variation in the genome that can code for a slightly different feature or function.[19]

An alternative technique to marker gene sequencing is called "shotgun" sequencing, or whole-genome sequencing (WGS), in which all of the DNA in a sample

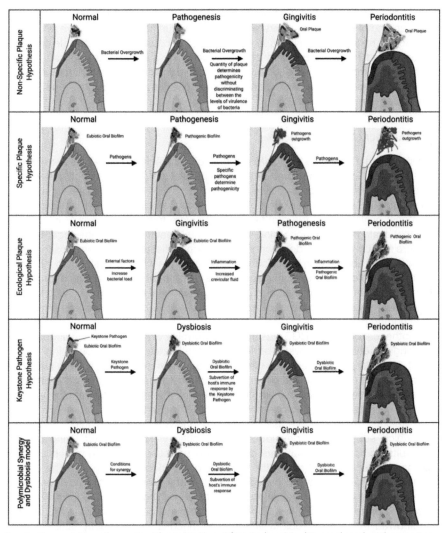

**Fig. 1.** Current Hypotheses For The Initiation Of Periodontitis. (*Reproduced with permission from* Radaic A, Kapila YL. The oralome and its dysbiosis: new insights into oral microbiome-host interactions. *Comp Struct Biotech J.* 2021; https://doi.org/10.1016/j.csbj.2021.02.010.)

is indiscriminately broken apart into millions of variably sized fragments which are then reassembled by connecting overlapping sequences using sophisticated mathematical algorithms.[22] Compared with NGS sequencing of the 16S rRNA gene which can only detect bacteria and archaea, WGS can identify all microbial inhabitants and can provide better quantitative data because PCR amplification-bias is eliminated.[21,22] Reassembled DNA sequences are longer with WGS, so taxonomic resolution is greater, and genes associated with microbiome function including virulence factors and antimicrobial resistance (AMR) can be detected.[21,22] Because WGS is more costly to perform and massive amounts of data must be processed, most microbiome studies to date have used NGS. Although gene sequencing technology has revolutionized our understanding of the microbial diversity in oral communities, in vitro culture remains a crucial tool in microbiology. New approaches to grow previously uncultivable bacterial species, called *culturomics,* have been devised that involves the application of a microbiome sample to a wide variety of media types, incubation in different atmospheres, at different temperatures, and for prolonged times, to encourage the growth of fastidious community members.[23]

## THE ORAL MICROBIOME OF DOGS

Initial studies that amplified the variable region of the 16S rRNA gene to determine the species present in the oral microbiome of "healthy dogs" did not categorize the samples according to periodontal disease status.[10,24–26] Of interest, however, was the early recognition that the oral microbiome of dogs was markedly different from that of humans; only16.4% of the oral taxa in dogs were found in humans.[10] In an NGS study that evaluated dogs according to periodontal health status, gram-negative species were most prevalent in dogs without periodontal disease, and gram-positive bacteria were most abundant in periodontitis, which was the exact opposite of the findings for humans (**Table 1**).[27] Gram-positive bacteria (*Streptococcus* sp.) are most prevalent in the healthy human oral cavity, and gram-negative, anaerobic bacteria such as *Porphyromonas gingivalis*, *Tannerella forsythia*, and *Treponema denticola* are often present in human periodontitis.[28]

In another canine study, NGS was used to determine which bacteria initially colonize supragingival enamel following professional teeth cleaning and polishing.[29] The earliest colonizers were gram-negative bacteria, dominated by the genera *Neisseria* and *Bergeyella*.[29] In a longitudinal study designed to identify microbiome changes that occurred over time without oral hygiene interventions, subgingival plaque samples were collected from selected teeth of 52 miniature Schnauzer dogs every 6 weeks for 60 weeks.[30] All teeth were associated with gingivitis at the beginning, and those teeth which subsequently developed periodontitis were compared using NGS.[30] The results demonstrated that periodontitis was not associated with the emergence of pathogenic species but rather the proportions of species changed as the clinical status of teeth deteriorated to periodontitis.[30] Another longitudinal study compared the microbiota from oral mucosal surfaces to supragingival plaque from 30 dogs before, and up to 5 weeks after (10 dogs), professional dental prophylaxis.[31] The results showed that the microbiota attached to mucosa was distinctly different from supragingival plaque, and 5 weeks after dental cleaning the relative proportion of species at both sites returned to pre-prophylaxis levels.[31]

In a study similar to the oral HMP, the microbiome from different niches within the canine oral cavity was examined.[32] Samples were collected from supragingival plaque, buccal mucosa, the dorsal surface of the tongue, and saliva from a cohort of 14 Labrador retriever dogs.[32] Similar to humans, different oral surfaces in dogs were colonized by distinct oral microbiomes. Supragingival plaque had the greatest species richness followed by mucosal surfaces (cheeks and tongue); canine saliva samples contained the fewest species.[32]

In the most recent NGS study to date, subgingival plaque samples from 587 dogs in 4 countries (UK, USA, China, and Thailand) were collected and analyzed according to oral health status to determine if the bacterial constituents were conserved across different geographic locations.[33] The authors reported that irrespective of geographic location, gram-negative bacteria from the phyla Bacteroidetes and Proteobacteria dominated the subgingival microbiome in health and in young dogs. Gram-positive

**Table 1**
Predominant subgingival oral bacterial taxa according to periodontal health status from dogs listed in order of decreasing abundance as determined by NGS

| | Davis, 2013[27] | | | Wallis, 2015[30] | | Wallis 2021[33] | |
|---|---|---|---|---|---|---|---|
| NO INFLAMMATION n=72 | GINGIVITIS n=77 | MILD PERIODONTITIS n=77 | GINGIVITIS Time=0 n=47 | MILD PERIODONTITIS Time= 6 weeks n=47 | NO INFLAMMATION G=0 n=587 | GINGIVITIS G=3 n=587 |
| *Porphyromonas cangingivalis* 10.47% | *Porphyromonas cangingivalis* 7.9% | *Porphyromonas cangingivalis* 4.5% | *Porphyromonas cangingivalis* 6.68% | *Porphyromonas cangingivalis* 6.83% | *Porphyromonas cangingivalis* 6.68% | *Peptostreptococcaceae* sp. 4.45% |
| *Moraxella* sp. 6.61% | *Moraxella* sp. 3.5% | *Peptostreptococcaceae* sp. 3.5% | *Moraxella* sp. 3.91% | *Porphyromonas canoris* 2.99% | *Bergeyella* sp. 2.95% | *Clostridiales* sp. 3.28% |
| *Bergeyella zoohelcum* 5.48% | *Bergeyella zoohelcum* 2.6% | *Peptostreptococcaceae* sp. 2.7% | *Bergeyella zoohelcum* 2.0% | *Treponema* sp. 2.78% | *Fusobacterium* sp. 2.00% | *Porphyromonas cangingivalis* 3.21% |
| *Neisseria shayeganii* 3.28% | *Neisseria shayeganii* 1.7% | *Clostridiales* sp. 2.2% | *Porphyromonas gulae* 1.95% | *Treponema denticola* 1.90% | *Pasturellaceae* sp. 1.74% | *Peptostreptococcaceae* sp. 2.99% |
| *Capnocytophaga* sp. 2.96% | *Peptostreptococcaceae* sp. 1.5% | *Lachnospiraceae* sp. 1.7% | *Porphyromonas canoris* 1.88% | *Porphyromonas gingivicanis* 1.88% | *Capnocytophaga* sp. 1.27% | *Treponema denticola* 1.64% |

PHYLA
Actinobacteria = ■
Bacteroidetes = □
Firmicutes = □
Fusobacteria= ■
Proteobacteria = □
Spirochetes = ──■──

bacteria from the phylum Firmicutes were most abundant in gingivitis and periodontitis, in small breeds, and in older dogs.[33]

## THE ORAL MICROBIOME OF CATS

In an early NGS study in cats, pooled samples from the gingiva, cheeks, and dental surfaces of 11 clinically healthy cats were analyzed to survey the oral microbiota.[34] A total of 273 genera from 18 bacterial phyla were detected, of which 47% of all sequences were shared among the 11 individuals. The predominant genera detected included *Pasteurella*, *Moraxella*, and *Thermomonas*, all of which are gram-negative bacteria.[34]

In an NGS diversity survey designed to establish a curated database of reference sequences of feline oral taxa, subgingival plaque samples were collected from 10 anesthetized cats with healthy oral tissues and from 10 cats with periodontitis.[11] A total of 171 species-level taxa from 11 phyla were detected.[11] In another study (**Table 2**), subgingival samples were collected from 20 cats with healthy oral tissues, 50 cats with gingivitis, and 22 cats with mild periodontitis.[35] Similar to dogs, these authors noted that approximately 75% of the subgingival bacteria in oral health were gram-negative bacteria. Percentage abundance of gram-positive bacteria increased as periodontal health status declined to gingivitis and periodontitis.[35]

NGS technology was recently used to compare the subgingival bacterial taxa in samples from 6 cats without oral inflammation, 20 cats with chronic periodontitis, 11 cats with aggressive (juvenile) periodontitis, and 7 cats with chronic gingivostomatitis.[36] Remarkably, the overall distribution of bacterial phyla was similar in healthy sites and inflamed sites. Putative pathogens were present in healthy sites and genera that predominated in health remained present but were reduced in abundance in diseased sites.[36] The authors suggested that inflammation might be responsible for the microbial population shifts that occurred in response to altered local environmental conditions and nutrient availability in inflamed sites.[36]

In the most recent study to date, WGS was used to detect subgingival community members and their functional potential from 6 cats with oral health compared to 14 cats with chronic periodontitis, 10 cats with aggressive periodontitis, and 9 cats with chronic gingivostomatitis.[37] This was the first veterinary study to use WGS rather than NGS to assess the oral microbiome, and although the data were preliminary, DNA from the samples permitted the detection of some functional genes.[37]

## CHANGES IN THE MICROBIOME DURING GINGIVITIS AND PERIODONTITIS

NGS oral diversity studies have been revelatory in determining which bacterial taxa are present in healthy and diseased sites and have exposed the differences between the oral taxa in humans and companion animals.[38] However, at the time of this writing, most oral microbiome studies in companion animals have relied on select variable regions of the 16S rRNA gene, which limits taxonomic discrimination. Studies of the contributions of archaea, fungi, protozoa, and viruses to oral health have been limited.[39–41] The use of WGS to expand the detection of taxa beyond bacteria and to determine the functional capacity of the oral microbiome has yet to be widely applied in dogs and cats.

The oral microbiome is attached to the various mucosal surfaces and teeth as a biofilm, which is a 3 dimensional, structured polymicrobial community that is enveloped within a self-produced, extracellular polymeric matrix (EPM) composed of polysaccharides, proteins, lipids, and extracellular DNA.[42,43] Biofilm formation occurs rapidly, as pioneer species attach to specific oral surfaces, followed by coaggregation of secondary colonizers, which then allows the biofilm to mature and expand.[47] Within biofilm, bacteria display genomic variation compared to planktonic forms of the same species, have altered metabolism, and interact with adjacent microbes including gene transfer. These changes, along with the physical protection conferred by EPM, result in a substantially reduced impact of antimicrobials and a greater chance of emergence of antibiotic resistance.[44,45] A biofilm protects the embedded microbial community from mechanical disruption, diffusion of disinfectants, and systemic antibiotics which cannot penetrate the EPM.[46] On oral mucosal surfaces, the attached biofilm provides a living barrier that helps protect against colonization by exogenous organisms (colonization resistance).[46,47] Gingiva and mucosal surfaces are regularly sloughed and replaced by cells from deeper layers, which are then recolonized by pioneer species. In contrast, biofilm attached to dental surfaces accumulates over time and becomes mineralized as calculus.[48] Calculus forms when the biofilm becomes saturated by calcium–phosphate salts present in saliva.[48] Viable biofilm covers calculus which then also becomes mineralized as calculus accumulates.[48,49]

Microbiota require attachment sites, a source of nutrients, moisture, waste removal, and an environment with the appropriate temperature, pH, and oxygen concentration.[42] However the conditions in the oral cavity are dynamic, not only related to host factors (age, health, diet, antimicrobials) but also due to changes within the microbiome itself (eg, increased metabolic waste, reduced oxygen levels, altered pH), which result in population shifts to species best adapted to survive.[47] Although health-related microbiota remain substantially present in microbiomes associated with inflamed tissue, the term "dysbiosis" has been applied to reflect that the microbial community is unbalanced and pathogens are increased in abundance.[44] However, evidence is mounting that inflammation may be primarily responsible for the increased abundance of more virulent species which then exacerbates the host response.[12,50–54]

Host neutrophils provide immune surveillance of oral tissues and continuously migrate to the gingiva and the gingival sulcus.[55–59] In humans, neutrophils appear histologically homogeneous but display functional heterogeneity, which can be assessed by cluster-of-differentiation (CD) cell-surface receptors.[57,58] In periodontal health, neutrophils display lower levels of CD marker genes which imply a reduced state of

**Table 2**
Predominant subgingival oral bacterial taxa according to periodontal health status from cats listed in order of decreasing abundance as determined by NGS or WGS

| Harris 2015[35] | | Rodrigues 2019[36] | | Rodrigues 2021[37] | |
|---|---|---|---|---|---|
| HEALTHY n=20 | PERIODONTITIS n=22 | HEALTHY n=6 | CHRONIC PERIODONTITIS n=20 | HEALTHY n=6 | CHRONIC PERIODONTITIS n=14 |
| *Fusobacterium* sp. 3.43% | *Peptostreptococcaceae* sp. 4.88% | *Enhydrobacter* sp. 7% | *Enhydrobacter* sp. 2.5% | *Porphyromonas* sp. 12.32% | *Porphyromonas* sp. 14.75% |
| *Porphyromonas circumdentaria* 3.24% | *Porphyromonas canoris* 3.09% | *Moraxella* sp. 6% | *Moraxella* sp. 2.4% | *Bacteroides* sp. 7.68% | *Bacteroides* sp. 9.95 |
| *Porphyromonas* sp. 3.21% | *Porphyromonas* sp. 2.78% | *Capnocytophaga* sp. 1.75% | *Fusibacter* sp. 1.9% | *Neisseria* sp. 6.88% | *Treponema* sp. 7.91% |
| *Moraxella* sp. 3.18% | *Treponema* sp. 2.69% | *Bergeyella* sp. 1.61% | NA | *Treponema* sp. 5.78% | *Neisseria* sp. 7.66% |
| *Capnocytophaga* sp. 3.04% | *Fillifactor villosus* 2.57% | *Corynebacterium* sp. 0.89% | NA | *Clostridium* sp. 4.12% | *Clostridium* sp. 4.27% |

———PHYLA
-Actinobacteria =
Bacteroidetes =
Firmicutes =
Fusobacteria =
Proteobacteria =
Spirochetes =

NA= Data not available

activation (called *para-inflammatory*) than proinflammatory neutrophils which have higher levels of CD markers.[55–57] Once within the gingival tissue and provided proinflammatory cytokines are at a low level, most of the neutrophils exit through the junctional epithelium at the apical extent of the gingival sulcus where they are transported by gingival crevicular fluid into the saliva to be swallowed.[56] This is thought to be a mechanism for disposal of large numbers of neutrophils without the risk of tissue damage caused by the release of potent neutrophilic enzymes.[56,57] However, if chemotactic cytokines are detected by neutrophil receptors, a host-mediated inflammatory reaction ensues.

Gingivitis is a reversible inflammatory response confined to the gingiva that is not associated with attachment loss. Gingivitis does not always progress to periodontitis, but gingivitis is commonly present in periodontitis.[60] In contrast, periodontitis is a complex inflammatory process during which irreversible damage occurs to the dental attachment apparatus which ultimately results in tooth exfoliation.[60] Tooth loss may be a host survival mechanism which resolves inflammation, limits the potential for sepsis, and restores homeostasis.[61]

## THE UTILITY OF ANTIMICROBIAL THERAPY IN THE TREATMENT OF PERIODONTAL DISEASE

Because periodontitis is an inflammatory disease that involves host factors and microbial communities rather than specific pathogenic bacteria, the utility of systemic antimicrobial therapy in the treatment of periodontitis is questionable. Complexities of the oral environment, variable penetration into biofilm, and reduced efficacy in debris-laden environments relegate antimicrobials to, at best, a subordinate role in periodontal treatment. Beyond efficacy, there is the growing global concern of AMR and adverse drug-induced side effects. Unfortunately, data indicating which veterinary patients are most likely to benefit from systemic antimicrobial therapy are lacking.

One of the most frequent uses (and overuse) of antimicrobials in veterinary medicine today is prophylaxis associated with dental procedures. Bacterial translocation and systemic sequelae such as bacterial endocarditis are a concern, but there has been limited study of systemic sequelae resulting from dental procedures. Individual case reports have described adverse events such as endocarditis and pericardial effusion after dental prophylaxis; however, the high frequency of dental procedures performed must be considered when interpreting sporadic case reports. One observational study identified a 6-fold increase in the incidence of endocarditis in dogs with severe periodontal disease than dogs with no or mild dental disease.[62] However, a retrospective case–control study of 76 dogs with endocarditis found no link to recent dental procedures.[63] Although high-level data are lacking, there is little to suggest that infective endocarditis is a common sequel to the dental treatment of dogs and cats.[64]

A 2019 updated policy statement by the American Veterinary Dental College (AVDC) recommended the use of antimicrobials to reduce bacteremia for *"animals that are immune compromised, have underlying systemic disease (such as certain clinically-evident cardiac disease [sub-aortic stenosis], or severe hepatic or renal disease) and/or when severe oral infection is present. Antibiotics should never be considered a monotherapy for the treatment of oral infections, and should not be used as preventive management of oral conditions."*[65] However, "immune compromised" and "clinically evident cardiac, hepatic and renal disease" could encompass a wide range of high and low-risk patients. Therefore, such statements provide little specific guidance and lead to unnecessary treatment. Other published guidelines have been similarly broad, such as recommending antimicrobial prophylaxis in patients with immune compromise, feline immunodeficiency virus infection, surgical implants, metabolic, hepatic, cardiac, pancreatic or renal disease,[66] or geriatric or debilitated animals, animals with preexisting heart or systemic disease or immunocompromise.[67] Such broad guidelines result in treatment of a relatively large percentage of patients and are inconsistent with current recommendations in human dentistry.[68] More restrictive criteria for prophylactic antimicrobial treatment in veterinary dentistry have been published, limiting treatment to high-risk patients such as those with patent ductus arteriosus, subaortic, or aortic stenosis, unrepaired cyanotic heart disease, previous infective endocarditis, and imbedded pacemaker leads.[69]

If antimicrobial prophylaxis is indicated, drug selection should be based on the most likely causes of infective endocarditis rather than putative periodontal pathogens. Gram-positive cocci, particularly *Streptococcus canis*, are commonly reported causes of infective endocarditis in dogs and cats, so prophylactic therapy should be targeted toward those species.[70] Enterobacterales (eg, *E. coli*) and other gram-negative bacteria have also been associated with infective endocarditis and so should also be covered. Ampicillin is highly effective against streptococci and is a reasonable consideration, although neither penicillins nor potentiated penicillins are particularly effective against Enterobacterales. In regions whereby injectable amoxicillin–clavulanic acid or ampicillin/sulbactam is available, these would be good choices to provide broader coverage, although amoxicillin/clavulanic acid is relatively ineffective against Enterobacterales.[71] Clindamycin provides excellent anaerobic and streptococcal coverage, but is ineffective against gram negatives. Cefazolin, a first-generation cephalosporin is a good option because of its efficacy against streptococci and most beta-lactamase-producing bacteria, and it is moderately effective against gram negatives. Treatment should be started 30 to 60 minutes before the procedure. For time-dependent drugs such as beta-lactams, antimicrobials should be redosed even 2 half-lives (eg, ~ every 2 hours for cefazolin). Treatment after the procedure is rarely indicated.

## SUMMARY

Microbiome research is still in its infancy and has just begun to clarify which microorganisms are present; their functional capabilities as individual taxa and as communities remain unclear. Despite decades of research, specific bacteria have not been shown to cause periodontitis, and although some taxa have virulent properties, that alone does not imply causation. Genomic studies are crucial to discovering new strategies to resolve oral inflammation without relying on systemic antimicrobial drugs that indiscriminately affect symbionts.

## CLINICS CARE POINTS

- The microbiome represents all of the genes and genomes of microbial inhabitants including bacteria, fungi, protozoa, and viruses present within a defined environment. To date, most microbiome studies have focused on bacteria.

- Gene sequencing technology has enabled the detection and taxonomic identification of microorganisms based upon their unique RNA or DNA sequences rather than standard culture techniques which can only detect those organisms that grow on artificial media.

- Gram positive bacteria predominate in the healthy human oral cavity and Gram negative species are most prevalent in periodontal disease. In dogs and cats, Gram negative species are most prevalent in health and Gram positive species are most prevalent in periodontal disease.

- Because periodontitis is associated with microbial communities rather than specific pathogenic species, systemic antimicrobial therapy for days before or for days dental treatment after is of questionable value.

- If antimicrobial prophylaxis is indicated, drug selection should be based upon the most likely bacteria associated with infective endocarditis rather than putative periodontal pathogens.

## DISCLOSURE

The authors have nothing to disclose.

## REFERENCES

1. Deo PN, Deshmukh R. Oral microbiome: unveiling the fundamentals. J Oral Maxillofac Pathol 2019;23:122–8.
2. Kumar PS, Dabdoub SM, Ganesan SM. Probing periodontal microbial dark matter using metataxonomics and metagenomics. Periodontol 2000 2021;85(1):12–27.
3. Belstrøm D. The oral microbiota as part of the human microbiota – links to general health. Nor Tannlegeforen Tid 2020;130:114–20.
4. Marchesi JR, Ravel J. The vocabulary of microbiome research: a proposal. Microbiome 2015;3:31.
5. Berg G, Rybakova D, Fischer D, et al. Microbiome definition re-visited: old concepts and new challenges. Microbiome 2020;8(1):103.
6. Turnbaugh P, Ley R, Hamady M, et al. The human microbiome project. Nature 2007;449(7164):804–10.
7. Gevers D, Knight R, Petrosino JF, et al. The human microbiome project: a community resource for the healthy human microbiome. PLoS Biol 2012;10:e1001377.

8. Chen T, Yu WH, Izard J, et al. The Human Oral Microbiome Database: a web accessible resource for investigating oral microbe taxonomic and genomic information. Database (Oxford) 2010;2010:baq013.

9. Escapa IF, Chen T, Huang Y, et al. New insights into human nostril microbiome from the Expanded Human Oral Microbiome Database (eHOMD): a resource for the microbiome of the human aerodigestive tract. mSystems 2018;3(6):e00187.

10. Dewhirst FE, Klein EA, Thompson EC, et al. The canine oral microbiome. PLoS One 2012;7(4):e36067.

11. Dewhirst FE, Klein EA, Bennett ML, et al. The feline oral microbiome: a provisional 16S rRNA gene based taxonomy with full-length reference sequences. Vet Microbiol 2015;175(2–4):294–303.

12. Curtis MA, Diaz PI, Van Dyke TE. The role of the microbiota in periodontal disease. Periodontol 2000 2020;83:14–25.

13. Woese CR, Fox GE. Phylogenetic structure of the prokaryotic domain: the primary kingdoms. Proc Natl Acad Sci U S A 1977;74:5088–90.

14. Liu YX, Qin Y, Chen T, et al. A practical guide to amplicon and metagenomic analysis of microbiome data. Protein Cell 2020. https://doi.org/10.1007/s13238-020-00724-8.

15. Wade WG, Prosdocimi EM. Profiling of oral bacterial communities. J Dent Res 2020;99(6):621–9.

16. Kroes I, Lepp PW, Relman DA. Bacterial diversity within the human subgingival crevice. Proc Natl Acad Sci U S A 1999;96:14547–52.

17. Schlaberg R. Microbiome diagnostics. Clin Chem 2020;66:68–76.

18. Comin M, Di Camillo B, Pizzi C, et al. Comparison of microbiome samples: methods and computational challenges. Brief Bioinform 2021;22:88–95.

19. Fuks G, Elgart M, Amir A, et al. Combining 16S rRNA gene variable regions enables high-resolution microbial community profiling. Microbiome 2018;6(1):17.

20. Johnson JS, Spakowicz DJ, Hong BY, et al. Evaluation of 16S rRNA gene sequencing for species and strain-level microbiome analysis. Nat Commun 2019;10(1):5029.

21. Yan Y, Nguyen LH, Franzosa EA, et al. Strain-level epidemiology of microbial communities and the human microbiome. Genome Med 2020;12(1):71.

22. Caselli E, Fabbri C, D'Accolti M, et al. Defining the oral microbiome by whole-genome sequencing and resistome analysis: the complexity of the healthy picture. BMC Microbiol 2020;20(1):120.

23. Lagier JC, Dubourg G, Million M, et al. Culturing the human microbiota and culturomics. Nat Rev Microbiol 2018;16:540–50.

24. Riggio MP, Lennon A, Taylor DJ, et al. Molecular identification of bacteria associated with canine periodontal disease. Vet Microbiol 2011;150:394–400.

25. Sturgeon A, Stull JW, Costa MC, et al. Metagenomic analysis of the canine oral cavity as revealed by high-throughput pyrosequencing of the 16S rRNA gene. Vet Microbiol 2013;162:891–8.

26. Oh C, Lee K, Cheong Y, et al. Comparison of the oral microbiomes of canines and their owners using next-generation sequencing. PLoS One 2015;10(7):e0131468.

27. Davis IJ, Wallis C, Deusch O, et al. A cross-sectional survey of bacterial species in plaque from client owned dogs with healthy gingiva, gingivitis or mild periodontitis. PLoS One 2013;8(12):e83158.

28. Willis JR, Gabaldón T. The human oral microbiome in health and disease: From sequences to ecosystems. Microorganisms 2020;8(2):308.

29. Holcombe LJ, Patel N, Colyer A, et al. Early canine plaque biofilms: characterization of key bacterial interactions involved in initial colonization of enamel. PLoS One 2014;9(12):e113744.
30. Wallis C, Marshall M, Colyer A, et al. A longitudinal assessment of changes in bacterial community composition associated with the development of periodontal disease in dogs. Vet Microbiol 2015;181:271–82.
31. Flancman R, Singh A, Weese JS. Evaluation of the impact of dental prophylaxis on the oral microbiota of dogs. PLoS One 2018;13(6):e0199676.
32. Ruparell A, Inui T, Staunton R, et al. The canine oral microbiome: variation in bacterial populations across different niches. BMC Microbiol 2020;20(1):42.
33. Wallis C, Milella L, Colyer A, et al. Subgingival microbiota of dogs with healthy gingiva or early periodontal disease from different geographical locations. BMC Vet Res 2021;17(1):7.
34. Sturgeon A, Pinder SL, Costa MC, et al. Characterization of the oral microbiota of healthy cats using next-generation sequencing. Vet J 2014;201(2):223–9.
35. Harris S, Croft J, O'Flynn C, et al. A pyrosequencing investigation of differences in the feline subgingival microbiota in health, gingivitis and mild periodontitis. PLoS One 2015;10(11):e0136986.
36. Rodrigues MX, Bicalho RC, Fiani N, et al. The subgingival microbial community of feline periodontitis and gingivostomatitis: characterization and comparison between diseased and healthy cats. Sci Rep 2019;9(1):12340.
37. Rodrigues MX, Fiani N, Bicalho RC, et al. Preliminary functional analysis of the subgingival microbiota of cats with periodontitis and feline chronic gingivostomatitis. Sci Rep 2021;11(1):6896.
38. Davis EM. Gene sequence analyses of the healthy oral microbiome in humans and companion animals: a comparative review. J Vet Dent 2016;33:97–107.
39. Wallis CV, Marshall-Jones ZV, Deusch O, et al. Canine and feline microbiomes. In: Singh RP, Kothari R, Koring PG, et al, editors. Understanding host-microbiome interactions - an omics approach. Singapore: Springer Nature; 2017. p. 279–326.
40. Patel N, Colyer A, Harris S, et al. The prevalence of canine oral protozoa and their association with periodontal disease. J Eukaryot Microbiol 2017;64(3):286–92.
41. Older CE, Diesel AB, Lawhon SD, et al. The feline cutaneous and oral microbiota are influenced by breed and environment. PLoS One 2019;14(7):e0220463.
42. Mark Welch JL, Dewhirst FE, Borisy GG. Biogeography of the oral microbiome: the site-specialist hypothesis. Annu Rev Microbiol 2019;73:335–58.
43. Proctor DM, Shelef KM, Gonzalez A, et al. Microbial biogeography and ecology of the mouth and implications for periodontal diseases. Periodontol 2000 2020; 82(1):26–41.
44. Radaic A, Kapila YL. The oralome and its dysbiosis: new insights into oral microbiome-host interactions. Comp Struct Biotech J 2021. https://doi.org/10.1016/j.csbj.2021.02.010.
45. Sadiq FA, Burmølle M, Heyndrickx M, et al. Community-wide changes reflecting bacterial interspecific interactions in multispecies biofilms. Crit Rev Microbiol 2021;1–21.
46. Rath S, Bal SCB, Dubey D. Oral biofilm: Development mechanism, multidrug resistance, and their effective management with novel techniques. Rambam Maimonides Med J 2021;12(1):e0004.
47. Duran-Pinedo AE. Metatranscriptomic analyses of the oral microbiome. Periodontol 2000 2021;85(1):28–45.
48. Akcali A, Lang NP. Dental calculus: the calcified biofilm and its role in disease development. Periodontol 2000 2018;76(1):109–15.

49. Karaaslan F, Demir T, Barış O. Effect of periodontal disease-associated bacteria on the formation of dental calculus: an in vitro study. J Adv Oral Res 2020;11(2):165–71.
50. Lamont RJ, Koo H, Hajishengallis G. The oral microbiota: dynamic communities and host interactions. Nat Rev Microbiol 2018;16(12):745–59.
51. Loos BG, Van Dyke TE. The role of inflammation and genetics in periodontal disease. Periodontol 2000 2020;83(1):26–39.
52. Van Dyke TE, Bartold PM, Reynolds EC. The nexus between periodontal inflammation and dysbiosis. Front Immunol 2020;11:511.
53. Bartold PM, Van Dyke TE. An appraisal of the role of specific bacteria in the initial pathogenesis of periodontitis. J Clin Periodontol 2019;46(1):6–11.
54. Kumar PS. Microbiomics: were we all wrong before? Periodontol 2000 2021; 85(1):8–11.
55. Rijkschroeff P, Loos BG, Nicu EA. Oral polymorphonuclear neutrophil contributes to oral health. Curr Oral Health Rep 2018;5:211–20.
56. Oveisi M, Shifman H, Fine N, et al. Novel assay to characterize neutrophil responses to oral biofilms. Infect Immun 2019;87(2):e00790.
57. Fine N, Tasevski N, McCulloch CA, et al. The neutrophil: constant defender and first responder. Front Immunol 2020;11:571085.
58. Hirschfeld J. Neutrophil subsets in periodontal health and disease: a mini review. Front Immunol 2020;10:3001.
59. Mikolai C, Branitzki-Heinemann K, Ingendoh-Tsakmakidis A, et al. Neutrophils exhibit an individual response to different oral bacterial biofilms. J Oral Microbiol 2020;13(1):1856565.
60. Stepaniuk K. Periodontology. In: Lobprise HB, Dodd JR, editors. Wiggs's veterinary dentistry: principles and practice. 2nd edition. Hoboken, NJ: Wiley Blackwell; 2019. p. 81–108.
61. Fine DH, Schreiner H, Velusamy SK. Aggregatibacter, a low abundance pathobiont that influences biogeography, microbial dysbiosis, and host defense capabilities in periodontitis: The history of a bug, and localization of disease. Pathogens 2020;9(3):179.
62. Glickman LT, Glickman NW, Moore GE, et al. Evaluation of the risk of endocarditis and other cardiovascular events on the basis of the severity of periodontal disease in dogs. J Am Vet Med Assoc 2009;234:486–94.
63. Peddle GD, Drobatz KJ, Harvey CE, et al. Association of periodontal disease, oral procedures, and other clinical findings with bacterial endocarditis in dogs. J Am Vet Med Assoc 2009;234:100–7.
64. Omobowale TO, Otuh PI, Ogunro BN, et al. Infective endocarditis in dogs: a review. Euro J Pharm Med Res 2017;4(8):103–9.
65. American Veterinary Dental College. The use of antibiotics in veterinary dentistry. https://avdc.org/download/30/position-statements/2873/antibiotic-use-april-2019.pdf. Accessed April 26, 2021.
66. Peak RM. Antibiotics in periodontal disease. In: Niemiec BA, editor. Veterinary periodontology. Ames (IA): John Wiley and Sons, Inc; 2013. p. 186–90.
67. Gorrel C. Veterinary dentistry for the general practitioner. Amsterdam (Netherlands): Elsevier; 2013.
68. Goff DA, Mangino JE, Glassman AH, et al. Review of guidelines for dental antibiotic prophylaxis for prevention of endocarditis and prosthetic joint infections and need for dental stewardship. Clin Infect Dis 2020;71:455–62.
69. Weese JS. Antimicrobials in veterinary dentistry. In: Gawor J, editor. The veterinary dental patient. Hoboken, NJ: Wiley-Blackwell; 2021. p. 87–107.

70. Sykes JE, Kittleson MD, Pesavento PA, et al. Evaluation of the relationship between causative organisms and clinical characteristics of infective endocarditis
in dogs: 71 cases (1992-2005). J Am Vet Med Assoc 2006;228:1723–34.
71. Clinical and Laboratory Standards Institute (CLSI). Vet01S performance standards for antimicrobial disk and dilution susceptibility testing for bacteria isolated
from animals 2020. USA.

# The Relationship Between Periodontal Infection and Systemic and Distant Organ Disease in Dogs

Colin Harvey, BVSc, FRCVS[a,b],*

## KEYWORDS

- Dog • Periodontal • Systemic • Distant organ • Prevention

## KEY POINTS

- Periodontal infection is common in dogs.
- Bacteremia is common in dogs with periodontal infection.
- Distant organ pathology associated with periodontal infection is seen in the kidneys, heart, and liver.
- Stress indicators (serum CRP, serum amyloid A, white blood cell count) increase as the severity of periodontal infection increases.
- Preventing accumulation of dental plaque is an important contributor to good health.

## INTRODUCTION

In addition to making the mouth more comfortable for the dog, good oral health ensures that the rest of the body does not suffer the consequences of distant organ abnormalities associated with bacteremia resulting from oral infections. When discussing the effects of oral infections, the term "periodontal disease" (PD) creates confusion for reasons noted later; when practical, I prefer to differentiate between *gingivitis* (inflammation of the gingival epithelium and connective tissue) and *periodontitis* (resorption of the connective tissue and bone that hold the tooth in the alveolus). When a general term covering both gingivitis and periodontitis is called for, I use "periodontal infection" in this review, and I distinguish between "distant organ" abnormalities (eg, renal or cardiac) and "systemic" abnormalities (eg, responses seen in changes in agents circulating in the blood).

---

[a] Colin Harvey LLC, 436 Covered Bridge Road, Cherry Hill, NJ 08034, USA; [b] School of Veterinary Medicine, University of Pennsylvania
* 436 Covered Bridge Road, Cherry Hill, NJ 08034.
*E-mail address:* Colin@ColinHarvey.info

Vet Clin Small Anim 52 (2022) 121–137
https://doi.org/10.1016/j.cvsm.2021.09.004
0195-5616/22/© 2021 Elsevier Inc. All rights reserved.

## BACTERIOLOGY AND PATHOPHYSIOLOGY OF GINGIVITIS AND PERIODONTITIS

The mouth is home to a rich bacterial biofilm on surfaces that are exposed to the external environment. In healthy individuals, this biofilm is in harmless balance with the local tissues, which are bathed in salivary fluid containing a rich mixture of antibacterial substances. Once something upsets this balance, bacteria in the biofilm proliferate and can cause local disease (gingivitis or periodontitis) and can be transported via the blood stream to other parts of the body.

The last 25 years have seen a massive increase in our understanding of the consequences of severe periodontal infection, although this is not new. One hundred and thirty years ago, W.D. Miller, MD, DDS, authored a paper titled "The Mouth as a Focus of Infection" in the *Dental Cosmos* (volume 33, pages 689–705, 1891); the paper includes these statements: *"The conviction has grown continually stronger, among physicians as well as dentists, that the human mouth, as a gathering-place and incubator of diverse pathogenic germs, performs a significant role in the production of varied disorders of the body … The evil results of allowing [periodontal infection] to gain the upper hand manifest themselves not only in the impairing or complete loss of the efficiency of the teeth as organs of mastication, but also, when a secretion of matter in the mouth becomes general, patients may suffer from fever, loss of appetite, stiffness, severe disturbances of the alimentary canal, insomnia, subictoritic discoloration of the skin, etc."*

The culprit in this story is the out-of-control dental plaque biofilm, resulting from poor oral hygiene. When allowed to develop unhindered by mechanical removal or chemical action, the dental plaque film increases in depth and complexity. Calcium carbonate and phosphate salts secreted by saliva become deposited on the plaque and mineralize to form dental calculus.[1] Dental plaque is attached to a nonvascularized surface (the enamel of the crown or the rough surface of dental calculus); as the thickness of dental plaque increases, ambient oxygen is reduced by bacterial metabolism in the deeper layers, producing an environment that allows anaerobic bacteria to thrive.

There is an extraordinarily wide range of bacterial species in the oral fluid and on the surfaces of teeth at any one time.[2,3] These species typically include organisms that are associated with infections in other parts of the body, such as staphylococci, streptococci, *Pseudomonas*, coliforms, and, particularly in cats, *Pasteurella*, as well as more mouth-specific anaerobic organisms and spirochetes.[2] Based on bacterial culture techniques, about 700 different bacterial species are known to grow in human mouths[4]; a similar number of species likely can grow in the mouths of carnivores, although the slightly alkaline pH of oral fluid in carnivores versus the slightly acidic pH in humans is likely responsible for some differences in the 2 floras. The bacterial flora is so broad that any attempt to culture a causative organism and select an antibiotic based on susceptibility tests for management of a particular clinical case is a waste of money.

Many of the bacteria considered to be periodontopathogens are anaerobic and will not grow under the aerobic conditions that are typically used for culturing clinical samples in veterinary clinical laboratories; some are fastidious, requiring specific culture media and full anaerobic conditions. The anaerobes thriving in the deeper levels of plaque and calculus are considered to be the primary periodontopathogens, initiating an inflammatory response that is recognized clinically as gingivitis.[1,5] Recent work using molecular biological techniques such as mRNA sequencing has identified many additional species in diseased areas of the mouth of dogs,[6–8] which has called into question our previous assumptions about periodontal pathogenicity.

The gingival tissues respond to periodontopathogens in the tooth-borne biofilm by becoming inflamed, as a result of release of a variety of biologically active agents such as bacterial lipopolysaccharide (LPS) endotoxins, chemotactic peptides, protein toxins, and organic acids. These agents stimulate the host to produce and release cytokines, including interleukin-1β, interleukin-8, prostaglandins, and tumor necrosis factor alpha (TNF-α).[9] The local result ranges from mild gingivitis to severe destructive periodontitis and eventual exfoliation of the tooth. This progression may be rapid in some dogs, may be slower in others, and may not occur in some.[1] Reasons for differences in the tissue response are variations in the thickness and bacterial constituents of plaque, oral hygiene modalities in use, and the immunologic health of the gingival tissues and body as a whole.

The pathophysiology of periodontal infection is similar to infections resulting from a bacteria-contaminated foreign body elsewhere in the body, although with some significant differences. The presence of a foreign body causes a pyogenic membrane to surround it in an attempt to wall off the seat of infection. The result is an abscess, which typically enlarges until it reaches an epithelial surface and bursts, allowing the abscess contents and the foreign body to drain; the inflamed tissues forming the wall of the abscess then clear up any remaining infection, and the abscess cavity resolves. In periodontal infection, there are 2 important differences. The foreign body is the tooth, which starts out being firmly attached to the alveolar bone. The enamel and any exposed cemental root surfaces are not vascularized, so the inflamed gingival tissues equivalent to the pyogenic membrane cannot completely surround the tooth. Periodontitis stimulated by the presence of the ongoing gingival infection results in a gradual loss of the bony attachment. A major difference from a foreign body abscess is that there is a path for drainage of purulent material along the surface of the tooth out to the oral environment; this limits the need for the severe infection to expand. Many months or more often years later, the periodontitis may be severe enough to have caused sufficient loss of attachment that the tooth becomes mobile and is eventually dislodged from the jaw. In this telling of the periodontal infection story, gingivitis and periodontitis can be "beneficial" in that the eventual result is ejection of the "foreign body"; however, the periodontal inflammatory response causes dilatation of blood vessels locally and the capillaries become more permeable. Significant bacteremic showers are frequent during chewing or tooth-brushing as a result of the inflamed soft tissues being squeezed against the alveolar bone.[10]

Bacterial culture of blood samples taken before, during, and after dental procedures shows that there is a bacteremic "shower" when a dirty mouth is scaled.[11,12] Bacteremia occurs several times a day as a result of a periodic increase in pressure on gingival tissue during chewing activity. In most dogs, the bacteria in the blood stream typically are cleared within 10 to 20 minutes[11] as they pass through the splenic filtering system, with activation of the reticuloendothelial system.

Because the cause of the infection (dental plaque bacteria) is removed during a dental scaling procedure, and bacteremia is typically short lived, antibiotic administration is not necessary for most dogs and cats undergoing dental scaling. Exceptions are as follows:

Ulcerative stomatitis (ulcers are located on buccal or lingual epithelia that lay against the inflamed gingiva).

Very severe gingivitis with spontaneous bleeding if a surgical procedure requiring gingival suturing at that site is to be performed.

If there is a distant organ condition that requires antibiotic prophylaxis.

When a clean surgical procedure will be performed elsewhere in the body during the same anesthetic episode.

It is not just whole bacteria that enter the blood stream during a bacteremic shower; bacterial degradation products, including LPS endotoxins, and locally produced tissue-destructive cytokines also leak into the capillaries. Depending on the frequency and severity of the bacteremia and the body's ability to respond to the bacteremic challenge, systemic and distant organ effects may occur.

## PREVALENCE OF PERIODONTAL INFECTION IN DOGS

Gingivitis and periodontitis are common in dogs. In 1899, Talbot[13] reported that in the mouths of dogs that were collected by dog pound staff in Chicago, 25% had gingivitis or more severe periodontal infection by 4 years of age, 80% from 8 to 10 years of age, and 95% greater than the age of 12 years. He also reported that 25% of the dogs aged 1 to 4 years exhibited at 3 large dog shows in Chicago had gingivitis, as did 75% of these dogs aged 4 to 8 years. A recent and detailed review of the prevalence of gingivitis and periodontitis in dogs[14] points out the challenges in stating an overall prevalence rate because of the methodological differences, particularly in the examination or scoring methods used.

Accumulation of plaque-covered calculus on the crown, whether or not associated with clinically evident gingivitis, is the most common clinical abnormality noted on physical examination,[15] depending on the criteria used to recognize periodontal infection. The range reported in the papers cited in this recent article[14] varied from 9% to 100% of dogs. One reason for the wide range in prevalence studies is the population of dogs studied; more detailed oral scoring is typically limited to studies of dogs presented to a veterinary dentist for treatment, which naturally have a higher prevalence of periodontal infection than is the case for the general population. Different breeds have different patterns of teeth affected (**Figs. 1 and 2**).[14,16–18] There is general agreement in reported studies that PD is more common and more severe in toy and small dogs (which tend to live longer than medium or large dogs), and in aging

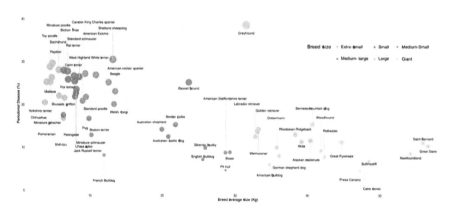

**Fig. 1.** Graphical representation of the prevalence of periodontal disease in 10 breeds of dog in each size category (extrasmall <6.5 kg, small 6.5–9 kg, medium-small 9–15 kg, medium-large 15–30 kg, large 30–40 kg, and giant >40 kg) that most frequently visited Banfield Pet hospitals (Wallis and colleagues, unpublished data). The color of the dots depicts the breed size category, and the size, the prevalence of periodontal disease (low prevalence small through to high prevalence large). Percentages on the x-axis are the prevalence of periodontal disease for each of the breeds of dog. (*Reprinted with permission from* Wallis C, Holcombe LJ. A review of the frequency and impact of periodontal disease in dogs. *J Small Anim Pract.* 2020;61:529–540.)

**A** Labrador retriever

**B** Miniature schnauzer

**C** Yorkshire terrier 37 weeks

**D** Yorkshire terrier 78 weeks

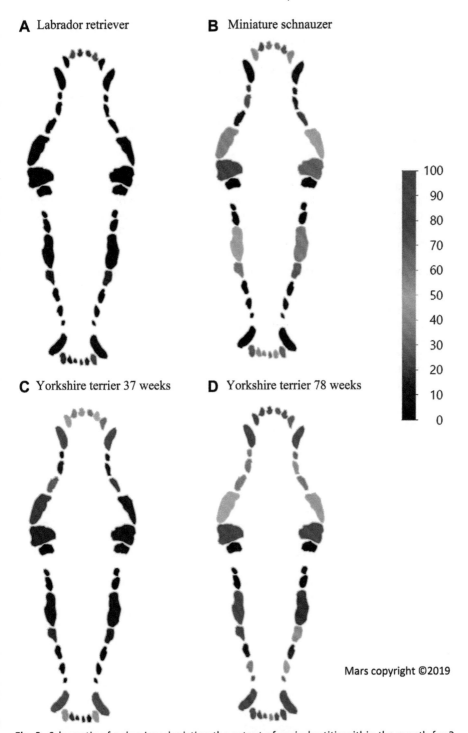

100
90
80
70
60
50
40
30
20
10
0

Mars copyright ©2019

**Fig. 2.** Schematic of a dog jaw depicting the extent of periodontitis within the mouth for 3 breeds of dog. (*A*) Labrador retriever. (*B*) Miniature schnauzer. (*C* and *D*) Yorkshire terrier. (*Reprinted with permission from* Wallis C, Holcombe LJ.A review of the frequency and impact of periodontal disease in dogs. *J Small Anim Pract.* 2020;61:529–540.)

dogs[14,15,19-23]; the result is that aging toy and small dogs are particularly at risk at a life stage at which they may be at a higher anesthetic risk if treatment is to be performed.

One likely reason for the high prevalence is that many pet dogs have little or no natural daily cleansing of the surfaces of their teeth; the home-cooked food or canned convenience foods that many owners feed their dogs may be excellent nutritionally but provide little effective chewing activity. The need to chew plays a critical role. Switching from a minced diet to one that contains the same ingredients but requires extensive masticatory activity, such as chewing whole bovine trachea and esophagus, causes measurable changes in gingival tissues within 24 hours.[24]

Another reason for differing general body reactions is that bacteria present vary from individual to individual, or the dogs' immune system competences vary. Examining the mouth when the dog is young (soon after completion of full eruption of the permanent teeth) is important because it is an opportunity to alert the owner to the need to pay careful attention to the mouth throughout life, particularly in dogs that have thick calculus deposits or gingivitis at a young age.

## PERIODONTAL–SYSTEMIC AND DISTANT ORGAN RELATIONSHIPS IN HUMANS

There are many studies reporting the relationship between periodontal infection and the rest of the body in humans; Refs.[25,26] provide recent summaries of this extensive bibliography. Abnormalities associated with chronic periodontitis include atherosclerotic cardiovascular disease and stroke, diabetes, adverse pregnancy outcomes, respiratory diseases, chronic kidney disease (CKD), rheumatoid arthritis, cognitive impairment, inflammatory bowel disease, obesity, metabolic syndrome, cancer, and increased acute-phase inflammatory responses (elevated C-reactive protein [CRP] in serum, increased white blood cell count).

## PERIODONTAL–SYSTEMIC AND DISTANT ORGAN ABNORMALITIES ASSOCIATED WITH GINGIVITIS-PERIODONTAL INFECTION IN DOGS

The first mention of a relationship between PD and abnormalities elsewhere in the body that I am aware of is in *Interstitial Gingivitis*,[13] a book published in 1899. This book includes detailed clinical and microscopic descriptions of gingivitis and periodontitis in dogs. Bodingbauer,[27] in 1946, described 3 dogs with "*general symptoms of illness, related to tooth infections, that were ameliorated or dissipated by extraction of the affected tooth.*" One of these dogs later died, and evidence of mitral endocarditis was found. The second one had fever, nephritis, and gastritis, and the third had fever and nephritis.

An observation commonly made by both owners and veterinarians following teeth scaling or more involved periodontal treatment or extraction is that the dog is "acting younger." Some unsupported comments in the literature or stated on product packaging or in advertisements are on the alarmist side; one could get the impression that dogs that do not have immaculately clean teeth are at risk of an early and ugly death from heart disease or renal disease! Although the evidence summarized in this article demonstrates that associations have been well documented and that these reports support the hypothesis that periodontal infection causes distant organ effects, we do not yet have the scientific data that are necessary to conclusively prove the cause and effect relationship. In summary, stating that "*dogs will live longer and healthier lives if their teeth are kept clean*" may be true but is not yet proven.

One of the challenges faced when trying to make sense of the risks posed by bacteremia is the credibility of the scoring systems used in statistical analysis. Although there are several published reports of distant organ conditions associated with PD, the periodontal scoring systems used vary greatly. The teeth of dogs and cats vary considerably in shape, size, and function, far more so than in human teeth.[28] The typical scores used in analyzing data from patients with periodontal infection are "mean mouth scores": the gingivitis scores or attachment loss measurements of all teeth are summed and divided by the number of teeth scored. In the typical mouth of a dog, even when there is severe PD affecting some teeth, there are usually other teeth in the mouth that have little or no periodontitis, with the result that the severity of disease in the most affected teeth is underreported. To address this issue, I developed a scoring system that is based on the size of the roots of each tooth, so that the mouth score is weighted based on tooth size[29,30]; an alternative weighted scoring system, using measurements of the circumference of the tooth at the gingival margin, is also available.[31]

A *second challenge* is that the progression of PD is not linear. Periods of severe inflammation and tissue destruction may be followed by periods when there is little or no active gingivitis. For example, if the teeth of a dog with periodontitis and severe gingivitis are scaled and polished, the bacteria causing the gingivitis will at least temporarily disappear; the gingivitis score will be significantly reduced, but the extent of periodontitis (loss of bony attachment) does not change. Thus there can be an apparent mismatch between the gingivitis score and the loss of attachment. When PD is to be scored, such as during a study of its association with systemic stress measurements, such as CRP or amyloid-A in serum, or distant organ health, the scoring should separately report gingivitis and attachment loss. Following scaling that removes the bacteria causing the gingivitis, the gingivitis score is expected to decrease, although the periodontitis score may not change. The episodic nature of periodontitis should be considered when drawing conclusions regarding the role of periodontal bacteremia as a cause of distant organ disease.[32]

A *third factor* that complicates attempts to unravel the role of periodontal infection as a cause of distant organ disease is the method used to identify periodontal bacteria. What was once a settled issue with regard to periodontopathogens, with bacterial species assigned to red (deep pockets, gingival bleeding), orange, yellow, green (healthy mouth), or purple (miscellaneous) groups,[33–35] and which led to the checkerboard DNA-DNA hybridization technique for identifying bacteria in plaque samples, is now in question as a result of use of molecular biological techniques such as mRNA analysis to identify bacteria. These new techniques have led to recognition of many bacterial species, some still unnamed, as being present in inflamed gingival pockets.[6–8] Although mRNA techniques provide quick, accurate indication of the species present, these techniques do not result in availability of pure cultures of specific species for antimicrobial susceptibility testing.

The body has a wonderful ability to accommodate minor abnormalities. It would be incorrect to say that the studies reviewed in this article prove that periodontal infection directly causes clinically important distant organ disease in dogs; we need to keep in mind that "association" does not necessarily equate with "cause and effect." There are 2 studies that could be considered as investigating cause and effect. In one,[36] body-wide and distant organ function scores improved after periodontal treatment; results are described in more detail later.

## MICROSCOPIC CHANGES IN DISTANT ORGANS

There are 2 studies performed in dogs that have shown that microscopic inflammatory or degenerative changes in distant organs, specifically the kidney, liver, and heart, increase with increasing severity of periodontal infection[31,37]; both studies use a weighted system to prevent the differences in tooth size undercounting of the extent of PD present.

In the first study,[37] 45 mixed breed laboratory dogs scheduled for euthanasia were evaluated using a combined gingivitis-periodontitis score. Histopathology was performed on samples of lung, myocardium, liver, kidney, tonsil, spleen, mandibular lymph node, and tracheobronchial lymph node. Mitral valves were evaluated grossly. Statistical analyses demonstrated that there was a positive association between periodontal infection and histopathologic changes in kidney, myocardium (papillary muscle), and liver; no statistically significant association was found for microscopic changes in lung, spleen, mandibular and tracheobronchial lymph nodes, and tonsil (**Table 1**).[37]

In the second study,[31] periodontal assessment, standard necropsy, and organ microscopic examinations were performed on 44 mature toy and miniature poodles that died naturally or were euthanized because of clinical disease. The PD burden was estimated from the total surface area of periodontal pocketing based on probe measurements of pocket depth and tooth circumference. Ordinal logistic regression (OLR) analysis established that for each square centimeter of attachment loss, there was a higher likelihood of greater changes being present in the left atrioventricular valves (OLR = 1.43). OLRs were also statistically significant for liver (OLR = 1.21) and kidney pathology (OLR = 1.42) (**Fig. 3**).[31]

**Table 1**
**Results of correlation analysis of severity of gingivitis and periodontitis with distant organ microscopic severity criteria**

| Tissue | Microscopic Criterion | Multiple Regression, P Value |
|---|---|---|
| Myocardium | Myocardial inflammation | 0.91 |
| | Monocyte degeneration, perimyseal fibrosis, thickening of myocardial vessels | 0.05[a] |
| Kidney | Glomerulus: mesangial thickening | 0.001[a] |
| | Tubules: degeneration | 0.30 |
| | Interstitium: lymphoplasmacytic inflammation, pyelitis | 0.04[a] |
| Liver | Parenchyma inflammation | 0.04[a] |
| | Portal inflammation | 0.69 |
| Lung | Peribronchitis, bronchiolitis | 0.45 |
| | Perivasculitis, alveolitis | 0.86 |
| | Pneumonia | 0.90 |
| Spleen | Follicular atrophy or hypoplasia | 0.68 |
| | Follicular hyperplasia | 0.55 |
| Tracheobronchial lymph node | Follicular hyperplasia, sinus histiocytosis, or inflammation | 0.28 |
| Mandibular lymph node | Follicular hyperplasia, sinus histiocytosis, or inflammation | 0.14 |
| Tonsil | Follicular hyperplasia, crypt inflammation, mucosal epithelial leukocyte migration | 0.79 |

Each item was scored on a 1–5 scale
[a] Statistically significant, $P < .05$.
Reprinted with permission from: DeBowes LJ, Mosier D, Logan E, et al. Association of periodontal disease and histologic lesions in multiple organs from 45 dogs. *J Vet Dent.* 1996;13:57-60.

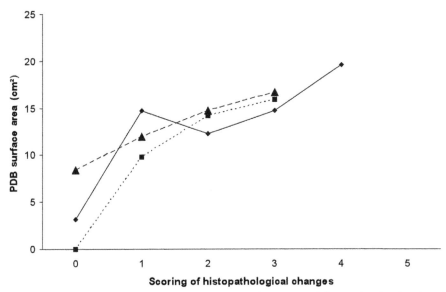

**Fig. 3.** Graph showing the relationships of estimated periodontal disease burden (PDB) and distant organ microscopic changes. (*Reprinted with permission from*: Pavlica Z, Petelin M, Juntes P, Erzen D, Crossley D, Skaleric U. Periodontal disease burden and pathologic changes in dogs. J Vet Dent. 2008;25:97–105.)

## CARDIAC CONDITIONS

Attachment of bacteria carried in the blood stream to the cardiac valves can potentially lead to endocarditis. Although both studies that examined a range of tissues microscopically following a detailed oral examination[31,37] demonstrated an increase in cardiac valve pathology with increasing severity of periodontal infection, the evidence for a link between periodontal infection and infective endocarditis in dogs is mixed.[38–42] The reported studies typically include too few dogs for statistical analysis given the number of variables that may affect the result, or the method of determining the diagnosis of endocarditis or scoring the periodontal data are too subjective to be reliable.

In a study of medical records[38] that reported an association between severity of periodontal infection and presence or absence of endocarditis, the digital medical records of 59,296 dogs examined in corporate veterinary practices with a history of PD were compared with an age-matched comparison group of 59,296 dogs with no recorded history of PD. Of the dogs recorded as having PD, 23,043 had stage 1 PD, 20,732 had stage 2 PD, and 15,521 had stage 3 PD; the PD stages were undefined. Significant associations were detected between the severity of PD and the subsequent risk of cardiovascular-related conditions, such as endocarditis and cardiomyopathy, but not between the severity of PD and the risk of a variety of other common noncardiovascular-related conditions.

Endocarditis is more common in larger dogs than in small or toy dogs,[41,42] which is contrary to the size relationship for periodontal infection.[14,19,43] One study reported that dental procedures such as scaling or extractions do not seem to be risk factors for endocarditis.[41] Another study[42] of 71 dogs with suspected or diagnosed endocarditis reviewed the clinical features of these dogs in depth; the only mention of oral disease was a listing of oral ulceration as one of several uncommon clinical findings in less than 10% of the dogs; 92% of these 71 dogs weighed greater than 15 kg.

In 2007, the American Heart Association and the American Dental Association (ADA) undertook a detailed meta-analysis of published studies relating to bacteremia and prophylactic antibiotic treatment and concluded that the risk of a human developing infective endocarditis is higher as a result of the low-key but daily bacteremia associated with tooth brushing and eating than due to occasional professional dental treatment; as a result, the ADA has significantly narrowed the circumstances considered to warrant prophylactic antimicrobial treatment in association with dental procedures.[44]

Thirty toy or small dogs presented for dental scaling were examined by auscultation, electrocardiography, echocardiography, and oral examination (in which each dog was scored as 1 = mild gingivitis, no periodontitis [20%], 2 = some teeth with mild periodontitis [30%], 3 = severe gingivitis, extensive periodontitis [50%]). Three of the dogs, all with a periodontal score of 3, had a bacteremia in a pretreatment blood sample. The 15 dogs with periodontal score = 3 were more likely to show mitral valve regurgitation, tricuspid valve regurgitation, aortic valve regurgitation, mitral valve thickening, mitral valve prolapse, and left atrial enlargement, with some electrocardiographic images suggesting endocarditis.[45]

## RESPIRATORY SYSTEM

The oral cavity may also serve as a reservoir for bacterial contamination of the lungs with subsequent development of bacterial pneumonia.[9]

## RENAL DISEASE

As noted earlier, 2 studies reported correlation of increasing severity of periodontitis/gingivitis with increasingly severe microscopic changes in renal tissues.[31,37] Several studies have shown an association between increasing clinical pathologic evidence of renal dysfunction and increasing severity of PD. In a study of 38 dogs that underwent periodontal treatment, which is described in greater detail later, there was a significant correlation of PD severity with increasing serum creatinine concentration.[36] In the renal panel (see **Table 1**), increasing microalbinuria and creatinine concentrations were significantly associated with increasing severity of gingivitis, but only increasing creatinine was significantly associated with increasing periodontitis.

In a retrospective longitudinal study,[46] the incidence of azotemic CKD was compared between a cohort of 164,706 dogs with PD (PD-American Veterinary Dental College stages 1, 2, or 3–4) and age-matched dogs with no record of PD. The hazard ratio for CKD increased with increasing severity of PD (PD stage 1 hazard ratio = 1.8, stage 2 hazard ratio = 2.0, stage 3/4 hazard ratio = 2.7, P trend = <0.0001) after adjustment for age, gender, neuter status, breed, body weight, number of hospital visits, and dental procedures. Increasing severity of periodontal infection was also associated with serum creatinine level greater than 1.4 mg/dL and blood urea nitrogen level greater than 36 mg/dL, independent of a veterinarian's clinical diagnosis of CKD.[46]

## HEPATIC DISEASE

As noted earlier, 2 studies report correlation of increasing severity of periodontitis/gingivitis with increasingly severe microscopic changes in hepatic tissues.[31,37] The liver is the site of production of the indicators of body-wide stress such as CRP and amyloid A that can be measured in serum.

## ASSOCIATIONS WITH COMPLETE BLOOD CELL COUNT PARAMETERS AND BODY STRESS RESPONSES

The LPS endotoxins and inflammation-inducing agents are released into the vascular system through the dilated porous gingival capillaries.[9] In one study,[43] dogs were assigned to a periodontal infection group (49 dogs with severe PD, 12 with moderate PD, and 7 had mild PD) or a periodontally healthy group (61 dogs). Dogs diagnosed as having distant organ diseases, such as renal, hepatic, or cardiac conditions, were excluded. The periodontal infection group was statistically significantly older than the periodontally healthy group. There were more small breed dogs (<10 kg) in the periodontal infection group. No influence of gender or reproductive status in PD progression was observed. Regarding systemic diseases, a statistically significant association ($P = .026$) was found between PD and cardiac disease.[43]

In a group of client-owned dogs, the weighted gingivitis and periodontitis scores[32] were compared with complete blood cell count (CBC) parameters and CRP concentration. There was a statistically significant relationship between the gingival bleeding index and white blood cell and polymorphonuclear leukocytes (PMN) counts and the CRP concentration. These data suggest that clinical laboratory data suggesting a systemic inflammatory response are associated with periods of active periodontal inflammation.[47] The absence of an association with periodontitis is likely due to the variable relationship between gingivitis scores (active or quiescent) and attachment loss (a permanent marker of past active attachment tissue destruction): a dog may be in a quiescent state with regard to gingivitis, but show extensive attachment loss from past active disease.[48]

Injury (including infection), indeed any stress anywhere in the body, has a measurable effect on the body as a whole. Typically acute-phase proteins, such as CRP and amyloid A that are released by the liver, are used to measure this stress effect. In one study,[36] dogs with PD were treated (by dental scaling and/or extraction as indicated), and their CRP concentrations before and several weeks after the periodontal treatment were measured; although the differences were moderate, CRP concentration correlated with the severity of PD and was reduced posttreatment.[36] The latter finding and a separate analysis of the effect of periodontal treatment on CRP concentration are the first data-driven reports that support the existence of a cause-and-effect relationship in dogs with naturally occurring periodontal infection.

In another study,[32] neutrophil to lymphocyte ratio (NLR), platelet to lymphocyte ratio, mean platelet volume to platelet ratio, and platelet large cell ratio index (PLCRi) were evaluated as biomarkers of a systemic inflammatory response in healthy dogs, dogs with gingivitis or periodontitis (G/P), and dogs with oropharyngeal tumors. No significant associations between CBC parameters and G/P were found. Both NLR and PLCRi were significantly higher in dogs with oral tumors when compared with healthy dogs and dogs with G/P.[32] In one of the articles cited earlier regarding the relationship between endocarditis and PD,[38] the investigators also reported a positive association between severity of PD and increased white blood cell count. Another study reported leukopenia in dogs with periodontal infection.[50]

An increase in severity of gingivitis is seen in pregnant humans and in one study of laboratory beagles,[48] but another study in laboratory beagles found no association between severity of gingivitis and pregnancy.[51] No statistically significant differences were found in severity of periodontal infection between male and female gender or intact and neutered status in dogs.[20]

## DIABETES MELLITUS

In humans, there is a clear association between diabetes and PD; people with diabetes are more likely to have PD than the rest of the population and diabetes is more labile in people with PD.[25] Recommending dental treatment if indicated and using an effective oral hygiene regimen are now standard in the management of human diabetic patients.

Four dogs with diabetes mellitus and chronic periodontitis, gingivitis, and dental calculus were evaluated using glycated albumin (GA) and fasting blood glucose (FBG) concentration as glycemic control markers. CRP and TNF-$\alpha$ were evaluated as inflammation markers, and reactive oxygen metabolites (d-ROM) and biological antioxidant potential (BAP) concentrations were evaluated as oxidant stress markers before and after periodontal treatment. There was a significant decrease in GA and CRP concentrations and a significant increase in BAP concentration following periodontal treatment. No significant difference in FBG and TNF-$\alpha$ and d-ROM concentrations was found. These results suggest that periodontal treatment could improve glycemic control in dogs with both diabetes mellitus and periodontal infection.[49]

Because of the variables involved and the additional challenges that come with the requirement for anesthesia for dental treatment in veterinary patients, a well-controlled study with a large enough number of subjects to fully investigate the periodontal-diabetes association in dogs in more detail will be difficult to conduct. The bottom line is obvious, though. Whether because of the perceived risk of systemic effects or to obtain a pet with a healthy mouth that encourages play, seeking good oral health is a winning strategy.

## RESULTS FROM STUDIES OF EXPERIMENTALLY INDUCED GINGIVITIS AND PERIODONTITIS IN DOGS

Beagles are commonly used subjects in periodontal research at dental schools. In the standard ligature model, braided suture material or gingival packing cord is placed around the tooth, or around an implant following tooth extraction, as a ligature at the neck of the tooth; the ligature encourages rapid accumulation of plaque bacteria and induces a severe gingivitis and rapid loss of attachment.

In 7 male beagle dogs, 4 rough-surfaced dental implants were placed on both sides of the mandible 14 weeks after tooth extraction, and an implant was placed 14 weeks later. Ligatures were placed around the implants 3 weeks later. Ligature removal and open flap debridement were performed 11 weeks later. The CBC values were compared with baseline after each procedure. Following experimental placement of the ligatures, statistically significant increases were noted for white blood cells, hemoglobin, red blood cells, mean corpuscular hemoglobin, platelets, and mean corpuscular hemoglobin concentration. These blood parameters returned to baseline values following ligature removal and open flap debridement.[52] In ligature-induced periodontitis in 12 dogs in another study, the atrial effective refractory period was shortened and atrial fibrillation inducibility increased, inflammatory cells were more generally found in the atrial myocardium, and CRP and TNF-$\alpha$ increased.[53]

As noted earlier, the data are not always supportive of periodontal infection as a cause of an increase in systemic stress factors. In one study[54] dental pulps in 10 dogs were exposed and infected with dental plaque to induce chronic apical periodontitis (CAP). In 3 of the 10 dogs, an intravenous challenge of *Porphyromonas gingivalis* was given after the development of CAP. Blood samples were drawn preoperatively and postinfection when CAP was seen radiographically. During the CAP period, the serum concentrations of CRP and amyloid A were not statistically different from pre-CAP concentrations; however, 3 dogs challenged by intravenous injection of *P gingivalis* showed elevated CRP concentrations, consistent with an acute-phase response.[54]

## SYSTEMIC OR DISTANT ORGAN

Systemic or distant organ conditions having an adverse effect on periodontal tissues in dogs

The earlier discussion concentrated on the effect of periodontal infection on distant organ or systemic stress response indicators. The opposite is also true: several distant organ conditions have an impact on oral tissues:

- *Hyperparathyroidism*, nutritional or renal, results in resorption of calcium from bones to maintain calcium homeostasis.[55] Calcium is resorbed by osteclastic activity in bones in a pronounced order, starting with alveolar bone, followed by cortical bone of the jaws and skull before the axial and then appendicular skeletal components are decalcified. The result is "rubber jaw." Serum ionized calcium concentrations were lower in older than in younger dogs and increasingly lower in dogs with increasingly severe periodontal infection.[23] When active periodontitis is underway, the weakened bone is more susceptible to resorption.
- *Renal failure* results in a high concentration of urea in saliva that becomes uric acid in the mouth, causing chemical burns on oral tissues where saliva puddles.
- *Diabetes mellitus* acts both ways; it is a risk factor for periodontal infection in humans[25,26] and in dogs,[49] and periodontal infection is a risk factor for diabetes mellitus. Treatment and subsequent prevention of periodontal infection assists management of diabetes in dogs.[49]

## PROGRESSION OF GINGIVITIS AND PERIODONTITIS

Most of the studies reviewed earlier were cross-sectional in nature. A few longitudinal studies showing the progression of periodontal infections in dogs are available. In 52 miniature schnauzer dogs aged between 1 and 7 years, with a total of 2155 teeth, who entered the study, gingivitis affected at least some teeth in every dog.[17] Of the 52 dogs 35 (67%) had at least 12 teeth that progressed to periodontitis within 60 weeks. Of the teeth that progressed to periodontitis, 54% were incisors, with the lingual aspect of the incisors being significantly more likely to be affected. The severity of gingivitis around periodontitis-affected teeth was variable. The rate of progression was significantly faster in older dogs. Only 1 dog (age 3.5 years) did not have any teeth progress to periodontitis after 60 weeks.[17]

## CONCLUSION AND THE IMPORTANCE OF PREVENTION

Although there are occasional studies that do not follow the trend, the bulk of the evidence in dogs reviewed earlier, as in man, points to their being a positive association between gingivitis and/or periodontitis and adverse effects elsewhere in the body. As Talbot noted 120 years ago: *"Prevent inflammation of the gum margin and pus infection cannot follow, no matter how many germs be in the mouth."* Reasons for not all studies showing approximately equivalent results are as follows:

- Variability in the quality and credibility of the measurement of gingivitis and periodontitis.
- Variability in the populations of dogs included in the study: age, body weight, and elimination of dogs with the target distant organ disease that show clinical evidence of the distant organ disease.
- Failure to include a sufficient number of dogs to permit statistical analysis given the variabilities noted earlier.

Even with these issues calling the specific conclusions of some studies into question, the overall conclusion is that allowing gingivitis and periodontitis to develop and then worsen is not good for the general health of the dog. Prevention of gingivitis is simple—control development of dental plaque, and its partner in enhancing an anaerobic environment, dental calculus. Preventing periodontitis is the same—prevent development and maturation of plaque and deposition of calculus.

Obtaining optimal oral health in our patients is a challenge, because they cannot brush or floss their own teeth. Although brushing remains the gold standard,[56] fortunately effective oral hygiene methods can include more than brushing. The Veterinary Oral Health Council ([VOHC] www.VOHC.org) provides a list of products that have met the preset VOHC standards for retarding accumulation of plaque and calculus (tartar); in addition to brushes and dental wipes, these products include dental diets, treats, water additives, gels, and toothpastes. The key is daily use, which is much easier to accomplish if the owner can find a way to make daily oral hygiene a fun interaction with her or his dog. Making use of more than one modality improves the result.

An oral care regime and twice-yearly veterinary dental health checks should be provided from an early age for breeds with high likelihood of developing periodontitis (see **Fig. 1**). While waiting for confirmation that the periodontal-systemic associations are indeed cause and effect, it would be prudent to practice prevention; this consists of the following 3 steps:[56]

1. Periodic, at least annual, oral examination (including "lifting the lip" every time a veterinarian see the patient for any reason) should be performed. Six-month intervals are recommended for dogs that early on are recognized as heavy plaque or calculus formers.
2. Effective daily oral hygiene,[21,57] starting from completion of eruption of the permanent teeth, is recommended. The options should be described to the owner and use of VOHC-accepted products should be demonstrated.
3. The teeth should be treated professionally when indicated, again starting from an early age.

## DISCLOSURE

There is no conflict of interest resulting from publication of this article.

## REFERENCES

1. Harvey CE. Periodontal disease in dogs: Etiology, pathogenesis and prevalence. Vet Clin North Am Small Anim Pract 1998;28:1111–28.
2. Harvey CE, Thornsberry C, Miller BL. Subgingival bacteria - comparison of culture results in dogs and cats with gingivitis. J Vet Dent 1995;12:147–50.
3. Harvey CE. Bacteriology of periodontal disease. In: Niemiec BA. *Veterinary Periodontology.* Wiley-Blackwell; 2013.
4. Tungland B. Human Microbiota in health and disease. Elsevier; 2018.

5. Hennet P, Harvey CE. Natural development of periodontal disease in the dog: A review of clinical, anatomical and histological features. J Vet Dent 1992;9:13–9.
6. McDonald J, Larsen N, Pennington A, et al. Characterising the canine oral microbiome by direct sequencing of reverse-transcribed rRNA molecules. PLoS ONE 2016;11(6):e0157046.
7. Davis IJ, Bull C, Horsfall A, et al. The unculturables: targeted isolation of bacterial species associated with canine periodontal health or disease from dental plaque. BMC Microbiol 2014;14:196.
8. Wallis C, Marshall M, Colyer A, et al. A longitudinal assessment of changes in bacterial community composition associated with the development of periodontal disease in dogs. Vet Microbiol 2015;181:271-282.
9. DeBowes LJ. The effects of dental disease on systemic disease. Vet Clin North Am Small Anim Pract 1998;28:1057–62.
10. Barkovskiĭ VS, Faĭziev I, Vlasova V. (Functional changes in the organic and systemic microcirculation in spontaneous periodontal lesions in dogs). Stomatologiia (Mosk) 1984;63:11–3.
11. Black AP, Crichlow AM, Saunders JR. Bacteremia during ultrasonic teeth cleaning and extraction in the dog. J Am Anim Hosp Assoc 1980;6:611–6.
12. Harari J, Besser TE, Gustafson SB, et al. Bacterial isolates from blood cultures of dogs undergoing dentistry. Vet Surg 1993;22:27–30.
13. Talbot ES. Interstitial Gingivitis: Or So-Called Pyorrhoea Alveolaris. Talbot, Eugene Solomon: 9781272502089: Amazon.com: Books. p. 63–65.
14. Wallis C, Holcombe LJ. A review of the frequency and impact of periodontal disease in dogs. J Small Anim Pract 2020;61:529–40.
15. Wallis C, Pesci I, Colyer A, et al. A longitudinal assessment of periodontal disease in Yorkshire terriers. BMC Vet Res 2019;15(1):207.
16. Wallis C, Patel KV, Marshall M, et al. A longitudinal assessment of periodontal health status in 53 Labrador retrievers. J Small Anim Pract 2018;59:560-569.
17. Marshall M, Wallis C, Milella A, et al. A longitudinal assessment of periodontal disease in 52 Miniature Schnauzer. Res Vet Sci 2014;10:166.
18. Lund EM, Armstrong PJ, Kirk CA, et al. Health status and population characteristics of dogs and cats examined at private veterinary practices in the United States. J Am Vet Med Assoc 1999;214:1336–41.
19. Harvey CE, Shofer F, Laster L. Association of age and body weight with periodontal disease in North American dogs. J Vet Dent 1994;11(3):94–105.
20. Stella JL, Bauer AE, Croney CC. A cross-sectional study to estimate prevalence of periodontal disease in a population of dogs (Canis familiaris) in commercial breeding facilities in Indiana and Illinois. PLoS ONE 2018;13(1):e0191395.
21. Garanayak V, Das M, Patra RC, et al. Effect of age on dental plaque deposition and its control by ultrasonic scaling, dental hygiene and chlorhexidine in dogs. Vet World 2019;12:1872–6.
22. Isogai H, Isogai E, Okamoto H, et al. Epidemiological study of periodontal diseases and some other dental disorders in dogs. Nihon Juigaku Zasshi 1989; 51:1151–62.
23. Carreira LM, Dias D, Azevedo P. Relationship between gender, age, and weight and the serum ionized calcium variations in dog periodontal disease evolution. Top Companion Anim Med 2015;30:51–6.
24. Egelberg J. Local effect of diet on plaque formation and development of gingivitis in dogs: I. Effect of hard and soft diets. Odontologisk Revy 1965;16:31–41.
25. Hegde R, Awan KH. Effects of periodontal disease on systemic health. Disease-a-Month. 2019;65:185–92.

26. Winning L, Linden GJ. Periodontitis and Systemic Disease. BDJ Team 2015;2: 15163.
27. Bodingbauer J. [*Septic infections of dental origin in the dog*]. Wiener Tierarzt Monat 1946;33:97–114.
28. Harvey CE. Shape and size of teeth of dogs and cats: Relevance to studies of plaque and calculus accumulation. J Vet Dent 2002;19:186–95.
29. Harvey CE, Laster L, Shofer FS. Scoring the full extent of periodontal disease in the dog: Development of a Total Mouth Periodontal Score (TMPS) system. J Vet Dent 2008;25:176–80.
30. Harvey CE, Laster L, Shofer F. Scoring the full extent of periodontal disease in the dog: Development of a Total Mouth Periodontal Score (TMPS) system. J Vet Dent 2008;25:176–80.
31. Pavlica Z, Petelin M, Juntes P, et al. Periodontal disease burden and pathological changes in dogs. J Vet Dent 2008;25:97–105.
32. Rejec A, Butinar J, Gawor J, et al. Evaluation of complete blood count indices in healthy dogs, dogs with periodontitis, and dogs with oropharyngeal tumors. J Vet Dent 2017;34:231–40.
33. Haffajee AD, Socransky SS. Introduction to microbial aspects of periodontal bio-film communities, development and treatment. Periodontol. 2000 2006;42:7–12.
34. Hardham J, Dreier K, Wong J, et al. Pigmented-anaerobic bacteria associated with canine periodontitis. Vet Microbiol 2005;106:119–28.
35. Socransky SS, Haffajee AD, Smith C, et al. Use of checkerboard DNA-DNA hy-bridization to study complex microbial ecosystems. Oral Microbiol Immunol 2004;19:352–62.
36. Rawlinson JE, Goldstein RE, Reiter AM, et al. Association of periodontal disease with systemic health indices in dogs and the systematic response to treatment of periodontal disease. J Am Vet Med Assoc 2011;238:601–9.
37. DeBowes LJ, Mosier D, Logan E, et al. Association of periodontal disease and histologic lesions in multiple organs from 45 dogs. J Vet Dent 1996;13:57–60.
38. Glickman L, Glickman N, Moore G, et al. Evaluation of the risk of endocarditis and other cardiovascular events on the basis of the severity of periodontal disease in dogs. J Am Vet Med Assoc 2009;234:486–94.
39. Ettinger SJ, Allen J, Barrrett K, et al. Questions validity of study on periodontal disease and cardiovascular events in dogs. Letter to Editor. J Am Vet Med Assoc 2009;234:1525–8, author reply 1526-1527.
40. Peddle G, Sleeper M, Ryan M, et al. Questions validity of study on periodontal disease and cardiovascular events in dogs. Letter to Editor. J Am Vet Med Assoc 2009;234:1525–8, author reply 1526-1527.
41. Peddle GD, Drobatz KJ, Harvey CE, et al. Association of periodontal disease, oral procedures and other clinical findings with bacterial endocarditis in dogs. J Am Vet Med Assoc 2009;234:100–7.
42. Sykes JE, Kittleson MD, Chomel BB, et al. Clinicopathological findings and outcome in dogs with infective endocarditis: 71 cases (1992-2005). J Am Vet Med Assoc 2006;228:1735–47.
43. Pereira Dos Santos JD, Cunha E, Nunes T, et al. Relation between periodontal disease and systemic diseases in dogs. Res Vet Sci 2019;125:136–40.
44. American Dental Association: Antibiotic prophylaxis prior to dental procedures. Antibiotic Prophylaxis Prior to Dental Procedures (ada.org)
45. Boutoille F, Dorizon A, Navarro A, Pellerin J-L, Gauthier O. Echocardiographic al-terations and periodontal disease in dogs: A clinical study. Proc. 15th Congress of Veterinary Dentistry, Cambridge, 2006.

46. Glickman LT, Glickman NW, Moore GE, et al. Association between chronic azotemic kidney disease and the severity of periodontal disease in dogs. Prev Vet Med 2011;99:193–200.
47. Kouki MI, Papadimitriou SA, Kazakos GM, et al. Periodontal disease as a potential factor for systemic inflammatory response in the dog. J Vet Dent 2013; 30:26–9.
48. Lindhe J, Rolf Attström A, Bjorn A-L. Influence of sex hormones on gingival exudation in gingivitis-free female dogs. J Perio Res 1968;3:273–8.
49. Oda H, Mori A, Saeki K, et al. J Pet Anim Nutr 2011;14:76–83.
50. Lonsdale T. Periodontal disease and leucopenia. J Small Anim Pract 1995;36: 542–6.
51. Basuki W, Rawlinson J, Lothamer C, et al. Evaluation of gingivitis in pregnant beagle dogs. J Vet Dent 2019;36:179–85.
52. Chaushu L, Tal H, Sculean A, et al. Peri-implant disease affects systemic complete blood count values: An experimental in vivo study. Clin Oral Investig 2020;24:4531–9.
53. Yu G, Yu Y, Li YN, et al. Effect of periodontitis on susceptibility to atrial fibrillation in an animal model. J Electrocardiol 2010;43:359–66.
54. Buttke TM, Shipper G, Delano EO, et al. C-reactive protein and serum amyloid A in a canine model of chronic apical periodontitis. J Endod 2005;31:728–32.
55. Svanberg G, Lindhe J, Hugoson A, et al. Effect of nutritional hyperparathyroidism on experimental periodontitis in the dog. Scand J Dent Res 1973;81:155–62.
56. Harvey CE. Management of periodontal disease: understanding the options. Vet Clin North Am Small Anim Pract 2005;35:819–36.
57. Harvey CE, Serfillipi L, Barnvos D. Effect of frequency of brushing teeth on plaque and calculus accumulation and gingivitis is dogs. J Vet Dent 2015;32:16–21.

# Management of Dental and Oral Developmental Conditions in Dogs and Cats

Stephanie Goldschmidt, BVM&S[a],*, Naomi Hoyer, DVM[b]

KEYWORDS

- Developmental abnormality • Juvenile • Veterinary dentistry • Malocclusion
- Cleft palate

KEY POINTS

- Developmental abnormalities are diagnosed at the first puppy/kitten examination or at 4 to 6 months as permanent teeth erupt and maxillofacial growth is more established.
- Practitioners should be aware of normal dental and oral appearance to allow identification of abnormalities early and implement treatment if required.
- Appropriate diagnosis and knowledge of developmental disorders is essential to determine if monitoring, such as in the case of a geminated tooth, or surgical treatment, such as in the case of a crowded supernumerary tooth, is recommended.
- Genetic, environmental, and idiopathic factors can result in developmental dental and oral abnormalities, thus genetic counseling may be appropriate given the history and exact defect.

## INTRODUCTION

Developmental abnormalities affecting the teeth and skull are present within the first 12 months of life. They may be apparent as early as the first puppy/kitten examination or not be clinically diagnosed until 4 to 12 months of age as the permanent teeth erupt, and maxillofacial growth progresses. The conditions are diverse ranging from cosmetic only to requiring advanced surgical intervention to alleviate pain and secondary complications. Overview of the clinical presentation, diagnosis, and appropriate treatment, when needed, of dental and oral developmental abnormalities will be discussed throughout this article.

[a] Dentistry & Oral Surgery, University of Minnesota, 1352 Boyd Avenue, C309 Veterinary Medical Center South, St Paul, MN 55108, USA; [b] Dentistry & Oral Surgery, Colorado State University, 300 W Drake, Fort Collins, CO 80523, USA
* Corresponding author.
*E-mail address:* Golds245@umn.edu

Vet Clin Small Anim 52 (2022) 139–158
https://doi.org/10.1016/j.cvsm.2021.09.002
0195-5616/22/© 2021 Elsevier Inc. All rights reserved.

## STRUCTURAL, SIZE, NUMERICAL, AND SHAPE ABNORMALITIES OF TEETH

In both dogs and cats, there is a dental formula and a standard appearance of any given tooth within that formula (**Table 1**).[1,2] Deviations from this standard are frequently recognized in domestic dogs and cats.

### Abnormalities in Tooth Number

Hyperdontia, also known as supernumerary teeth, is more commonly reported in the maxilla and more commonly noted in dogs, especially those with dolichocephalic head types.[3,4] Supernumerary teeth are a result of an additional tooth germ that develops. Treatment recommendations for supernumerary teeth depend entirely on whether their presence causes crowding that may predispose to periodontal disease. In these cases, if left undiagnosed and untreated, supernumerary teeth can result in significant pathology (**Fig. 1**).[5]

Tooth agenesis is the failure of a tooth bud to form. This results in either hypodontia, defined as lack of 6 or fewer teeth within the dentition, or oligodontia, defined as the absence of more than six teeth.[4,6,7] Agenesis is more common with permanent teeth, but if there is agenesis of the deciduous tooth, then agenesis of the permanent tooth bud should also be expected.[8–10]

### Abnormalities in Tooth Structure, Shape, and Size

Interruptions to normal odontogenesis (embryologic tooth development) in the form of genetic variations or febrile and inflammatory insults to the gravid female or young animal can result in abnormalities in the shape or structure of the tooth. In dogs, development of the permanent tooth structure and shape is complete by 8 weeks of age, so insults at any point from birth until 8 weeks can lead to abnormalities.

#### Abnormalities of crown morphology

Gemination is when a single tooth bud splits incompletely to form a double crowned single tooth (**Fig. 2**).[4,11] Geminated teeth should be monitored radiographically to ensure endodontic disease does not develop. They are likely to be at an increased risk for plaque retention because of the increased number of developmental grooves, so oral hygiene is critical to keep these teeth from developing periodontal disease. Complete gemination results in a supernumerary tooth that is the mirror image of its adjacent duplicate.

Fusion is the process where two adjacent tooth buds fuse to form a single tooth.[4,11] This results in a decrease in the number of teeth present in the dental arch, with an abnormal crown (**Fig. 3**). Fusion can occur in the crowns, roots, or both. These teeth should be examined radiographically to rule out endodontic disease, and similar to geminated teeth, oral hygiene is critical, as their crowns may be more plaque retentive. Concrescence is also a fusion of two teeth, but in this case, the crowns are completely separate, and the fusion occurs only within the cementum.[4,11] It is theorized to occur due to inflammation in the vicinity of nearby developing tooth roots. This abnormality is

| Table 1 | | |
|---|---|---|
| **Permanent and deciduous dental formulae for the domestic dog and cat** | | |
|  | **Deciduous Dental Formula** | **Permanent Dental Formula** |
| Dog | 2 × (I 3/3; C 1/1; P 3/3) = 28 | 2 × (I 3/3; C 1/1; P 4/4; M 2/3) = 42 |
| Cat | 2 × (I 3/3; C 1/1; P 3/2) = 26 | 2 × (I 3/3; C 1/1; P 3/2; M 1/1) = 30 |

*Abbreviations:* C, canine; I, incisor; M, molar; P, premolar.

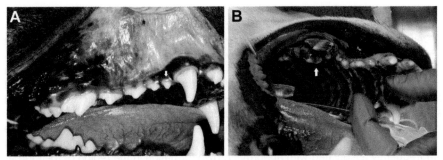

**Fig. 1.** Dogs; supernumerary right maxillary first premolar tooth causing no pathology (*A*) versus supernumerary right maxillary fourth premolar tooth causing crowding and periodontal disease (*B*).

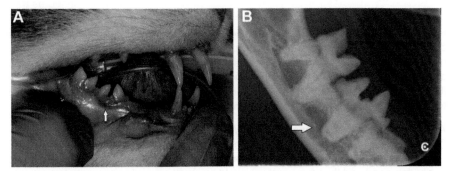

**Fig. 2.** Photograph (*A*) and radiograph (*B*) showing gemination of the right mandibular fourth premolar tooth in a cat.

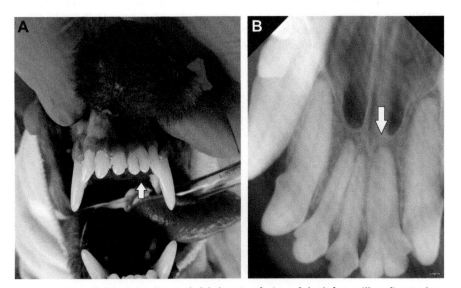

**Fig. 3.** Photograph (*A*) and radiograph (*B*) showing fusion of the left maxillary first and second incisor teeth in a dog, resulting in a crown with multiple cusps and a single root.

only detectable by radiographs and often requires no treatment. It will, however, be important to identify before attempting extraction of either of the teeth.

*Dens invaginatus*, also known as *dens in dente* (**Fig. 4**), is a crown abnormality that was previously presumed to be caused by invagination of a portion of the tooth crown into the developing tooth bud, analogous to the human condition.[4,11–13] However, a recent review of these lesions in mandibular first molar teeth in dogs showed several significant differences between the condition in dog and human teeth.[14] The histologic studies of the canine patients were more consistent with a condition called "molar incisor malformation" because the developmental origin of the invaginated tissue could not be determined. Regardless of the classification, these malformed teeth are frequently associated with abnormal crown formation in the region of their furcation and are thus predisposed to both periodontal and endodontic disease. These teeth may be challenging to treat endodontically because of their abnormal morphology, and extraction is often the most predictable treatment option if secondary pathology develops.[15]

### Abnormalities of root morphology

Root morphology abnormalities, including dilaceration and supernumerary roots, are often incidental radiographic findings but are important to appreciate, as they will make endodontic therapy and extraction more complicated. Dilaceration is an abnormal curvature of a root, often noted on the mandibular first molar tooth (**Fig. 5**).[11] Supernumerary roots are diagnosed most commonly in the two-rooted teeth, specifically the palatal aspect of maxillary third premolars.

### Abnormalities of enamel: enamel hypoplasia and hypomineralization

Although the terms hypoplasia and hypomineralization are used interchangeably, they represent different developmental abnormalities that both result in enamel that is easily damaged and thus frequently absent from teeth exposing the underlying dentin (**Fig. 6**). Both can lead to tooth sensitivity, increased susceptibility to fracture, susceptibility to caries, and endodontic infection. Focal or generalized enamel hypoplasia can occur in both dogs and cats with focal, related to trauma or inflammation of the developing tooth bud, being most common.[11] Generalized enamel hypoplasia can be due to pyrexia, especially when associated with canine distemper virus[16–18] or be hereditary, termed *amelogenesis imperfecta*, which has been described in poodles and Italian greyhounds.[19,20]

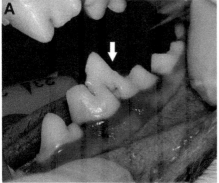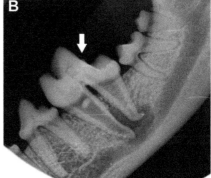

**Fig. 4.** Photograph (*A*) and radiograph (*B*) of mandibular molar malformation (previously known as dens invaginatus) at the left mandibular first molar tooth in a dog.

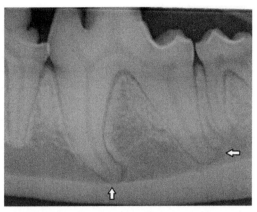

**Fig. 5.** Dilaceration of the roots of the left mandibular first molar tooth of a dog.

### Abnormalities of dentin

Both dentinogenesis imperfecta and dentinal dysplasia have been reported in dogs[6,21,22] and are associated with extremely abnormal crown appearance and root hypoplasia. Dentin disorders are typically confirmed with radiographs and should be monitored for evidence of endodontic disease.

### Abnormalities in Eruption and Exfoliation

There are clinically recognized variations in the standard eruption times (**Table 2**) based on breed. Abnormalities that fall outside of normal breed-related variation are persistent deciduous teeth and unerupted permanent teeth.

Deciduous teeth are considered persistent if they are still in the oral cavity when the permanent teeth have erupted, regardless of the existence of a permanent successor.[6,7,23] Persistent deciduous teeth must be extracted to prevent crowding, malocclusion, and periodontitis of the permanent successor. Persistent deciduous teeth for which there is no permanent successor may be maintained in the oral cavity but will need to be monitored, as they are predisposed to root resorption and fracture.

Permanent teeth that fail to erupt into occlusion can be classified as either primary retention, defined as a developmentally normal tooth with no apparent impediment that fails to erupt, or impaction, defined as occurring secondary to an obstruction

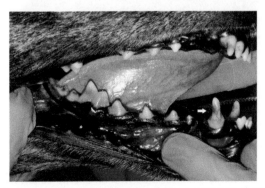

**Fig. 6.** Generalized enamel hypomineralization of the permanent dentition in a German shepherd dog.

**Table 2**
**Eruption times for the deciduous and permanent dentition in the dog and cat**

| | Deciduous Teeth (wk) | | Permanent Teeth (mo) | |
|---|---|---|---|---|
| | Dog | Cat | Dog | Cat |
| Incisors | 3–4 | 2–3 | 3–5 | 3–4 |
| Canines | 3 | 3–4 | 4–6 | 4–5 |
| Premolars | 4–12 | 3–6 | 4–6 | 4–6 |
| Molars | — | — | 5–7 | 4–5 |

such as soft tissue, bone, or contact with other teeth. Teeth that fail to erupt must be treated. When the failure to erupt is secondary to a fibrous gingival obstruction, and the tooth has not lost its eruptive potential, an operculectomy can be performed to allow eruption to complete.[24] Teeth that have primary retention and still maintain their eruptive potential can be treated orthodontically. Teeth that are impacted within bone, or have lost their eruptive potential, must be extracted to prevent dentigerous cyst formation (**Fig. 7**).[25–28]

## DENTAL AND SKELETAL MALOCCLUSION

Malocclusions are a developmental abnormality seen in both dogs and cats, though it is more frequently reported in dogs.[6,7,29–31] Occlusion should be evaluated as early as 6 weeks of age to identify traumatic malocclusions early and maximize the chance for successful interventions if possible. The features of normal deciduous occlusion are as follows: the incisive edge of mandibular incisors should sit at the level of the cingulum at the palatal aspect of the maxillary incisors. The mandibular canine tooth should be centered between the maxillary third incisor and canine tooth. The premolar teeth should interdigitate with a scissor bite. The skeletal structures should be symmetric. In the permanent dentition, the dental structures are oriented in the same way. In addition, the central cusp of the mandibular first molar tooth should occlude palatal to the maxillary fourth premolar tooth, and the distal cusp of the mandibular first molar tooth should occlude with the occlusal surface of the maxillary first molar tooth. Normal occlusion is termed class 0. There are 4 classes of malocclusion:

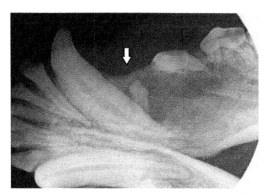

**Fig. 7.** Dentigerous cyst formation associated with an unerupted left mandibular first premolar tooth in a dog. Note the bone loss distal to the canine tooth and root resorption and displacement of the adjacent second and third premolar teeth.

- Class 1: Dental malocclusion with a normal relationship of the upper and lower dental arches, but one or more teeth are malpositioned (**Fig. 8**).
- Class 2: Skeletal malocclusion that results in a longer upper jaw relative to the lower jaw (**Fig. 9**). Class 2 malocclusions are frequently traumatic because of the location of contact of the mandibular canine and incisor teeth and the palatal tissue.
- Class 3: Skeletal malocclusion that results in a longer lower jaw relative to the upper jaw (**Fig. 10**), also known as underbite, undershot, mandibular prognathism, or maxillary brachygnathism. Class 3 malocclusions are frequently identified in dogs with brachycephalic skull types.
- Class 4: Skeletal malocclusion that is asymmetrical in either a side to side, dorsoventral, or rostrocaudal direction, also known as a wry bite.

Malocclusions require treatment if they result in traumatic occlusion between the teeth or causing soft tissue trauma. Depending on the malocclusion, treatment options include selective extractions, crown reductions with endodontic therapy, or orthodontic movement.

## CONGENITAL LIP AND PALATE DEFECTS

Orofacial clefts arise from abnormalities in the normal embryologic development of the face (**Table 3**).[32–35] Pending on the severity of the defect they can be classified as:

- Cleft lip: Defect in the lip, alveolus, or incisive bone. These are also referred to as clefts of the primary palate.
- Cleft palate: Defect in the hard palate and/or soft palate caudal to the incisive papilla/palatine fissures. These are also referred to as clefts of the secondary palate.
- Cleft lip and palate: Defect of both the primary and secondary palate.

Orofacial clefts are described as complete or incomplete and unilateral or bilateral (**Fig. 11**). Clefts can also be separated into syndromic and nonsyndromic, meaning they are, or are not, associated with other congenital abnormalities. In humans, approximately one-third of clefts are syndromic, with over 300 different associated

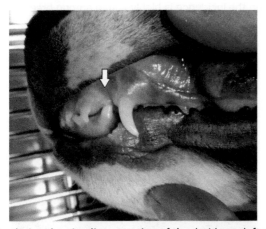

**Fig. 8.** Class 1 malocclusion showing linguoversion of the deciduous left mandibular canine tooth in a dog. Note the normal occlusal relationship of the incisor teeth.

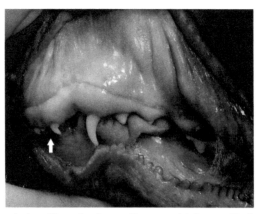

**Fig. 9.** Class 2 malocclusion. Note the linguodistoverted left mandibular deciduous canine tooth causing bite trauma to the hard palate mucosa in a dog.

syndromes reported.[36] The incidence of syndromic cleft palates in dogs is unknown, but one small study found that of 9 dogs with orofacial clefts, all had at least 1 additional craniomaxillofacial anomaly, with the most common affecting the tympanic bullae.[37]

### Etiology

The etiology of orofacial clefts is complex and can be secondary to genetics, environmental factors, or a combination of the two. Boxers, Nova Scotia Duck Tolling Retrievers, and Pyrenees shepherds have documented autosomal recessive inheritance.[38–40] Established environmental factors that have been implicated in cleft palate formation in mice and humans include hypervitaminosis A, folic acid deficiency, glucocorticoids, alcohol, smoking, and select drugs and toxins.[41,42] To the authors' knowledge, no robust environmental etiologic studies have been performed in dogs.

### Incidence/Risk Factors

The reported incidence in canine cohort studies is anywhere from 1.1 to 30 per 1000 live births. However, the incidence is highly varied among breeds, ranging from none

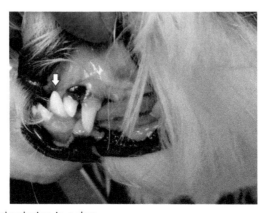

**Fig. 10.** Class 3 malocclusion in a dog.

**Table 3**
**Embryologic events involved in lip and palate formation**

| Embryologic Event | Forms | Result of Failure |
|---|---|---|
| Fusion of the bilateral medial nasal processes | Philtrum and part of the upper lip | May result in midline cleft lip and bifid nose; full effect of failure unknown |
| Fusion of medial nasal processes with maxillary processes | Upper lip, incisive bone, and alveolar processes | Cleft lip aka cleft of the primary palate |
| Fusion of the palatal shelves of the maxillary processes | Hard and soft palate | Cleft palate aka cleft of the secondary palate |

to 140 cases per 1000 live births depending on the breed.[34,43] Cleft palate occurs more commonly than cleft lip and cleft lip/palate combination, with a recent canine survey-based study reporting 59% of orofacial clefts were cleft palate, 26% were cleft lip, and 15% were cleft lip/cleft palate.[43] Overrepresented breeds include Boston terriers, French bulldogs, Cavalier King Charles spaniels, and English bulldogs. There is an increased odds risk for cleft development for dogs belonging to the Mastiff/terrier genetic cluster as well as dogs with brachycephalic skull type. It is rare for dolichocephalic breeds to present with orofacial clefts.[35,43]

### Cleft Lip Presentation, Diagnosis, and Treatment

A cleft lip can refer to a spectrum of abnormalities spanning from an incomplete cleft causing only a notch in the lip to a complete defect at the level of the maxillary third incisor tooth and extension into the nose (**Fig. 12**).[35,44] Cleft lip is often diagnosed

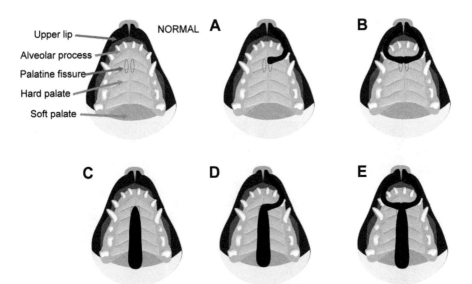

**Fig. 11.** Classification of orofacial clefts. Unilateral complete cleft lip (A), bilateral complete cleft lip (B), complete cleft palate (C), complete unilateral cleft lip and palate (D), and complete bilateral cleft lip and palate (E).

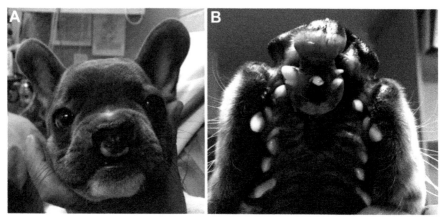

**Fig. 12.** External (*A*) and intraoral (*B*) view of bilateral cleft lip in a dog. Note the communication between the nose and oral cavity occurs mesiopalatal to all the third incisor teeth.

at birth. Depending on the severity, these may be cosmetic-only or may be associated with clinical signs of rhinitis, or rarely aspiration pneumonia, if there is an associated defect in the incisive bone. If an oronasal communication is present, surgical fixation is recommended. Repair should ideally be delayed until 4 to 6 months of age to allow the patient's maxillofacial growth to slow and the permanent teeth to erupt. Repair is focused on the reconstruction of the floor of the nasal cavity as the primary goal and esthetic reconstruction of the lip as a secondary goal. For a review of repair techniques, the author refers the reader to this published article.[44]

### Midline Cleft Lip and Bifid Nose Presentation, Diagnosis, and Treatment

Rarely, there will be a midline cleft affecting the lip. Midline facial clefts may also present as a bifid nose (**Fig. 13**). The exact etiology of midline cleft lip and bifid nose is unknown, but it is believed to occur from lack of fusion of the medial nasal processes.[45] These are exceedingly rare in dogs, with only one report in the literature.[46] The severity of symptoms, for example, if there is severe moist dermatitis in the groove of the bifid nose and/or presence of oronasal communication, will dictate if surgical repair is required.[46]

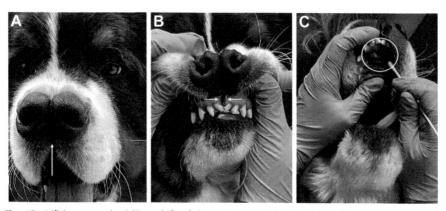

**Fig. 13.** Bifid nose and midline cleft of the primary palate (*A–C*) in a dog.

## Cleft Palate Presentation, Diagnosis, and Treatment

Clinical signs of cleft palate are often noticed soon after birth and include drainage of milk from the nose, gagging or coughing while eating, and failure to thrive. Repair is recommended to prevent complications including rhinitis and aspiration pneumonia. Numerous surgical techniques are described with the most common being the Van Langenbeck technique, bipedicle flap technique, and the overlapping flap technique (**Fig. 14**).[47,48] For more complex clefts, or those that have undergone previous repair, double-layer techniques are more appropriate as they better combat the adverse local factors in the oral cavity including tongue movements, mastication, and microbial contamination.[49]

Functional success after cleft palate repair is reported at 85%.[47] However, multiple surgeries are often required for the successful closure of the defect. A recent study reported that oronasal fistula persisted after initial surgery in 50% of dogs.[47] Number of tissue layers used for closure, surgical technique used, if the procedure was staged, and the defect severity did not affect outcome.[47]

There are varying recommendations in the literature regarding the ideal time to perform surgery, but most recommend waiting until 3 to 4 months of age unless highly symptomatic.[47,48] Waiting until maxillofacial growth has slowed helps to minimize the adverse effects of palatoplasty on midface growth.[50–52] Surprisingly, waiting longer to perform the repair does not seem to carry a benefit, with one study revealing a worse outcome when the repair was performed in patients more than 8 months of age.[47]

To allow delay in repair, patients often require orogastric tube feeding or placement of a temporary prosthesis or specialized teat while being bottle fed.[53,54] Use of a temporary prosthetic obturator can also be helpful in preventing aspiration pneumonia during staged procedures.[49] In specific cases, obturators can also be used in place of surgical repair.[55,56]

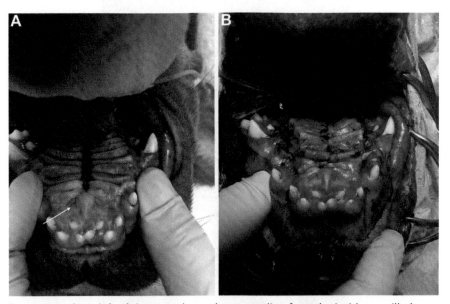

**Fig. 14.** Complete cleft of the secondary palate extending from the incisive papilla (*arrow*, *A*) through the entire hard and soft palate. The cleft was surgically repaired using the Von Langenbeck technique (*B*).

## Hypoplastic Soft Palate

Soft palate hypoplasia can be unilateral or bilateral (**Fig. 15**) and clinically present similar to those with midline clefts. The etiology of hypoplastic palates is unknown but is theorized to be a failure of fusion between the lateral aspect of the palatine process and the tissues that will form the tonsillar crypt. These are more technically challenging to surgically repair compared with midline clefts. However, the exact success rate is not reported in the literature, and most case studies, albeit small, report good to excellent outcomes.[57–59]

## Presurgical Considerations for Orofacial Clefts

CT scan is recommended before surgical intervention for surgical planning as well as to identify other maxillofacial abnormalities (syndromic clefts).[37] CBC/chemistry and thoracic radiographs are recommended before general anesthesia.

### DEVELOPMENTAL ABNORMALITIES RESULTING IN BONY PROLIFERATION

When an immature dog or cat presents with a firm bony abnormality (**Fig. 16**), bone fracture with proliferative bone healing, osteomyelitis, a cystic lesion such as a dentigerous cyst or odontoma, and developmental bony abnormalities are the top differentials. Developmental bony abnormalities in dogs, also known as hyperostotic conditions, present with osseous proliferation of the bones of the skull (**Fig. 17**; **Table 4**).[60–70] Dogs may be asymptomatic or present with increased salivation, signs of oral pain, episodic pyrexia, or an inability to masticate or fully open/close the mouth. Bony proliferation stops when the growth period is over; thus, treatment consists of symptomatic care, if needed, with anti-inflammatories and other analgesics until

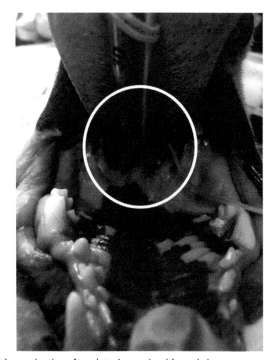

**Fig. 15.** Bilateral hypoplastic soft palate in a mixed breed dog.

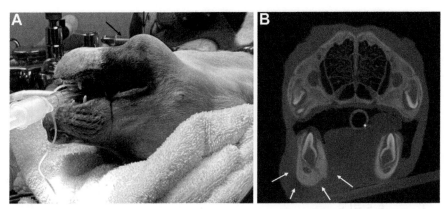

**Fig. 16.** Clinical image of an anesthetized juvenile dog with a unilateral (*right*) firm mandibular swelling (*A, black arrow*) and corresponding CT image revealing bony proliferation (*B, white arrows*).

skeletal maturity. If bone biopsy was obtained, or there are active signs of infection, then antibiotic therapy may also be indicated.[66] Surgical intervention is occasionally required for craniomandibular osteopathy to manage secondary complications such as temporomandibular joint (TMJ) ankylosis or otitis media.[61] Rarely, euthanasia is indicated if the quality of life is severely compromised.[65]

Craniomandibular osteopathy, periostitis ossificans, and calvarial hyperostotic syndrome have never been reported in the cat. Recently, a case report described a 2-month-old cat that presented for severe periosteal proliferation of both the long bones and mandible, concluding this was most consistent with Caffey disease (infantile

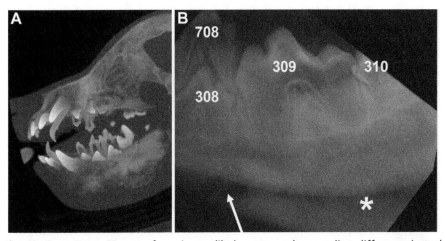

**Fig. 17.** Cone Beam CT scan of craniomandibular osteopathy revealing diffuse periosteal bone proliferation on the mandible in a dog (*A*). Dental radiographs of a dog with periostitis ossificans (*B*) highlighting bony proliferation and the space between the "double cortex" created (*arrow, asterisk*). (*From* Blazejewski SW, Lewis JR, Gracis M, et al. Mandibular periostitis ossificans in immature large breed dogs: 5 cases (1999-2006). *J Vet Dent.* 2010; 27: 148-159); reprinted with permission.)

**Table 4**
**Developmental abnormalities resulting in bony proliferation in dogs**

| | Breed Predilection | Age at Presentation | Etiology | Bones Affected | Long Bones Affected | Unilateral vs Bilateral | Pain | Diagnostic Imaging |
|---|---|---|---|---|---|---|---|---|
| Craniomandibular osteopathy | West Highland White terriers, Scottish terriers, Cairn terriers overrepresented, but reported in numerous breeds | 3–12 mo | Believed to be a genetic abnormality (defect in the SLC37A2 gene documented in affected terriers; recently diagnosed in 16 pure-bred Deutsch Drahthaar dogs with connected lineage | Mandible, occipital bone, tympanic bulla | Rarely | Normally bilateral and symmetric | Yes | Spiculated periosteal new bone |
| Periostitis ossificans | Large breed dogs | 3–5 mo | Possibly due to local trauma/infection/ inflammation of a dental follicle; lifting of vital periosteal layers resulting in new periosteum being laid down (creation of multiple cortical bone layers) | Mandible | No | Unilateral | No | "Double cortex" due to multiple cortical bone layers produced, most commonly seen on the ventral mandible |
| Calvarial hyperostotic syndrome | Mastiffs | 5–10 mo | Believed to be genetic in Mastiffs (previously believed to be a sex-linked abnormality) | Frontal, occipital, parietal, temporal, but no mandibular involvement | No | Unilateral | Yes | Periosteal proliferation, appearing very similar to CMO |

cortical hyperostosis).[71] Like other hyperostotic conditions, the disease in that case was self-limiting.

In all cases of bony proliferation, diagnostic imaging with radiography or CT scan as well as a bone biopsy are recommended. Although histopathology will be similar for all described developmental bony abnormalities (proliferative woven bone), biopsy will help to rule out other fibro-osseous or neoplastic bony disorders.

## OPEN-MOUTH JAW LOCKING

Open-mouth jaw locking occurs when the coronoid process is trapped on the ventrolateral surface of the zygomatic arch. Although not a developmental disorder in itself, it is theorized to occur because of abnormal skull morphology allowing the coronoid to flare laterally at times of widest mouth opening (such as during yawning). Specifically, TMJ dysplasia, soft tissue abnormalities of the TMJ (lateral ligament laxity, joint capsule disease), spasticity of the pterygoid muscles, flattening of the zygomatic arch, excessive mandibular symphyseal laxity, and breed-specific conformations have all been implicated.[72,73] Open-mouth jaw locking has been reported in numerous canine and feline breeds but appears to be more common in brachycephalics.

Animals will present severely distressed and physically unable to close the mouth. Diagnostic imaging with skull radiography, or ideally CT scan, can confirm diagnosis as well as fully evaluate the TMJ for predisposing abnormalities (**Fig. 18**). Initial treatment focuses on sedation to open the mouth wider while simultaneously manipulating the coronoid medially to return it to a normal position. However, this is unlikely to prevent recurrence. Thus, surgical treatment with partial zygomectomy and/or partial coronoidectomy is recommended. Other surgical options that have been reported include maxillomandibular fixation to limit jaw motion and strengthen the TMJ joint capsule, lateral ligament imbrication on the contralateral or ipsilateral side, condylectomy, and symphysiotomy, symphysiectomy, and intermandibular arthrodesis.[72,73]

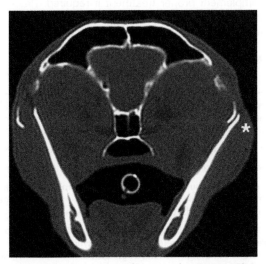

**Fig. 18.** Computed tomography (CT) image of a cat with open-mouth jaw locking, showing the left coronoid process displaced on the ventrolateral aspect of the zygomatic arch (*asterisk*). (*From* Soukup JW, Snyder CJ, Gengler WR. Computed tomography and partial coronoidectomy for open-mouth jaw locking in two cats. *J Vet Dent.* 2009; 26: 226-233; reprinted with permission.)

## DEVELOPMENTAL SOFT TISSUE ABNORMALITIES
### Tight Lip Syndrome

Tight lip syndrome is when there is no or very little oral vestibule in the rostral lower jaw, with the lower lip tightly curled over the mandibular incisor ± canine teeth. This abnormality allows the lip to be traumatized by the teeth and may also lead to linguo-version of the mandibular incisors because of excess lip pressure. In theory, the lip can also restrict mandibular growth because of excessive pressure. To the authors' knowledge, this condition has only been reported in the Shar Pei dog and appears to be unique to this breed. Owing to discomfort associated with this condition as well as the risk of malocclusion, a surgical procedure to deepen the mandibular vestibule should be performed.[74,75]

### Congenital Abnormalities of the Tongue

Congenital abnormalities of the tongue are rare, although they may be underreported, as puppies may be euthanized because of an inability to successfully nurse. Conditions that may be seen include:[76–78]

- Microglossia: Tongue is too small. No surgical option. Alternative feeding routines and/or euthanasia may be considered.
- Ankyloglossia (tongue-tie): Frenulum is adhered to the floor of the mouth, limiting tongue movement. Frenulectomy is curative for this condition.
- Macroglossia: Tongue is too large. This is most common in brachycephalic breeds and may be related to airway obstruction. Surgery to decrease the size of the tongue has not been reported, but this may be considered in cases with severe symptoms.

## SUMMARY

Developmental abnormalities of the teeth and oral cavity are varied and require an early diagnosis to implement proper treatment if required. Practitioners should be aware of normal anatomy and be able to recognize which of these abnormalities are cosmetic and/or self-limiting, thus not requiring treatment.

## CLINICS CARE POINTS

- Developmental abnormalities of teeth can be identified in either deciduous or permanent dentition. Once identified, those abnormalities must be explored with an anesthetized oral exam and radiographs.
- Abnormalities of tooth eruption and exfoliation may require surgical intervention.
- Malocclusions require early screening and must be evaluated for associated trauma.
- Congenital cleft palate can result in severe secondary complications including rhinitis and aspiration pneumonia and should be repaired at ideally 4-6 months of age. Functional success with repair is up to 85% but may require multiple surgeries.
- Developmental causes of bony proliferation include craniomandibular osteopathy (CMO), periostitis ossificans, or calvarial hyperostotic mastiffs syndrome. Most of the time, these disease processes are self-limiting when the dogs reach skeletal maturity, rarely symptomatic therapy (NSAIDS, antibiotics if biopsied) or surgical intervention (CMO only) is required.
- Open mouth jaw lock occurs due to underlying developmental skeletal abnormalities and is most often treated by coronoidectomy.

## DISCLOSURE

The authors declare that the research was conducted in the absence of any commercial or financial relationships that could be construed as a potential conflict of interest.

## REFERENCES

1. Lemmons M, Beebe D. Oral anatomy and physiology. In: Lobprise HB, Dodd JR, eds. Wigg's veterinary dentistry: principles and practice, 2nd edition. Hoboken, NJ: Wiley-Blackwell: 2019. p. 1–25.
2. Bellows J. Small animal dental equipment, materials, and techniques. Hoboken, NJ: Wiley-Blackwell: 2004. p. 87–112.
3. Dole RS, Spurgeon TL. Frequency of supernumerary teeth in a dolichocephalic canine breed, the greyhound. Am J Vet Res 1998;59:16–7.
4. Shope BH, Mitchell PQ, Carle D. Developmental pathology and pedontology. In: Lobprise HB, Dodd JR, eds. Wigg's veterinary dentistry: principles and practice, 2nd edition. Hoboken, NJ: Wiley-Blackwell: 2019. p. 63–82.
5. Skrabalak DS, Looney AL. Supernumerary tooth associated with facial swelling in a dog. J Am Vet Med Assoc 1993;203:266.
6. Fiani N, Arzi B. Diagnostic imaging in veterinary dental practice. J Am Vet Med Assoc 2009;235:271–3.
7. Hale FA. Junvenile veterinary dentistry. Vet Clin North Am Small Anim Pract 2005;35:789–817.
8. Dupont GA, DeBowes LJ. Atlas of dental radiography in dogs and cats. St Louis, MO: Saunders-Elsevier: 2009. p. 195–207.
9. Andrews AH. A case of partial anodontia in the dog. Vet Rec 1972;90:144–5.
10. Vieira ALS, Ocoarino NM, Beoloni JN, et al. Congenital oligodontia of the deciduous teeth and anodontia of the permanent teeth in a cat. J Feline Med Surg 2009;11:156–8.
11. Boy S, Crossley D, Steenkamp G. Developmental structural tooth defects in dogs – experience from veterinary dental referral practice and review of the literature. Front Vet Sci 2016;3:9.
12. Duncan HL. Diagnostic imaging in veterinary dental practice. Dens invaginatus leading to arrested maturation of the right and left mandibular first molar teeth. J Am Vet Med Assoc 2010;237:1251–3.
13. Stein KE, Marretta SM, Eurell JA. Dens invaginatus of the mandibular first molars in a dog. J Vet Dent 2005;22:21–5.
14. Ng KK, Rine S, Choi E, et al. Mandibular carnassial tooth malformations in 6 dogs - Micro-computed tomography and histology findings. Front Vet Sci 2019;6:464.
15. Coffman CR, Visser CJ, Visser L. Endodontic treatment of dens invaginatus in a dog. J Vet Dent 2009;26:220–5.
16. Dubielzig RR. The effect of canine distemper virus on the ameloblastic layer of the developing tooth. Vet Pathol 1979;16:268–70.
17. Bittegeko SB, Arnberg J, Nyka R, et al. Multiple dental developmental abnormalities following canine distemper infection. J Am Anim Hosp Assoc 1995;31:42–5.
18. Boutoille FF, Hennet PR. Diagnostic imaging in veterinary dental practice. Enamel hypoplasia. J Am Vet Med Assoc 2011;238:1251–3.
19. Mannerfelt T, Lindgren I. Enamel defects in standard poodle dogs in Sweden. J Vet Dent 2009;26:213–5.
20. Gandolfi B, Liu H, Griffioen L, et al. Simple recessive mutation in ENAM is associated with amelogenesis imperfecta in Italian greyhounds. Anim Genet 2013;44:569–78.

21. Gold R, Pool RR, Edwards EE. Osteogenesis and dentinogenesis imperfecta in a four-month-old English mastiff. Vet Rec 2019;7(3).
22. Smithson CW, Smith MM, Gamble DA. Multifocal odontoblastic dysplasia in a dog. J Vet Dent 2010;27:242–7.
23. Hobson P. Extraction of retained primary canine teeth in a dog. J Vet Dent 2005; 22:132–7.
24. Carle DS, Shope BS. Soft tissue impaction in a 7-month old Bedlington Terrier. J Vet Dent 2014;31:96–105.
25. Taney KG, Smith MM. Surgical extraction of impacted teeth in a dog. J Vet Dent 2006;23:168–77.
26. Baxter CJ. Bilateral mandibular dentigerous cysts in a dog. J Small Anim Pract 2004;45:210–1.
27. Gioso MA, Carvalho VG. Maxillary dentigerous cyst in a cat. J Vet Dent 2003;20: 28–30.
28. Surgeron TW. Surgical exposure and orthodontic extrusion of an impacted canine tooth in a cat: a case report. J Vet Dent 2000;17:81–5.
29. Lobprise H. Occlusion and orthodontics. In: Lobprise HB, Dodd JR, eds. Wigg's veterinary dentistry: principles and practice, 2nd edition. Hoboken, NJ: Wiley-Blackwell: 2019. 411–438.
30. Hoyer NK, Rawlinson JE. Prevalence of malocclusion of deciduous dentition in dogs: an evaluation of 297 puppies. J Vet Dent 2019;36:251–6.
31. AVDC nomenclature. Available at: https://avdc.org/avdc-nomenclature/. Accessed April 19, 2021.
32. Shkoukani MA, Lawrence LA, Liebertz DJ, et al. Cleft palate: a clinical review. Birth Defects Res C Embryo Today 2014;102:333–42.
33. Freiberger K, Hemker S, McAnally R, et al. Secondary palate development in the dog (Canis lupus familiaris). Cleft Palate Craniofac J 2021;58:230–6.
34. Pankowski F, Paśko S, Max A, et al. Computed tomographic evaluation of cleft palate in one-day-old puppies. BMC Vet Res 2018;14(1):316.
35. Peralta S, Fiani N, Kan-Rohrer KH, et al. Morphological evaluation of clefts of the lip, palate, or both in dogs. Am J Vet Res 2017;78:926–33.
36. Setó-Salvia N, Stanier P. Genetics of cleft lip and/or cleft palate: association with other common anomalies. Eur J Med Genet 2014;57:381–93.
37. Nemec A, Daniaux L, Johnson E, et al. Craniomaxillofacial abnormalities in dogs with congenital palatal defects: computed tomographic findings. Vet Surg 2015; 44:417–22.
38. Moura E, Cirio SM, Pimpão CT. Nonsyndromic cleft lip and palate in boxer dogs: evidence of monogenic autosomal recessive inheritance. Cleft Palate Craniofac J 2012;49:759–60.
39. Wolf ZT, Brand HA, Shaffer JR, et al. Genome-wide association studies in dogs and humans identify ADAMTS20 as a risk variant for cleft lip and palate. Plos Genet 2015;11(3):e1005059.
40. Kemp C, Thiele H, Dankof A, et al. Cleft lip and/or palate with monogenic autosomal recessive transmission in Pyrenees shepherd dogs. Cleft Palate Craniofac J 2009;46:81–8.
41. Abbott BD. The etiology of cleft palate: a 50-year search for mechanistic and molecular understanding. Birth Defects Res B Dev Reprod Toxicol 2010;89:266–74.
42. Murray JC. Gene/environment causes of cleft lip and/or palate. Clin Genet 2002; 61:248–56.
43. Roman N, Carney PC, Fiani N, et al. Incidence patterns of orofacial clefts in purebred dogs. PLoS One 2019;14(11):e0224574.

44. Fiani N, Verstraete FJ, Arzi B. Reconstruction of congenital nose, cleft primary palate, and lip disorders. Vet Clin North Am Small Anim Pract 2016;46:663–75.
45. Kolker AR, Sailon AM, Meara JG, et al. Midline cleft lip and bifid nose deformity: description, classification, and treatment. J Craniofac Surg 2015;26:2304–8.
46. Arzi B, Verstraete FJ. Repair of a bifid nose combined with a cleft of the primary palate in a 1-year-old dog. Vet Surg 2011;40:865–9.
47. Peralta S, Campbell RD, Fiani N, et al. Outcomes of surgical repair of congenital palatal defects in dogs. J Am Vet Med Assoc 2018;253:1445–51.
48. Marretta SM. Cleft palate repair techniques. In: Verstraete FJM, Lommer MJ, editors. Oral and maxillofacial surgery in dogs and cats. Edinburgh, UK: Saunders Elsevier; 2012. p. 351–62.
49. Peralta S, Nemec A, Fiani N, et al. Staged double-layer closure of palatal defects in 6 dogs. Vet Surg 2015;44:423–31.
50. Bakri S, Rizell S, Lilja J, et al. Vertical maxillary growth after two different surgical protocols in unilateral cleft lip and palate patients. Cleft Palate Craniofac J 2014; 51:645–50.
51. Maluf I Jr, Doro U, Fuchs T, et al. Evaluation of maxillary growth: is there any difference using relief incision during palatoplasty? J Craniofac Surg 2014;25: 772–4.
52. Barutca SA, Aksan T, Usçetin I, et al. Effects of palatine bone denudation repair with periosteal graft on maxillary growth: an experimental study in rats. J Craniomaxillofac Surg 2014;42:e1–7.
53. Conze T, Ritz I, Hospes R, et al. Management of cleft palate in puppies using a temporary prosthesis: a report of three cases. Vet Sci 2018;5(3):61.
54. Martínez-Sanz E, Casado-Gómez I, Martín C, et al. A new technique for feeding dogs with a congenital cleft palate for surgical research. Lab Anim 2011;45(2): 70–80.
55. Edstrom E, Smith M. Prosthetic appliance for oronasal communication obturation in a dog. J Vet Dent 2014;31:108–12.
56. Hale F, Sylvestre A, Miller C. The use of a prosthetic appliance to manage a large palatal defect in a dog. J Vet Dent 1997;14(2):61–4.
57. Mullins RA, Guerin SR, Pratschke KM. Use of a split-thickness soft palate hinged flap and bilateral buccal mucosal rotation flaps for one-stage repair of a bilateral hypoplastic soft palate in a dog. J Am Vet Med Assoc 2016;248:91–5.
58. Headrick JF, McAnulty JF. Reconstruction of a bilateral hypoplastic soft palate in a cat. J Am Anim Hosp Assoc 2004;40:86–90.
59. White RN, Hawkins HL, Alemi VP, et al. Soft palate hypoplasia and concurrent middle ear pathology in six dogs. J Small Anim Pract 2009;50:364–72.
60. Alexander JW. Selected skeletal dysplasias: craniomandibular osteopathy, multiple cartilaginous exostoses, and hypertrophic osteodystrophy. Vet Clin North Am Small Anim Pract 1983;13:55–70.
61. Beever L, Swinbourne F, Priestnall SL, et al. Surgical management of chronic otitis secondary to craniomandibular osteopathy in three West Highland white terriers. J Small Anim Pract 2019;60:254–60.
62. Vagt J, Distl O. Complex segregation analysis of craniomandibular osteopathy in Deutsch Drahthaar dogs. Vet J 2018;231:30–2.
63. Hytönen MK, Arumilli M, Lappalainen AK, et al. Molecular characterization of three canine models of human rare bone diseases: caffey, van den Ende-Gupta, and Raine Syndromes. Plos Genet 2016;12(5):e1006037.
64. Pettitt R, Fox R, Comerford EJ, et al. Bilateral angular carpal deformity in a dog with craniomandibular osteopathy. Vet Comp Orthop Traumatol 2012;25:149–54.

65. Ratterree WO, Glassman MM, Driskell EA, et al. Craniomandibular osteopathy with a unique neurological manifestation in a young Akita. J Am Anim Hosp Assoc 2011;47(1):e7–12.
66. Blazejewski SW, Lewis JR, Gracis M, et al. Mandibular periostitis ossificans in immature large breed dogs: 5 cases (1999-2006). J Vet Dent 2010;27:148–59.
67. Fukuda M, Inoue K, Sakashita H. Periostitis ossificans arising in the mandibular bone of a young patient: report of an unusual case and review of the literature. J Oral Maxillofac Surg 2017;75(9):1834.e1–8.
68. Pastor KF, Boulay JP, Schelling SH, et al. Idiopathic hyperostosis of the calvaria in five young bullmastiffs. J Am Anim Hosp Assoc 2000;36:439–45.
69. McConnell JF, Hayes A, Platt SR, et al. Calvarial hyperostosis syndrome in two bullmastiffs. Vet Radiol Ultrasound 2006;47:72–7.
70. Mathes RL, Holmes SP, Coleman KD, et al. Calvarial hyperostosis presenting as unilateral exophthalmos in a female English Springer Spaniel. Vet Ophthalmol 2012;15:263–70.
71. Allevi G, Serafini F. Polyostotic cortical hyperostosis in an 8-week-old cat with a 3-year follow-up. J Small Anim Pract 2021;62:59–64.
72. Soukup JW, Snyder CJ, Gengler WR. Computed tomography and partial coronoidectomy for open-mouth jaw locking in two cats. J Vet Dent 2009;26:226–33.
73. Reiter AM. Symphysiotomy, symphysiectomy, and intermandibular arthrodesis in a cat with open-mouth jaw locking–case report and literature review. J Vet Dent 2004;21:147–58.
74. Holmstrom SE. Inferior labial frenoplasty and tight lip syndrome. In: Verstraete FJM, Lommer MJ, editors. Oral and maxillofacial surgery in dogs and cats. Edinburgh, UK: Saunders Elsevier; 2012. p. 515–8.
75. Eisner ER. Vestibule deepening procedure for tight lip syndrome in the Chinese Shar-pei dog. J Vet Dent 2008;25:284–9.
76. Temizsoylu MD, Avki S. Complete ventral ankyloglossia in three related dogs. J Am Vet Med Assoc 2003;223:1443–5, 1433.
77. Jones BA, Stanley BJ, Nelson NC. The impact of tongue dimension on air volume in brachycephalic dogs. Vet Surg 2020;49:512–20.
78. Wiggs RB, Lobprise HB, de Lahunta A. Microglossia in three littermate puppies. J Vet Dent 1994;11(4):129–33.

# Management of Severe Oral Inflammatory Conditions in Dogs and Cats

Jamie G. Anderson, DVM, MS[a],*, Philippe Hennet, DV[b]

## KEYWORDS

- Canine • Feline • Oral diseases • Chronic ulcerative stomatitis
- Chronic gingivostomatitis • Eosinophilic lesions • Wegener's granulomatosis
- Pyogenic granuloma

## KEY POINTS

- Oral inflammatory diseases in dogs and cats are common, sometimes poorly understood, and therefore challenging.
- CCUS is an immunoinflammatory disease with improved understanding and medical treatment options.
- Feline chronic gingivostomatitis is the most common severe oral inflammatory condition encountered in cats.
- Oral squamous cell carcinoma is an important differential for severe inflammatory conditions in cats.
- Microscopic analysis is critical in determining a definitive diagnosis.

## SEVERE ORAL INFLAMMATORY CONDITIONS IN DOGS
### Introduction

To begin the discussion of management of severe oral inflammatory disease in dogs, it is helpful to have a generalized approach and to make the correct diagnosis. As for most inflammatory diseases in dogs, whether it is pancreatitis, prostatitis, hepatitis, or chronic ulcerative stomatitis, it makes sense to begin with a complete physical examination. Depending on the dog's age and the nature of the inflammation, routine clinicopathologic evaluation including complete blood count, chemistry analysis, thyroid evaluation and urinalysis are essential. These steps are foundational in the assessment of any inflammatory disorder. The next step is to make the correct diagnosis, for which then management strategies can be formulated. The DAMNIT scheme is a useful approach to the diagnosis of oral lesions and allows a schematic differential list of etiologies (**Fig. 1**).[1,2] As current research in veterinary dentistry becomes more

[a] Department of Oral Medicine, University of Pennsylvania, 8605 Mace Boulevard, Dixon, CA 95620, USA; [b] Unité de dentisterie et chirurgie oromaxillofaciale, ADVETIA Centre Hospitalier Vétérinaire, 9 avenue Louis Breguet, Vélizy-Villacoublay 78140, France
* Corresponding author.
*E-mail address:* jgadvm@gmail.com

Vet Clin Small Anim 52 (2022) 159–184
https://doi.org/10.1016/j.cvsm.2021.09.008

vetsmall.theclinics.com

sophisticated, the list of idiopathic disorders in this schema are becoming better understood.[3–6]

Management of severe oral inflammatory diseases including canine chronic ulcerative stomatitis (CCUS), eosinophilic granuloma complex, and Wegener's granulomatosis (WG) will be discussed. For each disease state, a brief introductory paragraph will start the discussion. Then, specifics will be given relative to how to approach the comprehensive oral health assessment and treatment (COHAT), how to obtain useful histopathology samples as well as culture/microbiome samples. A third section, based on a definitive diagnosis, will detail successful treatment regimens. As the current literature advises, an attempt will be made to address why the particular drug protocols are optimally effective.

### Canine Chronic Ulcerative Stomatitis

As the name implies, ulcerative stomatitis is a chronic inflammatory disease. Recent research has identified breed predispositions and has outlined the associated clinical and radiographic findings.[3] A canine ulcerative stomatitis disease activity index (CUS-DAI) was developed to determine objectively how a patient responds to therapy. Additional research defined the types of leukocytes involved in the stomatitis lesion including B cells, T cells, CD3 negative IL17+ cells, macrophages, and mast cells.[7] Interestingly, the leukocytes found infiltrating CCUS tissue were different from normal healthy control tissue and from the advanced periodontitis lesion. We were able to conclude that CCUS is an immune-mediated inflammatory disease. Comparatively, many of the leukocytes in the CCUS lesion were different from those found in feline chronic gingivostomatitis (FCGS),[8] implying different underlying immune mechanisms. Because CCUS has previously been thought to be a result of contact with plaque and or plaque retentive surfaces, and perhaps was the impetus for the extraction of teeth, a next-generation sequencing analysis of the oral microbiome was undertaken. This analysis revealed a unique biofilm on the CCUS mucosal lesion which was different from that on the opposing tooth surface, from that of normal healthy mucosa, and

# DAMNIT Algorithm

- **D**   degenerative, developmental

- **A**   auto-immune, allergic, anatomic

- **M**   metabolic, mechanical

- **N**   nutritional, neoplastic

- **I**   infectious, inflammatory, idiopathic, immune mediated

- **T**   toxic, traumatic

**Fig. 1.** DAMNIT algorithm assists in the differential diagnosis for oral lesions. (*Courtesy of* Dr Anderson.)

from severe periodontitis.[9] The results of this study do not support the extraction of healthy teeth in treating CCUS.

### Management at Comprehensive Oral Health Assessment and Treatment

With the patient under general anesthesia and before any interventions, such as rinsing or chlorhexidine application, a CUSDAI score should be assigned. As well, at this time, collect biofilm samples with sterile endodontic paper points for commercial next generation sequencing analysis of the microbiome. Oral irrigation, oral/dental charting, and full mouth dental radiography are performed routinely. CCUS patients with severe mucosal lesions are generally quite painful. Appropriate premedication and local anesthesia are warranted. Given the evidence that ulcerative lesions persist after extraction in 40% of dogs with CCUS,[3] that the bacterial microbiome is not similar between the opposing tooth surface and the lesions,[9] and that periodontal disease stage does not correlate with the severity of CCUS,[3] this author (JGA) recommends the extraction of "hopeless" teeth only.

Common differential diagnoses for CCUS include autoimmune disorders such as pemphigus vulgaris (PV), bullous pemphigoid (BP), systemic lupus erythematosus as well as erythema multiforme and ulcerative neoplasms. Biopsy and histopathology are warranted if there is concern that the lesions do not look typical.[3] Generally, the lesions are mucosal and easily sampled. To help differentiate from autoimmune disorders, take a perilesional sample with normal tissue included. A larger deep sample would be 8 to 12 mm and include the submucosal and connective tissue. Closure of the biopsy site may be warranted. A good sample is only as good as the pathologist assessing it. Choose a pathologist with expertise in veterinary oral pathological condition. Clinical photographs should be sent with your biopsy, and a requisition form with a complete clinical history can be very helpful.

### "CLINICS CARE POINTS"
### Management Post-COHAT

- Analgesics
- Oral home care
  - Healthy Mouth water additive
  - Tooth brushing after lesion resolution
- Pentoxifylline + doxycycline + niacinamide (PDN)
  - Pentoxifylline 20 mg/kg orally twice daily
  - Doxycycline 5 mg/kg orally twice daily
    - Can switch out doxycycline for metronidazole 15 mg/kg orally once daily
  - Niacinamide 200 to 250 mg orally twice daily
  - Side effects are mostly gastrointestinal: poor appetite, vomiting
  - Taper Pentoxifylline; first give q 24 hours, then every other day as clinical remission allows
- Cyclosporine (CyA) and metronidazole
  - Atopica 5 mg/kg orally once daily
  - Metronidazole 15 mg/kg orally once daily
  - Both cytochrome P450 inhibitors
    - Drugs are synergistic
    - Decrease doses in hepatic disease
  - Laboratory monitoring for hepatotoxicity
  - Cyclosporine blood levels
    - Commercial laboratory
    - 0.5 mL of whole blood (EDTA)

- ○ Cyclosporine pharmacodynamic assay (CPA)
  - ▪ Heparinized cyclosporine samples
  - ▪ Shipped frozen to Mississippi State University College of Veterinary Medicine Pharmacodynamic Laboratory
  - ▪ IL-2 monitoring of immune suppression
- ○ Side effects are primarily gastrointestinal and hepatic; nausea, vomiting, and diarrhea
- ○ Taper off CyA as clinical remission allows

### Therapeutic Considerations (Thoughts on Why These Drugs Work in CCUS)

*Pentoxifylline* has long been known to be a potent inhibitor of inflammatory damage. In 1995, 2 main mechanisms of action were described: (a) reduction of the production of inflammatory cytokines (especially TNF) by phagocytes stimulated with a variety of microbial products (eg, endotoxin); and (b) reversal of the effect of these cytokines on phagocytes.[10] In conditions such as CCUS, whereby inflammatory cytokines and phagocytes likely contribute to tissue damage, pentoxifylline is helpful. Although the specific cytokines in CCUS are not yet known, we do know that IL17 and FoxP3 heavily infiltrate the tissues.[3,7] This dysregulated inflammatory response in combination with a dysbiotic microbiome allows us to begin to understand pathogenesis in CCUS. Research reveals that pentoxifylline inhibits, in particular, the production of proinflammatory interleukin 17 (IL-17), interleukin 2 (IL-2), and interferon-gamma.[11] Pentoxifylline also reduces lymphocyte proliferation, increases leukocyte deformability, and inhibits neutrophil adhesion and activation. Working as an anticlaudication drug, it increases erythrocyte flexibility and dilates blood vessels. Finally, pentoxifylline also has potent antioxidant effects.[12] In human oral medicine practice, pentoxifylline is consistently used for recurrent apthous ulcers,[13] medication-related osteonecrosis, and radiation-induced oral mucositis.[14] The incidence of adverse reactions to pentoxifylline in people have been shown to be less than 1%. Digestive and central nervous system side effects are dose related.

*Doxycycline* is a broad-spectrum antimicrobial agent and remains an inexpensive alternative for the treatment of community-acquired respiratory infections and urinary tract infections. At antimicrobial doses, it is the drug of choice for treating infections caused by *Borrelia*, *Ehrlichia,* and *Rickettsia*. In the 1980s, investigations led to a shift in the pathogenesis and treatment of periodontitis called "host-modulation therapy." Whereby it was once believed that anaerobic bacteria caused periodontitis, it became recognized that bacteria operated as the trigger for destructive host immune response mechanisms.[15,16] Tetracycline antibiotics became part of the host-modulation therapy, as they could inhibit the matrix metalloproteinases (MMP) that caused periodontal tissue breakdown.[17] Nonantibacterial tetracycline formulations such as subantimicrobial dose doxycycline (SDD) have been recognized to be useful host modulators in a wide variety of oral and systemic disorders including diabetes mellitus, arthritis and postmenopausal bone loss ion people.[18] More recent canine research suggests that SDD provides an adjunct to nonsurgical periodontal therapy.[19,20] Another beneficial action of tetracyclines is their ability to act as reactive oxygen species scavengers.[17] Though the SDD research in canines is limited, it may be that an intermediate dose of doxycycline stabilizes the inflammatory response by promoting the suppression of proinflammatory cytokines and increases the anti-inflammatory cytokines working through non-antibacterial mechanisms in CCUS.

*Niacinamide*, vitamin B3, is an essential water-soluble nutrient. In the body, it is converted to the co-factors NADH and NADPH that are involved in many cellular metabolic pathways. As NAD+ is thought to be at the intersection of cell metabolism and cell signaling, vitamin supplementation has become an important therapeutic.[21] As well as providing nutrient value, vitamins including B3 are known to have immunologic functions[22] and play an important role in homeostasis between physiologic normalcy and pathologic conditions of especially the oral and gastrointestinal mucosa.

*Cyclosporine* is an effective immunosuppressive agent which inhibits T-cell function and suppresses cell-mediated immune responses.[23] Its mechanism of action is by binding to intracellular cyclophilin A, forming a cyclosporine-cyclophilin complex, which inhibits calcineurin, an enzyme critical to the synthesis of cytokines such as IL-2, IL-4, TNF alpha and INF gamma by T-cells.[24–26] Cyclosporin is also known to inhibit the production of IL-17 by memory Th17 cells.[27] Although current research has not defined the cytokines important in CCUS, we do know that CD3+ T cells, T regulatory cells, and IL-17+ cells are important. As cyclosporine effectively inhibits T-cell function and cell-mediated immunity,[24] this might be the proposed mechanism of action in CCUS.

*Metronidazole* is a commonly used antibiotic in veterinary medicine, although it also has important anti-inflammatory and immunosuppressive actions.[28] Metronidazole decreases leukocyte-endothelial cell adhesion and migration from the bloodstream into tissue.[29] It dampens down the proliferation of lymphocytes by causing damage to lymphocyte DNA.[30] It also reduces the number and function of macrophages.[31] The described important infiltrating leukocytes in CCUS include moderate to large numbers of T cells (CD3, CD4, CD8, FoxP3), B cells (CD20, Mum1), IL17+ cells, macrophages (CD204) and mast cells. Because metronidazole decreases the levels of IL-2 and INF gamma produced by T cells and significantly inhibits antibody production by B lymphocytes, this provides a proposed mechanism to control CCUS. Neurotoxicity has been reported with high-dose metronidazole use in some dogs.[32] Additionally, metronidazole's antibiotic activity may better inhibit the bacterial microbiome of the CCUS lesion. The lesion is found to have a unique, species-specific bacterial community including *Porphyromonas cangingivalis* and *P. gingivalis*, 2 canine species related to *P. gingivalis* of people, *Neisseria weaveri*, *Fusobacterium spp.*, and a *Tannerella forsythia*-like phylotype (JA microbiome).[9]

## EOSINOPHILIC STOMATITIS

Oral eosinophilic inflammatory lesions are thought to be a hypersensitivity reaction to environmental, ingested material including coat dander, parasitic infections, and other external antigens. Oral eosinophilic granuloma complex of cats is common and easily recognized in part because of its proliferative yellow gritty appearance due to the mineralization of its collagen and eosinophil-derived proteins. In canines, eosinophilic ulcers are more common, and appear flat and ulcerated (**Fig. 2**). Although Cavalier King Charles spaniels and Siberian husky breeds have been reported to commonly be affected,[33–35] numerous other breeds will display these lesions. Peripheral eosinophilia is reported with a 33% to 60% frequency. Lesions are located on the palate (65.4%), tongue (26.9%), and other oral locations (7.7%).[36] Histologic descriptions are well presented[37] in the textbook by Murphy, Bell and Sokup.[38] Immunohistochemistry of this lesion has not yet been evaluated and may inform pathogenesis and direct specific treatment. In one study of 24 dogs, 70% of asymptomatic dogs resolved without medication.[36] As well, a statistically significant correlation was noted between lesion location and body weight; but no associations were noted with peripheral eosinophilia, between lesion location and breed, signalment and response to therapy, or the use of prednisone and lesion resolution.[36]

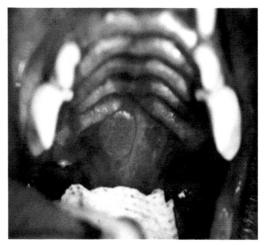

**Fig. 2.** Eosinophilic granuloma on the palate of a 5-year-old Dachshund. (*Courtesy of* Dr Anderson.)

### Management

Eosinophilic lesions are often identified during the oral examination portion of the COHAT. The dog may not be symptomatic, even with multiple lesions. Making the correct diagnosis is tantamount to treatment and sound clinical practice. For eosinophilic lesions, it is important to rule out allergic causation in addition to parasitic, fungi, and bacterial infections. A complete blood count and chemistry panel are warranted, though peripheral eosinophilia may not indicate a diagnosis. As well, lesion cytology cannot be used as a confirmatory test. An incisional or excisional biopsy is necessary.

### "CLINICS CARE POINTS"
### Management Post-COHAT

Options are limited in part due to the unclear pathogenesis in these lesions.

- Wait and watch, especially if asymptomatic
- Treat for 6 to 8 weeks if symptomatic
- Glucocorticoids
  - Prednisone, Budesonide, Triamcinolone local injection
  - Dosages and regimens vary widely
- Surgical excision in selected lesions

### WEGENER'S GRANULOMATOSIS

WG also known as granulomatosis with polyangiitis is an uncommon canine autoimmune inflammatory disorder affecting the gingiva, oral mucosa, and underlying alveolar bone. Complement system inhibition with C5a has an important role in pathogenesis.[39,40] As such, C5a inhibitors are being investigated as possible glucocorticoid sparing treatment in people.[41] A recent review outlines therapeutic options for people with ANCA-associated vasculitis.[42] An excellent case report by Krug and colleagues documents the clinical, radiographic and specific histologic findings.[43] WG can be a challenging diagnosis to make if the clinician is not aware of this entity, its specific clinical and radiographic appearance, and histologic peculiarities.

Clinically, the gingival lesion can be multifocal, bruised, and erythematous in appearance, expansile, and friable. In all regards, it looks like a neoplasm. Radiographically the lesion is associated with severe alveolar bone loss. The key to a correct diagnosis is in the presence of granulomatous inflammation that is, not secondary to fungal or infectious disease. Reasonable differential diagnoses are traumatic granuloma, necrotizing ulcerative stomatitis, pyogenic granuloma, neoplasia, and immune-mediated conditions. The veterinary literature for WG is sparse and the confirmatory autoimmune test to assess for antineutrophil cytoplasmic antibodies is only available in research settings.

### Management

For WG, making the correct diagnosis can be a challenge. As for other severe oral inflammatory disorders, a full clinicopathologic evaluation is needed. Bacterial and fungal cultures will assist in ruling out more common differentials. Risk factors have been identified in people and include trimethoprim-sulfamethoxazole and minocycline.[44] Risk factors in dogs have not been reported. Diagnosis is based on indirect immunofluorescence, antineutrophil cytoplasmic antibodies-associated vasculitis,[45,46] and routine histopathology. Biopsy of this lesion should be incisional and include bone if involved. A second perilesional sample might prove useful to distinguish it from other immune-mediated diseases. Consultation with a specialist in dermatopathology may be helpful.

### "CLINICS CARE POINTS"
### Management Post-COHAT

Management of dogs with mucosal WG is multi-modal and includes:

- Oral home care
- Prednisone 1.5 to 2.0 mg/kg orally twice daily for 10 days or until lesion remission
- Gastroprotective support
- Hepatoprotective support
- With lesion regression
  - Prednisone taper 1 mg/kg orally q24 hr and add in Cytoxan[43] 50 mg orally q24 hr × 4 days, rest Cytoxan for 3 days, repeat cycle[43]
  - Consider oncology referral
  - Consider metronomic therapy with Cytoxan[47,48]
  - Cytoxan treatment monitor for severe hemorrhagic cystitis
- If refractory
  - Consider dermatology consultation and/or referral for continued care
  - Consider monoclonal antibody treatment, such as rituximab (RTX)[42]

### SEVERE ORAL INFLAMMATORY CONDITIONS IN CATS
### Introduction

Severe oral inflammatory conditions are frequent in cats. They may be focal or diffuse lesions affecting a single area or widely spread within the oral cavity. As squamous cell carcinoma is the most prevalent oral tumor in cats and may show various ulcerative and proliferative clinical appearances, differentials are of fundamental importance and require microscopic analysis of the tissue.[49–51] In 2 recent retrospective histologic studies of oral lesions in dogs and cats in the USA and in Eastern Europe, it was shown that 51% (37/73) to 58% (85/146) of the lesions, respectively, biopsied in cats had an inflammatory origin.[49,50] In a 2020 retrospective study of 297 feline oral cavity lesions diagnosed by histopathology in Portugal, inflammatory and neoplastic lesions accounted for 187 (63%) and 110 (37%) of the studied cases, respectively. FCGS was the most common histologic diagnosis (39.1%), followed by squamous cell carcinoma (16.5%) and eosinophilic granuloma complex (11.1%).[51]

### Feline Chronic Gingivostomatitis/Caudal Stomatitis

FCGS is a painful and debilitating feline oral condition characterized by a severe immune mediated chronic bilateral inflammation of the gingiva, alveolar, labio-buccal mucosa, and caudal oral mucosa (retromolar area lateral to the palatoglossal folds).[8,52–57] Cats affected by FCGS are often presented with severe dysorexia/anorexia, oral pain, weight loss, ptyalism, halitosis, and lack of grooming.[56,58–61] The lesions are ulcerative in nature and clinically present with an ulcerative or ulcero-proliferative pattern.[8,57,58,61,62] Lingual ulcers may also be present in some cats.[56,58,61] In addition, FCGS has been shown to be associated with more widely distributed and severe periodontitis and with a higher prevalence of external inflammatory root resorption and retained roots than other oral diseases.[53] Nevertheless, the presence of caudal stomatitis distinguishes FCGS from other feline oral conditions (**Fig. 3**).[52,53,58,63] Histologic findings show a complex, chronic and destructive inflammatory process affecting the epithelium and lamina propria with frequent extension into submucosal tissues.[4,8,56,62] The number of plasma cells, neutrophils and CD3+ T lymphocytes correlate with the severity of inflammation. T cells are present in the superficial mucosa and submucosa, whereas B cells and Mott cells are restricted to the submucosa.[8] The inflammatory response showing a predominance of CD8+ (cytotoxic) T cells over CD4+ (helpers) T cells suggest a cytotoxic cell-mediated immune response to antigenic stimulation that may be associated with viral infections.[8,62] Additionally, the CD4/CD8 ratio in the peripheral blood of FCGS cats is dysregulated due to an increasing number of CD8+ cells in circulation.[4,8]

Different infectious and noninfectious causes have been suspected: bacteria, fungi, viral infection, dental diseases, and allergic reactions.[64–68] Feline calicivirus (FCV) has been identified as a causative agent of upper respiratory tract infection and ulcerative lesions in the oral cavity since the seventies.[69,70] After initial infection, many cats become oral chronic carriers and the virus may be detected in cats without clinical signs.[65,66] Though no direct causal relationship between FCV and FCGS has been established, various experiments support its involvement.[60,63–67,71] In a very recent

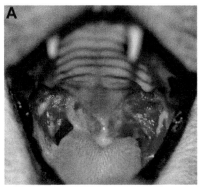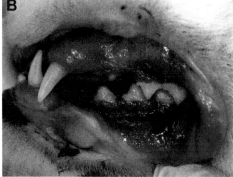

**Fig. 3.** Cats with chronic gingivostomatitis showing typical lesion of ulceroproliferative caudal mucositis (*A*) and gingivitis and alveolar/labial/buccal ulcerative mucositis (*B*). (*Courtesy of* Dr Hennet.)

shotgun metagenomic study of the feline oral microbiome, it was shown that FCV was the only microbe strongly associated with FCGS; FCV was not identified in healthy cats and in cats with periodontitis. Additionally, FCGS cats presented an upregulation of genes promoting antiviral activity than control cats, an event which is compatible with the hypothesis of antigenic stimulation of viral origin contributing to FCGS.[63] Environmental and stress factors may also play a role. FCGS is more prevalent in multi-cat than in single-cat environments and in cats, with no access to outdoors.[60,72] The risk correlates with the number of cohabiting cats.[72] Multi-cat housing may allow chronic carriers shedding viruses to facilitate the cyclic reinfection of susceptible individuals, which immune function may be impaired by the stress of living in a multi-cat environment.[72]

## "CLINICS CARE POINTS"

- COHAT
  - Make the correct clinical oral diagnosis (bilateral caudal stomatitis ± alveolar/labial/buccal/sublingual mucositis)
  - CBC, chemistry panel, and viral testing
  - Perform full oral examination including full-mouth dental radiographs
  - Score the lesions (location, nature, extent, and depth)
  - Take biopsy if lesions are atypical and/or asymmetrical
- Management at COHAT
  - Multimodal analgesia
  - Extract premolar/molar teeth and all root tips
  - Extract incisors and canine teeth if affected by periodontitis, endodontic disease, dental resorption, or alveolar/labial/buccal/sublingual mucositis
  - Perioperative management and care (hospitalization, fluids, multimodal analgesia, appetite stimulant ± feeding tube placement)
- Management post-COHAT
  - Medical treatment
    - Antimicrobials (antimicrobials, oral antiseptics)
    - Pain management (NSAID, opioids, gabapentinoids)
    - Appetite stimulant (mirtazapine)
  - Revaluation at 3 to 4 weeks
  - Classify cats as good responder, mild responder or poor responder
  - Adapt medical treatment according to response to dental extraction
  - Consider immunomodulating treatment of a poor responder (refractory cases)
  - Recheck refractory cases every month until improvement to adapt supporting medical treatment and immunomodulating treatment

## *Medical Management*

Medical treatment alone is unrewarding and has been shown to only provide temporary improvement.[55,57–59,61,73–75] It is mainly based on the alleviation of symptoms through the use of anti-inflammatory drugs and painkillers as well as the control of secondary bacterial infection through the use of antimicrobials and topical antiseptic treatments. In a retrospective study of 104 cats with FCGS, 56% of them received SAIDs (alone or with antibiotics) and 31% NSAIDs (alone or with antibiotics) at the time of referral. No difference in the severity of the lesions between groups was observed preoperatively showing that one protocol was not more efficient than another one.[61] In 2 groups of 5 cats whereby a bovine lactoferrin oral spray and piroxicam oral medication were used, clinical signs of FCGS were improved in 77% of the cats, and the combination of the oral spray and the NSAIS was more effective than the NSAID alone in reducing clinical signs.[76] Two protocols of near infra-red laser therapy have been studied in 2 groups of 5 cats with FCGS after dental treatment and concurrent adjunct medical treatment. Though the protocol with the lower energy per surface area showed greater and faster improvement, the small size of the groups, the lack of standardization of adjunct treatments, and the lack of a control group are making results inconclusive.[77] Most of the studies on the sole medical treatment of FCGS are based on anecdotal reports and small series or poorly designed studies. Medical treatment is mainly used in combination with or after surgical treatment of the management of refractory cases. In a recent pilot study in 5 cats, mesenchymal stem cell (MSC) therapy was shown ineffective in reducing clinical signs and in inducing immunomodulation when used before surgical treatment/dental extractions in opposite to what has been shown for the treatment of refractory cases after dental extractions.[78]

### Surgical Treatment (Dental Extractions)

Dental extractions as a possible treatment of cats presenting with chronic gingivitis and ulcerative caudal stomatitis (called "faucitis" at that time) and refractory to medical treatment was proposed by Gaskell and Gruffydd-Jones in 1977.[70] Extraction of all teeth or premolar and molar teeth is the currently accepted standard of care for the primary management of FCGS.[54,55,58,59,61] The rational for dental extraction is the suppression of chronic antigenic stimulation caused by dental plaque and by dental inflammatory or infectious diseases. Root remnants and teeth facing areas of mucosal inflammation are extracted as well as teeth presenting with advanced periodontitis, dental resorption, dental fracture with pulpal necrosis (unless proper endodontic treatment can be performed).[54,58,61] Substantial improvement or complete remission has been reported in 67% to 80% of FCGS cats.[54,58,59] Cats showing little or no improvement (refractory cases) also required continuous medical treatments. Provided extraction criteria are considered, no difference has been shown between full-mouth extraction and subtotal-mouth extraction (premolar/molar teeth ± additional teeth).[54,61] Therefore, full-mouth extraction cannot be recommended as a general approach as it involves a longer, more painful invasive procedure.

In a large retrospective study in the USA on the outcome of 95 cats with FCGS treated with dental extractions, 28.4% showed clinical cure, 38.9% showed substantial improvement and 32.6% were little or not improved.[54] 68.8% of cats showing clinical cure or substantial improvement required extended medical treatment (antimicrobials, anti-inflammatory drugs and/or analgesics) after dental extractions (**Fig. 4**). Cats showing resolution of abnormal behavior, decrease in oral inflammation and no further need for antimicrobials at the time of the first recheck examination (median time = 16 days) were more likely to have a more positive long-term outcome.[54] In a recent retrospective study of 56 FCV-positive cats with FCGS that were followed postoperatively at the same institution in France, clinical cure (defined as the absence of pain and complete healing of oral lesions) was achieved in 32% of cats within a median time of 33.5 days, significant improvement (persistence of some degree of pain and oral lesion without the need for medication) was achieved in 29% of the cats within a median time of 49 days, and slight to no improvement requiring continuous medication in 39% of the cats. 60.7% of the owners considered their cat either cured or significantly improved.[61] Neither the severity of caudal stomatitis lesion nor the load of FCV was correlated to the outcome. But cats showing a lower degree of inflammation of mucosa facing the teeth seemed to improve more rapidly than cats with a higher score.[61]

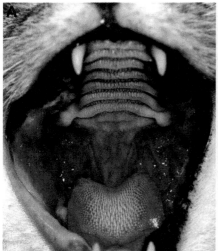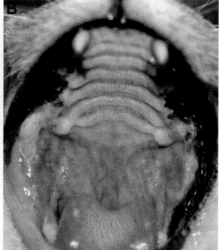

**Fig. 4.** Cat with FCGS cured following dental extractions and adjunctive medical treatment. At the time of extractions (*A*) and after complete healing (*B*). (*Courtesy of* Dr Hennet.)

## *Perioperative Pain Management*

As FCGS is a chronic debilitating disease-inducing severe pain and impairing food intake, pain control is mandatory, preoperatively and perioperatively. A recent study on postoperative pain in cats undergoing dental extractions showed that postoperative pain scores in cats with multiple extractions were higher than preoperative pain scores indicating that the surgical procedure itself induced pain despite the use of multimodal analgesia including local anesthetic blocks, NSAIDs, and an opioid.[79] Multimodal analgesia may include local anesthetic agents, opioids, NSAIDs, alpha-2 adrenoceptor agonists, NMDA-receptor antagonists, and gabapentinoids.[80] Oral surgery, including dental extraction procedures, greatly benefit from the use of locoregional anesthesia. Drugs and techniques have been well documented.[81,82]

Cats with multiple extractions for the treatment of FCGS should be hospitalized for proper pain management, as they may require administration of an opioid for pain relief up to 72 hours after surgery. As the pain scores following multiple extractions may still be higher than those of cats with minimal oral diseases up to 6 days, analgesia needs to be continued after discharge. Cats with severe disease and more intensive oral surgery may take longer to eat after dental extractions, and as hard food may induce pain, soft food should be recommended for at least 1 week after surgery.[79] The Feline Grimace scale has recently been shown to be a reliable parameter to evaluate postoperative pain after dental extractions in cats.[83,84]

Buccal administration of a proprietary injectable solution of 0.02 mg/kg of buprenorphine to cats suffering from chronic gingivostomatitis has been shown to produce a significant analgesic effect than a placebo and showed low interindividual variability in plasma concentration.[85] A pharmacokinetic study has shown that oral administration (0.03 mg/kg) of a compounded formulation of buprenorphine (dissolution in liquid of a 2 mg tablet to give a 0.3 mg/mL solution) resulted in a lesser absorption than the commercially available aqueous formulation (0.3 mg/mL).[86] A recent prospective, blinded, randomized clinical trial has shown that a long-acting (24h) buprenorphine solution provided similar analgesic effects than a regular buprenorphine solution injected thrice a day in cats undergoing dental extractions but elicited less resentment.[87]

### Management of Refractory Cases

Refractory cases are defined as FCGS cats that are still presenting significant oral lesions associated with pain and impairment of food intake 1 month after dental extractions despite the use of adjunct medical treatment to alleviate pain, inflammation, and superinfection. Studies have shown that 30% to 40% of cats show little or no improvement after dental extractions and may be considered refractory cases.[54,61] Medical adjunct treatment of refractory cases includes antimicrobials, anti-inflammatory drugs, analgesics, and immunomodulating agents.

*Antimicrobials* are used to control secondary infection and subsequent worsening of oral inflammatory lesions. Clinical signs associated with secondary infection include halitosis, thick/purulent saliva, and crusting around the oral cavity. There is a great diversity of bacteria associated with dental diseases and FCGS. Based on the environmental conditions, opportunistic bacteria develop, and no specific genera or species has been recognized to play a major role.[5,88] The most prevalent bacterial phyla are Bacteroidetes, Firmicutes, Spirochaetes, and fusobacteria. Most of the genera found to be more abundant in various forms of periodontitis and in FCGS are gram-negatives and anaerobes.[5,68] Antimicrobials commonly used include amoxicillin-clavulanate, clindamycin, and metronidazole.[54,61,62] Recently, fungi have been identified in the oral cavity of healthy cats and FCGS cats and interactions between bacteria and fungi have been shown.[68] Nevertheless, predominant fungi identified are suspected commensals of the oral cavity, and the significant higher fungal diversity found in cats with FCGS than healthy cats is not in favor of a major pathogenic role played by a specific fungus.[68]

*Glucocorticoids* are often administrated to decrease inflammation and stimulate food intake. Retrospective studies on FCGS have shown that glucocorticoids are often used by clinicians before referral for comprehensive treatment.[54,58,59,61] Based on the clinician's habits and the cat's behavior, short-acting or long-acting glucocorticoids are used. Injectable long-acting glucocorticoids should only be reserved for fractious cats, as they do not allow easy modification of treatment, they may be associated with side effects, and resolution of the disease cannot be expected. Personal experience indicates that efficacy decreases with time resulting in more frequent injections and potential risk of abuse. In a double-blinded, randomized controlled study, cats in the control group were given a 3-week course of clindamycin (11 mg/kg/d) associated with 1 mg/kg/d oral prednisolone for the first 7 days, followed by 1 mg/kg/d every other day for the 7 following days, and then followed by 0.5 mg/kg/d every other day for the 7 last days. No significant effect was observed during the course of treatment or after it was stopped.[52]

*NSAIDs* have become popular for the control of inflammation and analgesia. Meloxicam, tolfenamic acid, and robenacoxib have shown similar analgesic effects for the control of postoperative pain in cats.[89,90] Metacam was not shown to affect renal function when used preoperatively at 0.2 mg/kg for dental surgery in cats.[91] Though renal excretory function was not affected, gastro-intestinal adverse effects and proteinuria were increased in cats with chronic kidney disease given a low-dose meloxicam (0.02 mg/kg/d) during a 6-month period.[92] Nevertheless, the WSAVA-Global pain council supports the long-term use of the lowest effective doses of meloxicam and robenacoxib for chronic pain management in cats with stable compromised renal function (minimal changes in bodyweight and creatinine over a period of at least 2 months).[93] Meloxicam is marketed as a liquid oral formulation which can be precisely dosed. Chronic pain management in FCGS cats can benefit from the use of the labeled dose for the first few days followed by progressive dose reduction to the least effective dose.

## Immunomodulating Agents

Recent studies have shown that the oromucosal administration of interferon-omega, oral administration of cyclosporine, and IV injection of stem cells may provide some improvement or even a cure for refractory cats.[4,52,94,95]

### Recombinant Feline Interferon-Omega (rFeIFN-ω)

Interferons (IFNs) are a family of cytokines generated by cells in response to viral infection and which have the ability to impede viral replication and induce apoptosis of infected cells.[96,97] IFN-ω has also been shown to have immunomodulating effects through the regulation of the innate, nonspecific-immune response.[97] A *recombinant feline interferon-omega (rFeIFN-ω)* has been marketed for parvovirus infection in dogs and retroviruses in cats and has been shown to share the typical characteristics of type I human IFN and to have antiviral activity against feline herpesvirus, FCV and feline coronavirus.[98,99] Recombinant human IFN-α (rHuIFN-α) has been used in cats by parenteral administration (IV, IM, SC), but this results in the production of neutralizing antibodies with the inhibition of the therapeutic effects of the active principle. The same event happens with oral administration high but not low-dose rHuIFN-α in cats.[100] The administration of a species-specific feline IFN (rFeIFN) has been shown to prevent this event.[101] Mucosal administration of IFN has also been investigated. The therapeutic effect of IFN after the oromucosal administration is due to immunomodulatory activity through the oropharyngeal lymphoid tissues and via paracrine activity, as this glycoprotein is destroyed during transit through the digestive tract.[102,103] Oral administration of type I IFN may potentiate T-helper 1 (Th1) response.[104] In a randomized, controlled, double-blinded study in cats evaluating direct oral administration of 0.1 MU rFeIFN-ω to refractory cases of FCGS over a 3-month period, 55% of the cats were cured or improved (10% cured, 35% markedly improved, and 10% moderately improved). Pain scores, wellbeing scores, and stomatitis significantly decreased from D0 to D90.[52] rFeIFN-ω has been successfully used to control clinical signs in two cats with type II diabetes mellitus and concurrent FCGS, in which glucocorticoids were contraindicated.[104] Recently, subcutaneous injection of 1 MU/kg rFeIFN-ω was investigated in FCV positive cats presenting FCGS. A significant decrease in clinical signs and stomatitis was observed between D0 and D21. A moderate positive correlation was shown between clinical improvement and decreased viral load, suggesting an effect of systemic administration of rFeIFN-ω on virus replication.[105]

### Cyclosporine (Ciclosporin)

*Cyclosporine* is a calcineurin inhibitor licensed for the management of chronic allergic dermatitis in cats and dogs.[106] It exerts its immunomodulatory effect on the cell-mediated immune system through the inhibition of T lymphocyte function and proliferation and has been shown to induce apoptosis of lymphocytes.[107] A randomized, controlled, double-blinded study of refractory cases of FCGS (FCV status unknown) showed that cats receiving cyclosporine over a 6-week period (n = 9) presented a significant clinical improvement than placebo (n = 7). 77.8% (7/9) of the cats when receiving cyclosporine showed a mean improvement of 52.7% of clinical parameters than 14.3% (1/7) of the cats receiving the placebo. At 6 weeks, the mean improvement of clinical parameters was 52.7% in the cyclosporine group and 12.2% in the placebo group. Based on these promising results, cats in the placebo group were offered the cyclosporin treatment of a new 6 weeks period and showed the same good clinical improvement. The study was extended, and 11 cats received cyclosporin for at least 3 months. 45.5% of them (5/11) showed clinical cure.[94]

*Mesenchymal stem cells*

*Mesenchymal stem cells (MSCs)* are multipotent, fibroblast-like, stromal cells, of non-hematopoietic origin, with self-renewal capacity, present in connective tissue throughout the body. In veterinary medicine, MSCs are obtained mainly from adipose tissue and bone marrow. Frequency in fat is about 10-fold higher than in bone marrow. MSCs regulate immune responses such as altering antibody production by B-lymphocytes, inhibiting T-cell proliferation and shifting T-lymphocyte subtypes, and inducing immune tolerance to allogeneic transplants. They release more than 200 bioregulatory products that have antimicrobial, immunomodulatory, antifibrotic, antiapoptotic, hematopoietic stem cell support, chemoattraction, angiogenesis, neuro-protective, and mitogenic functions.[108–110] The efficacy of both autologous and allogeneic, fresh, adipose-derived MSCs administered intravenously has been studied in cats with refractory FCGS.[4,78,95]

Treatment with 2 intravenous injections, 1 month apart, of fresh autologous adipose-derived MSCs (5 million per kg) in 7 cats with refractory FCGS resulted in complete clinical remission in 3 cats (42.8%) or substantial clinical improvement in 2 others (29.5%) within 1 and 4 months after the first injection. Minimal to no response was observed in 2 cats (29.5%).[4] Improvement of clinical signs was associated with a decrease of oral mucosal lesions. In a similar study investigating the effect of intravenous injections of fresh allogeneic MSCs in 7 cats, 4 cats (57%) showed substantial clinical improvement, and 2 cats had minimal to no improvement at 6 months. 2 of the 4 responders showed clinical cure by 18 to 20 months, whereas 2 of the 3 nonresponders were euthanized at 6 to 12 months. A multi-center clinical trial in the USA reported the result of either autologous (n = 13) or allogeneic (n = 5) adipose-derived MSCs injections in 18 cats with refractory FCGS.[95] Of the 18 cats, 5 (27.8%) showed clinical cure, 8 (44.4%) substantial clinical improvement and 5 (27.8%) no improvement. Clinical response was observed between 3 and 6 months after MSCs therapy. Cats with a low CD4/CD8 ratio and less than 15% cytotoxic CD8 T cells with low expression of CD8 (CD8$^{lo}$) at the start of the study seemed more responsive to the therapy.[4,95] Clinical improvement or cure were less frequent (60% vs 77%) in cats receiving allogeneic than autologous MSCs. Nevertheless, the authors stated that they stopped using autologous adipose-derived MSCs due to the deleterious effect of feline foamy virus on MSCs culture and are now favoring allogeneic adipose-derived MSCs obtained from specific pathogen-free (SPF) cats.[95,111]

## ORAL EOSINOPHILIC LESIONS

Eosinophilic granuloma complex (EGC) comprises 3 different forms of related cutaneous and oral lesions: indolent ulcers, eosinophilic plaque and eosinophilic granuloma.[112–114] Eosinophilic granuloma of the oral cavity appears as pink raised irregular nodules, sometimes ulcerative, which can be located in different areas: dorsum of the tongue, sublingual mucosa, hard palate, soft palate, and palatoglossal folds.[112] The lesions often show whitish/yellowish granules on their surface and have a gritty consistency, which is assumed to be the degenerative collagen observed histopathologically (**Fig. 5**). It has been described to mainly occur in cats less than 2 years of age and may disappear spontaneously in very young cats.[112] In some cats, circulating eosinophilia or other cutaneous manifestation of EGC may also be present.[112,113] Eosinophilic granuloma has been reported to be caused by an underlying hypersensitivity. But other causes such as low-grade bacterial infection, chronic trauma caused by excessive grooming, immunologic factors have also been

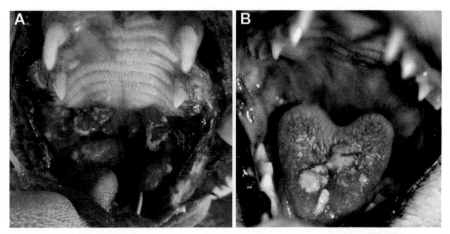

**Fig. 5.** Oral eosinophilic granuloma in cats. Palatal (*A*) and lingual lesions (*B*). (*Courtesy of Dr Hennet.*)

suggested.[112,113] A genetic cause has been suggested based on the observation of a high incidence of eosinophilic granuloma in some littermates, in some breeding colonies including one closed breeding colony composed of interrelated specific-pathogen-free cats. In this latter colony, no evidence of allergic disease, autoimmune disease, exposure to specific bacteria or parasites was demonstrated; dietary trial and various medications (except glucocorticoids) did not alter the progression of lesions in affected cats.[112] Bacteria and viruses have been suggested as potential causes. As any raised, ulcerated lesion in the oral cavity is quickly colonized by bacteria, evidence of bacteria might be due to secondary infection.[114] In most cases, the exact cause of oral eosinophilic granuloma remains undetermined.

A complete dermatologic evaluation must be completed to rule out an identifiable cause of hypersensitivity. In young cats (less than 2 years old) with no allergic condition diagnosed, the possibility of a genetic predisposition and spontaneous regression may be considered. For many years, treatment of recurrent oral eosinophilic granuloma has been based on glucocorticoids.[112] Prednisolone or methylprednisolone is used as the first choice and may be substituted by dexamethasone if no improvement is observed.[115] Fractious cats may benefit from long-acting glucocorticoids.[116,117] For cats nonresponsive to corticosteroid therapy or when glucocorticoids are contraindicated, cyclosporin may be used at the label dosage of 7 mg/kg for 4 to 6 weeks. If a good response is observed, the dosage is tapered down or alternate-day therapy is used, then twice weekly therapy is continued until complete resolution of the lesion.[117,118] Ciclosporin at the recommended daily dose is well tolerated by most cats, with the main adverse effects limited to mild gastro-intestinal disturbances (anorexia, vomiting, soft stool or diarrhea).[106,119,120]

## "CLINICS CARE POINTS"

- COHAT
  - Presumptive diagnosis based on clinical appearance and location
  - CBC and chemical screening
  - Biopsy to confirm diagnosis (eosinophilic infiltration with degranulation and observation of flame figures, which are distinct deposits of collagen coated

with amorphous to granular eosinophilic debris) and rule out neoplasms, foreign body reaction, or chronic stomatitis
- Management at COHAT
  ○ Complete dermatologic evaluation to rule out an identifiable cause of hypersensitivity
  ○ Strict ectoparasite control through the administration of **dinotefuran**, fipronil, imidacloprid, selamectin, or an isoxazoline to all cats of the household and through environmental treatment
  ○ Initiate corticosteroid treatment (**Table 1**)
- Management post-COHAT
  ○ Evaluate glucocorticoids treatment after first week and tapering schedule if effective (see **Table 1**)
  ○ Change to cyclosporin if glucocorticoids are ineffective or are associated with severe side-effects
  ○ Avoid cyclosporin in patients with malignant neoplasia[119] and in FIV and FeLV positive cats[106]
  ○ Control CBC, serum chemistry profile and urinalysis

## PYOGENIC GRANULOMA

The so-called oral pyogenic granuloma in cats appears as a focal, broad-based, or exophytic proliferative lesion of the buccal oral mucosa, apical to the mucogingival line. It has a pink to red appearance, sometimes with a yellowish surface, and is often ulcerated and bleeds easily.[121,122] The term "pyogenic granuloma" is a misnomer, as the lesion is unrelated to bacteria, neither producing pus, nor being strictly speaking a granuloma.[123] It is considered a reactive tumor-like lesion arising in response to various stimuli such as chronic low-grade local irritation. Trauma has been suggested as a cause of the lesion.[124] Most of the lesions in cats arise on the buccal mucosa next to the mandibular first molar tooth, though other sites such as the maxillary fourth pre-molar tooth and maxillary canine tooth may also be observed.[121,122] The lesion may develop very quickly within a few weeks, is bilateral in 50% of the cases and most of the time associated with a traumatic occlusion of the opposite maxillary fourth pre-molar tooth (**Fig. 6**).[121,122]

Histologically, the exophytic mass is composed of granulation tissue with variable degrees of edema and neutrophilic inflammation; the surface is ulcerated and

| Table 1 | | | |
|---|---|---|---|
| Use of glucocorticoids in cats with allergic disease[11,112,115,116] | | | |
| **Drug** | **Route** | **Induction** | **Maintenance** |
| Prednisolone | PO | 2–4 mg/kg q24 h in 1st wk | 2–4 mg/kg q48 h in 2nd wk, then 25% dose reduction each wk for 4 wk |
| Methylprednisolone | PO | 2 mg/kg q24 h in 1st wk | 2 mg/kg q48 h in 2nd wk, then 25% dose reduction each wk for 4 wk |
| Dexamethasone | PO | 0.1–0.2 mg/kg q24 h in 1st wk | 0.05–1 mg/kg q48 h in 2nd wk, then 25% dose reduction each wk for 4 wk |
| Methylprednisolone acetate* | IM | 4 mg/kg q 3 wk | Repeat every 3 wk for a maximum of 3 times |

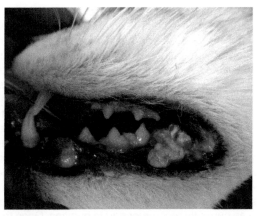

**Fig. 6.** Large pyogenic granuloma associated with traumatic occlusion of the left maxillary fourth premolar tooth in cat. (*Courtesy of* Dr Hennet.)

covered by a thin layer of fibrin or necrotic cellular debris with occasional bacterial colonization on its surface.[121] The clinical and histologic aspects are consistent with the nonlobular capillary hemangioma (non-LCH type of pyogenic granuloma) described in humans, which consists of highly vascular proliferation that resembles granulation tissue.[122–124]

In a retrospective study of 26 cats presenting with an oral pyogenic granuloma, successful treatment was achieved in all cases by removing the occlusal traumatic contact by dental extraction (88%) or coronal reduction of the tooth (coronoplasty/odontoplasty) with a fine abrasive bur under irrigation (12%), possibly associated with lesion excision.[122] In another study of 8 cats, surgical resection of the lesion alone resulted in 100% recurrence.[121] In the author's (PH) experience, coronoplasty is not appropriate in most cases as, once the proliferative lesion is developed, the cusp of the maxillary fourth premolar tooth deeply engages it, and conservative treatment would require amputating most of the main cusp (paracone) of the tooth with subsequent pulpal exposure and need for endodontic treatment. Severe periodontitis with gingival recession and bone loss on the buccal aspect of the mandibular fist molar may result from chronic trauma and may require extraction of this tooth as well.

### "CLINICS CARE POINTS"

- Exophytic proliferative lesion of the buccal oral mucosa next to the mandibular first mandibular tooth with traumatic occlusion of the opposite maxillary fourth premolar
- Perform oral examination including full-mouth dental radiographs
- Biopsy to confirm the diagnosis (granulation tissue with variable degrees of edema and neutrophilic inflammation), and rule out neoplasm
- Extraction of the tooth inducing traumatic occlusion (eg, maxillary fourth premolar tooth) and resection of the lesion

### AUTOIMMUNE CONDITIONS WITH ORAL MANIFESTATIONS
#### Pemphigus Vulgaris

PV is a chronic autoimmune blistering dermatosis that affects the mucosal, mucocutaneous junction and/or skin; the mucosal and/or skin lesions evolve from flaccid blisters (vesicles and/or bullae) to deep erosions and are associated with pain, especially when the lesions develop in the oral cavity. Histopathology shows an intraepithelial suprabasal acantholysis, and either a positive direct immunofluorescence test or the serologic detection of autoantibodies against epithelial cell surface antigens is diagnostic.[125] It is one of the rarest autoimmune skin diseases encountered in animals accounting for 0.1% and 0.2% of canine and feline dermatoses, respectively.[126] In a recent comprehensive review of the literature pertaining to deep pemphigus described in dogs, cats, and horses, PV was identified in only 4 domestic shorthair cats described by the same author.[125] None of these cats had detectable circulating autoantibodies. Lesions were confined to the head/face, and ulcers were the only lesion described. All cats had oral cavity, lips, and nasal planum involvement. One of the cats had nearly the entire oral cavity affected and presented lymphadenopathy, halitosis, and hypersalivation.[126] To have the best chance of achieving a histopathological diagnosis, biopsies should include one-third of the erosion/ulcer and two-thirds of the perilesional mucosa as currently recommended in humans. Once the diagnosis is obtained, treatment is based on high doses of prednisolone (at least 3 mg/kg twice daily) or with a combination of a lower dose of prednisolone and another immunosuppressant such as ciclosporin.[125]

### Bullous Pemphigoid and Mucous Membrane Pemphigoid

BP is an autoimmune blistering dermatosis of humans characterized by autoantibodies specific for collagen XVII epitopes and a clinical presentation of vesicles predominating on haired skin.[127] Contrary to BP whereby the lesion predominates on nonmucosal skin, mucous membrane pemphigoid (MMP), also known as cicatricial pemphigoid, is a rare autoimmune disease of humans in which lesions occur on mucosae or at mucocutaneous junctions because of autoantibodies directed against various basement membrane proteins.[127] These two blistering diseases were first described in 2 cats presenting with vesiculating, erosive, ulcerative and/or crusting dermatitis affecting mainly the lips, soft or hard palate, ear pinnae, and digits.[128] One of these 2 cats and another cat in a subsequent study were diagnosed with MMP based on clinical presentation and immunologic testing.[128,129] Cats with MMP presented predominantly bilateral mucocutaneous and mucosal erythematous, erosive or ulcerative lesions localized on the periorbital, auricular (concave hairless surface of ear pinnae) and perioral (lip commissure) regions.[128,129] Histopathology revealed subepidermal vesicles rich in eosinophils and neutrophils in BP and with few inflammatory cells in MMP.[127] Detection of basement membrane-fixed immunoglobulin G (IgG) autoantibodies is best made from paraffin-embedded specimens submitted for histopathology and tested with direct immunofluorescence or immunoperoxidase methods. Nevertheless, the identification of the targeted autoantigens (eg, collagen XVII or laminin-5) necessitates advanced immunologic methods such as immunoblotting or ELISA tests.[127]

Treatment of MMP in humans is 2-fold, topical to treat localized manifestations and systemic to control autoimmune disorder. Systemic glucocorticoids, frequently administered in combination with immunosuppressive agents such as azathioprine, mycophenolate mofetil, and methotrexate, remain the mainstay of treatment. Intravenous immunoglobulins, plasmapheresis, rituximab, or other anti-CD20 monoclonal antibodies may be considered in patients with resistant or recurrent manifestations.[130] As MMP is a very rare disease in cats, information on treatment is scarce. In the 2 documented feline cases, response to oral glucocorticoids was observed. In one case, lesions recurred when the dose was reduced. In the other case, treatment consisted of 2 mg/kg twice a day of prednisolone for 1 month, then the dose was reduced by half monthly and discontinued after 6 months, and the cats remained free of lesion for the next 6 months.[128,129] Based on the treatment of MMP in humans and treatment of other autoimmune disorders in cats, the combination of glucocorticoids and another immunosuppressant may also be considered.

## CLINICS CARE POINTS

- Auto-immune diseases with oral manifestations are very rare in cats and dogs.
- Pemphigus vulgaris, bullous pemphigoid, and mucous membrane pemphigoid are autoimmune blistering dermatosis described in cats and dogs.
- Diagnosis is made through histopathology and direct immunofluorescence test.
- Treatment is based on high doses of prednisolone (at least 3 mg/kg twice daily) or with a combination of a lower dose of prednisolone and another immunosuppressant.

## DISCLOSURE

J.G. Anderson and P. Hennet have no commercial or financial conflicts of interest to disclose.

## REFERENCES

1. Arzi B, Anderson JG, Verstraete FJ. Oral manifestations of systemic disorders in dogs and cats. J Vet Clin Sci 2008;1(4):112–24.
2. Anderson JG. Approach to diagnosis of canine oral lesions. Compend Contin Educ 1991;13:1215–26.
3. Anderson JG, Peralta S, Kol A, et al. Clinical and histopathologic characterization of canine chronic ulcerative stomatitis. Vet Pathol 2017;54:511–9.
4. Arzi B, Clark KC, Sundaram A, et al. Therapeutic efficacy of fresh, allogeneic mesenchymal stem cells for severe refractory feline chronic gingivostomatitis. Stem Cells Transl Med 2017;6:1710–22.
5. Rodrigues MX, Bicalho RC, Fiani N, et al. The subgingival microbial community of feline periodontitis and gingivostomatitis: characterization and comparison between diseased and healthy cats. Sci Rep 2019;9(1):12340.
6. Soukup JW, Bell CM. The canine furcation cyst, a newly defined odontogenic cyst in dogs: 20 cases (2013-2017). J Am Vet Med Assoc 2020;256:1359–67.
7. Anderson JG, Kol A, Bizikova P, et al. Immunopathogenesis of canine chronic ulcerative stomatitis. PLoS One 2020;15(1):e0227386.
8. Vapniarsky N, Simpson DL, Arzi B, et al. Histological, immunological, and genetic analysis of feline chronic gingivostomatitis. Front Vet Sci 2020; 7:310.
9. Anderson JG, Paster BJ, Kokaras A, et al. Characterization of the oral microbiome in canine chronic ulcerative stomatitis. J Immun Res 2021;7(1): 1037.
10. Mandell GL. Cytokines, phagocytes, and pentoxifylline. J Cardiovasc Pharmacol 1995;25(Suppl 2):S20–2.
11. Thanhauser A, Reiling N, Bohle A, et al. Pentoxifylline: a potent inhibitor of IL-2 and IFN-gamma biosynthesis and BCG-induced cytotoxicity. Immunology 1993; 80:151–6.
12. Siegel AN, Rodrigues N, Nasri F, et al. Novel therapeutic targets in mood disorders: Pentoxifylline (PTX) as a candidate treatment. Prog Neuropsychopharmacol Biol Psychiatry 2021;104:110032.

13. Thornhill MH, Baccaglini L, Theaker E, et al. A randomized, double-blind, placebo-controlled trial of pentoxifylline for the treatment of recurrent aphthous stomatitis. Arch Dermatol 2007;143:463–70.

14. Cavalcante RC, Tomasetti G. Pentoxifylline and tocopherol protocol to treat medication-related osteonecrosis of the jaw: A systematic literature review. J Craniomaxillofac Surg 2020;48:1080–6.

15. Golub LM, Lee HM. Periodontal therapeutics: Current host-modulation agents and future directions. Periodontol 2000 2020;82:186–204.

16. Hajishengallis G, Chavakis T, Lambris JD. Current understanding of periodontal disease pathogenesis and targets for host-modulation therapy. Periodontol 2000 2020;84:14–34.

17. Griffin MO, Ceballos G, Villarreal FJ. Tetracycline compounds with non-antimicrobial organ protective properties: possible mechanisms of action. Pharmacol Res 2011;63:102–7.

18. Golub LM, Elburki MS, Walker C, et al. Non-antibacterial tetracycline formulations: host-modulators in the treatment of periodontitis and relevant systemic diseases. Int Dent J 2016;66:127–35.

19. Kim SE, Hwang SY, Jeong M, et al. Clinical and microbiological effects of a sub-antimicrobial dose of oral doxycycline on periodontitis in dogs. Vet J 2016; 208:55–9.

20. Kim SE, Kim S, Jeong M, et al. Experimental determination of a subantimicrobial dosage of doxycycline hyclate for treatment of periodontitis in Beagles. Am J Vet Res 2013;74:130–5.

21. Makarov MV, Trammell SAJ, Migaud ME. The chemistry of the vitamin B3 metabolome. Biochem Soc Trans 2019;28(47):131–47.

22. Suzuki H, Kunisawa J. Vitamin-mediated immune regulation in the development of inflammatory diseases. Endocr Metab Immune Disord Drug Targets 2015;15: 212–5.

23. Bennett WM, Norman DJ. Action and toxicity of cyclosporine. Annu Rev Med 1986;37:215–24.

24. Archer TM, Boothe DM, Langston VC, et al. Oral cyclosporine treatment in dogs: a review of the literature. J Vet Intern Med 2014;28:1–20.

25. Kobayashi T, Momoi Y, Iwasaki T. Cyclosporine A inhibits the mRNA expressions of IL-2, IL-4 and IFN-gamma, but not TNF-alpha, in canine mononuclear cells. J Vet Med Sci 2007;69:887–92.

26. Matsuda S, Koyasu S. Mechanisms of action of cyclosporine. Immunopharmacology 2000;47(2–3):119–25.

27. Zhang C, Zhang J, Yang B, et al. Cyclosporin A inhibits the production of IL-17 by memory Th17 cells from healthy individuals and patients with rheumatoid arthritis. Cytokine 2008;42:345–52.

28. Pradhan S, Madke B, Kabra P, et al. Anti-inflammatory and Immunomodulatory Effects of Antibiotics and Their Use in Dermatology. Indian J Dermatol 2016;61: 469–81.

29. Arndt H, Palitzsch KD, Grisham MB, et al. Metronidazole inhibits leukocyte-endothelial cell adhesion in rat mesenteric venules. Gastroenterology 1994; 106:1271–6.

30. Reitz M, Rumpf M, Knitza R. Metronidazole induces DNA strand-breaks in cultures of human lymphocytes and phytohemagglutinin-stimulated human lymphocytes. Arzneimittelforschung 1991;41(1):65–9.

31. Fararjeh M, Mohammad MK, Bustanji Y, et al. Evaluation of immunosuppression induced by metronidazole in Balb/c mice and human peripheral blood lymphocytes. Int Immunopharmacol 2008;8:341–50.
32. Tauro A, Beltran E, Cherubini GB, et al. Metronidazole-induced neurotoxicity in 26 dogs. Aust Vet J 2018;96:495–501.
33. Bredal WP, Gunnes G, Vollset I, et al. Oral eosinophilic granuloma in three cavalier King Charles spaniels. J Small Anim Pract 1996;37:499–504.
34. Madewell BR, Stannard AA, Pulley LT, et al. Oral eosinophilic granuloma in Siberian husky dogs. J Am Vet Med Assoc 1980;177:701–3.
35. Vercelli A, Cornegliani L, Portigliotti L. Eyelid eosinophilic granuloma in a Siberian husky. J Small Anim Pract 2005;46:31–3.
36. Mendelsohn D, Lewis JR, Scott KI, et al. Clinicopathological features, risk factors and predispositions, and response to treatment of eosinophilic oral disease in 24 dogs (2000-2016). J Vet Dent 2019;36:25–31.
37. Singh BB, Baker R, Boshell J, et al. Observations on the eosinophilic granules in the dorsal papillae of the dog tongue. J Oral Pathol 1980;9:99–105.
38. Murphy B, Bell CM, Soukup JW. Veterinary oral and maxillofacial pathology. City and state. Hoboken (NJ): Wiley Blackwell; 2020. p. 243.
39. Huugen D, van Esch A, Xiao H, et al. Inhibition of complement factor C5 protects against anti-myeloperoxidase antibody-mediated glomerulonephritis in mice. Kidney Int 2007;71:646–54.
40. Schreiber A, Xiao H, Jennette JC, et al. C5a receptor mediates neutrophil activation and ANCA-induced glomerulonephritis. J Am Soc Nephrol 2009;20: 289–98.
41. Zipfel PF, Wiech T, Rudnick R, et al. Complement Inhibitors in Clinical Trials for Glomerular Diseases. Front Immunol 2019;10:2166.
42. Carpenter S, Tervaert JW, Yacyshyn E. Advances in therapeutic treatment options for ANCA-associated vasculitis. Expert Opin Orphan Drugs 2020;8: 127–36.
43. Krug W, Marretta SM, de Lorimier LP, et al. Diagnosis and management of Wegener's granulomatosis in a dog. J Vet Dent 2006;23:231–6.
44. Woodring T, Abraham R, Frisch S. A case of probable trimethoprim-sulfamethoxazole induced circulating antineutrophil cytoplasmic antibody-positive small vessel vasculitis. Dermatol Online J 2017;23(8). 13030/qt3j9537pg.
45. Phatak S, Aggarwal A, Agarwal V, et al. Antineutrophil cytoplasmic antibody (ANCA) testing: Audit from a clinical immunology laboratory. Int J Rheum Dis 2017;20:774–8.
46. Savige J, Trevisin M, Pollock W. Testing and reporting antineutrophil cytoplasmic antibodies (ANCA) in treated vasculitis and non-vasculitic disease. J Immunol Methods 2018;458:1–7.
47. Mutsaers AJ. Metronomic chemotherapy. Top Companion Anim Med 2009;24: 137–43.
48. Matsuyama A, Woods JP, Mutsaers AJ. Evaluation of toxicity of a chronic alternate day metronomic cyclophosphamide chemotherapy protocol in dogs with naturally occurring cancer. Can Vet J 2017;58:51–5.
49. Wingo K. Histopathologic diagnoses from biopsies of the oral cavity in 403 dogs and 73 cats [published correction appears in. J Vet Dent 2018;35:7–17, 2018;35:307.

50. Mikiewicz M, Paździor-Czapula K, Gesek M, et al. Canine and feline oral cavity tumours and tumour-like lesions: a retrospective study of 486 cases (2015-2017). J Comp Pathol 2019;172:80–7.

51. Falcão F, Faísca P, Viegas I, et al. Feline oral cavity lesions diagnosed by histopathology: a 6-year retrospective study in Portugal. J Feline Med Surg 2020;22: 977–83.

52. Hennet PR, Camy GA, McGahie DM, et al. Comparative efficacy of a recombinant feline interferon omega in refractory cases of calicivirus-positive cats with caudal stomatitis: a randomised, multi-centre, controlled, double-blind study in 39 cats. J Feline Med Surg 2011;13:577–87.

53. Farcas N, Lommer MJ, Kass PH, et al. Dental radiographic findings in cats with chronic gingivostomatitis (2002-2012). J Am Vet Med Assoc 2014;244: 339–45.

54. Jennings MW, Lewis JR, Soltero-Rivera MM, et al. Effect of tooth extraction on stomatitis in cats: 95 cases (2000-2013). J Am Vet Med Assoc 2015;246: 654–60.

55. Winer JN, Arzi B, Verstraete FJ. Therapeutic management of feline chronic gingivostomatitis: A systematic review of the literature. Front Vet Sci 2016;3:54.

56. Rolim VM, Pavarini SP, Campos FS, et al. Clinical, pathological, immunohistochemical and molecular characterization of feline chronic gingivostomatitis. J Feline Med Surg 2017;19:403–9.

57. Lee DB, Verstraete FJM, Arzi B. An Update on Feline Chronic Gingivostomatitis. Vet Clin North Am Small Anim Pract 2020;50:973–82.

58. Hennet P. Chronic gingivo-stomatitis in cats: Long-term follow-up of 30 cases treated by dental extractions. J Vet Dent 1997;14(1):15–21.

59. Bellei E, Dalla F, Masetti L, et al. Surgical therapy in chronic feline gingivostomatitis (FCGS). Vet Res Commun 2008;32(Suppl 1):S231–4.

60. Dolieslager SMJ. Studies on the aetiopathogenesis of feline chronic gingivostomatitis [PhD Thesis]. Glasgow (Scotland): University of Glasgow; 2013.

61. Druet I, Hennet P. Relationship between *Feline calicivirus* load, oral lesions, and outcome in feline chronic gingivostomatitis (caudal stomatitis): Retrospective study in 104 cats. Front Vet Sci 2017;4:209.

62. Harley R, Gruffydd-Jones TJ, Day MJ. Immunohistochemical characterization of oral mucosal lesions in cats with chronic gingivostomatitis. J Comp Pathol 2011; 144:239–50.

63. Fried WA, Soltero-Rivera M, Ramesh A, et al. Use of unbiased metagenomic and transcriptomic analyses to investigate the association between feline calicivirus and feline chronic gingivostomatitis in domestic cats. Am J Vet Res 2021;82: 381–94.

64. Lommer MJ, Verstraete FJ. Concurrent oral shedding of feline calicivirus and feline herpesvirus 1 in cats with chronic gingivostomatitis. Oral Microbiol Immunol 2003;18:131–4.

65. Dowers KL, Hawley JR, Brewer MM, et al. Association of Bartonella species, feline calicivirus, and feline herpesvirus 1 infection with gingivostomatitis in cats. J Feline Med Surg 2010;12:314–21.

66. Quimby JM, Elston T, Hawley J, et al. Evaluation of the association of Bartonella species, feline herpesvirus 1, feline calicivirus, feline leukemia virus and feline immunodeficiency virus with chronic feline gingivostomatitis. J Feline Med Surg 2008;10:66–72.

67. Dolieslager SM, Riggio MP, Lennon A, et al. Identification of bacteria associated with feline chronic gingivostomatitis using culture-dependent and culture-independent methods. Vet Microbiol 2011;148:93–8.
68. Krumbeck JA, Reiter AM, Pohl JC, et al. Characterization of oral microbiota in cats: Novel insights on the potential role of fungi in feline chronic gingivostomatitis. Pathogens 2021;10(7):904.
69. Povey C. Viral diseases of cats: Current concepts. Vet Rec 1976;98:293–9.
70. Gaskell RM, Gruffydd-Jones T. Intractable feline stomatitis. Vet Annu 1977;17:195–9.
71. Reubel GH, Hoffmann DE, Pedersen NC. Acute and chronic faucitis of domestic cats. A feline calicivirus-induced disease. Vet Clin North Am Small Anim Pract 1992;22:1347–60.
72. Peralta S, Carney PC. Feline chronic gingivostomatitis is more prevalent in shared households and its risk correlates with the number of cohabiting cats. J Feline Med Surg 2019;21:1165–71.
73. Johnessee J, Hurvitz A. Feline plasma cell gingivitis-pharyngitis. J Am Anim Hosp Assoc 1983;19:179–81.
74. White SD, Rosychuk RA, Janik TA, et al. Plasma cell stomatitis-pharyngitis in cats: 40 cases (1973-1991). J Am Vet Med Assoc 1992;200:1377–80.
75. Harley R, Helps CR, Harbour DA, et al. Cytokine mRNA expression in lesions in cats with chronic gingivostomatitis. Clin Diagn Lab Immunol 1999;6:471–8.
76. Hung YP, Yang YP, Wang HC, et al. Bovine lactoferrin and piroxicam as an adjunct treatment for lymphocytic-plasmacytic gingivitis stomatitis in cats. Vet J 2014;202:76–82.
77. Squarzoni P, Bani D, Cialdai F, et al. NIR laser therapy in the management of feline stomatitis. SM Dermatolog J 2017;13(3):1021.
78. Arzi B, Taechangam N, Lommer MJ, et al. Stem cell therapy prior to full-mouth tooth extraction lacks substantial clinical efficacy in cats affected by chronic gingivostomatitis. J Feline Med Surg 2021;23:604–8.
79. Watanabe R, Doodnaught G, Proulx C, et al. A multidisciplinary study of pain in cats undergoing dental extractions: A prospective, blinded, clinical trial. PLoS One 2019;14(3):e0213195.
80. Steagall PV, Monteiro-Steagall BP. Multimodal analgesia for perioperative pain in three cats. J Feline Med Surg 2013;15:737–43.
81. Castejón-González AC, Reiter AM. Locoregional anesthesia of the head. Vet Clin North Am Small Anim Pract 2019;49:1041–61.
82. de Vries M, Putter G. Perioperative anaesthetic care of the cat undergoing dental and oral procedures: key considerations. J Feline Med Surg 2015;17:23–36.
83. Evangelista MC, Benito J, Monteiro BP, et al. Clinical applicability of the Feline Grimace Scale: real-time versus image scoring and the influence of sedation and surgery. Peer J 2020;8:e8967.
84. Watanabe R, Doodnaught GM, Evangelista MC, et al. Inter-rater reliability of the Feline Grimace Scale in cats undergoing dental extractions. Front Vet Sci 2020;7:302.
85. Stathopoulou TR, Kouki M, Pypendop BH, et al. Evaluation of analgesic effect and absorption of buprenorphine after buccal administration in cats with oral disease. J Feline Med Surg 2018;20:704–10.
86. Gulledge BM, Messenger KM, Cornell KK, et al. Pharmacokinetic comparison of two buprenorphine formulations after buccal administration in healthy male cats. J Feline Med Surg 2018;20:312–8.

87. Watanabe R, Marcoux J, Evangelista MC, et al. The analgesic effects of bupre-norphine (Vetergesic or Simbadol) in cats undergoing dental extractions: A ran-domized, blinded, clinical trial. PLoS One 2020;15(3):e0230079.
88. Older CE, Gomes MOS, Hoffmann AR, et al. Influence of the FIV status and chronic gingivitis on feline oral microbiota. Pathogens 2020;9(5):383.
89. Murison PJ, Tacke S, Wondratschek C, et al. Postoperative analgesic efficacy of meloxicam compared to tolfenamic acid in cats undergoing orthopaedic sur-gery. J Small Anim Pract 2010;51:526–32.
90. Speranza C, Schmid V, Giraudel JM, et al. Robenacoxib versus meloxicam for the control of peri-operative pain and inflammation associated with orthopaedic surgery in cats: a randomised clinical trial. BMC Vet Res 2015;11:79.
91. Kongara K, Cave N, Weidgraaf K, et al. Effect of non-steroidal anti-inflammatory drugs on glomerular filtration rate and urinary N-acetyl-β-D-glucosaminidase ac-tivity in cats after dental surgery. Vet Anaesth Analg 2020;47:631–6.
92. KuKanich K, George C, Roush JK, et al. Effects of low-dose meloxicam in cats with chronic kidney disease. J Feline Med Surg 2021;23:138–48.
93. Monteiro B, Steagall PVM, Lascelles BDX, et al. Long-term use of non-steroidal anti-inflammatory drugs in cats with chronic kidney disease: from controversy to optimism. J Small Anim Pract 2019;60:459–62.
94. Lommer MJ. Efficacy of cyclosporine for chronic, refractory stomatitis in cats: A randomized, placebo-controlled, double-blinded clinical study. J Vet Dent 2013; 30:8–17.
95. Arzi B, Peralta S, Fiani N, et al. A multicenter experience using adipose-derived mesenchymal stem cell therapy for cats with chronic, non-responsive gingivos-tomatitis. Stem Cell Res Ther 2020;11(1):115.
96. Leal RO, Gil S. The use of recombinant feline interferon omega therapy as an immune-modulator in cats naturally infected with feline immunodeficiency virus: New perspectives. Vet Sci 2016;3(4):32.
97. Li SF, Zhao FR, Shao JJ, et al. Interferon-omega: Current status in clinical appli-cations. Int Immunopharmacol 2017;52:253–60.
98. Yamamoto JK, Okuda T, Yanai A. Antifeline herpesvirus and calicivirus effects of feline interferon. J Interfer Res 1990;10:S114.
99. Ueda Y, Sakurai T, Kasama K, et al. Pharmacokinetic properties of recombinant feline interferon and its stimulatory effect on 2',5' oligoadenylate synthetase ac-tivity in the cat. J Vet Med Sci 1993;55:1–6.
100. Gomez-Lucia E, Collado VM, Miró G, et al. Follow-up of viral parameters in FeLV- or FIV-naturally infected cats treated orally with low doses of human interferon alpha. Viruses 2019;11(9):845.
101. Zeidner NS, Myles MH, Mathiason-DuBard CK, et al. Alpha interferon (2b) in combination with zidovudine for the treatment of presymptomatic feline leuke-mia virus-induced immunodeficiency syndrome. Antimicrob Agents Chemoth 1990;34:1749–56.
102. Cummins JM, Krakowka S, Thompson CD. Systemic effects of interferons after oral administration in animals and humans. Am J Vet Res 2005;66:164–76.
103. Tovey M, Maury C. Oromucosal interferon therapy: marked antiviral and anti-tumor activity. J Interferon Cytokines Res 1999;19:145–55.
104. Leal RO, Gil S, Brito MT, et al. The use of oral recombinant feline interferon omega in two cats with type II diabetes mellitus and concurrent feline chronic gingivostomatitis syndrome. Ir Vet J 2013;66(1):19.
105. Matsumoto H, Teshima T, Iizuka Y, et al. Evaluation of the efficacy of the subcu-taneous low recombinant feline interferon-omega administration protocol for

feline chronic gingivitis-stomatitis in feline calicivirus-positive cats. Res Vet Sci 2018;121:53–8.

106. Colombo S, Sartori R. Ciclosporin and the cat: Current understanding and review of clinical use. J Feline Med Surg 2018;20:244–55.

107. Cridge H, Kordon A, Pinchuk LM, et al. Effects of cyclosporine on feline lymphocytes activated in vitro. Vet Immunol Immunopathol 2020;219:109962.

108. Clark KC, Fierro FA, Ko EM, et al. Human and feline adipose-derived mesenchymal stem cells have comparable phenotype, immunomodulatory functions, and transcriptome. Stem Cell Res Ther 2017;8(1):69.

109. Dias IE, Pinto PO, Barros LC, et al. Mesenchymal stem cells therapy in companion animals: useful for immune-mediated diseases? BMC Vet Res 2019; 15(1):358.

110. Taechangam N, Iyer SS, Walker NJ, et al. Mechanisms utilized by feline adipose-derived mesenchymal stem cells to inhibit T lymphocyte proliferation. Stem Cell Res Ther 2019;10(1):188.

111. Arzi B, Kol A, Murphy B, et al. Feline foamy virus adversely affects feline mesenchymal stem cell culture and expansion: implications for animal model development. Stem Cells Dev 2015;24(7):814–23.

112. Power HT, Ihrke PJ. Selected feline eosinophilic skin diseases. Vet Clin North Am Small Anim Pract 1995;25:833–50.

113. Bloom PB. Canine and feline eosinophilic skin diseases. Vet Clin North Am Small Anim Pract 2006;36(1):141–vii.

114. Wildermuth BE, Griffin CE, Rosenkrantz WS. Response of feline eosinophilic plaques and lip ulcers to amoxicillin trihydrate-clavulanate potassium therapy: a randomized, double-blind placebo-controlled prospective study. Vet Dermatol 2012;23(2):110, e25.

115. Noli C. Flea biology, allergy and control. In: Noli C, Colombo S, editors. Feline dermatology. Cham: Springer; 2020. p. 437–49.

116. Ganz EC, Griffin CE, Keys DA, et al. Evaluation of methylprednisolone and triamcinolone for the induction and maintenance treatment of pruritus in allergic cats: a double-blinded, randomized, prospective study. Vet Dermatol 2012;23(5): 387, e72.

117. Buckley L, Nuttall T. Feline eosinophilic granuloma complex(ities): some clinical clarification. J Feline Med Surg 2012;14:471–81.

118. Palmeiro BS. Cyclosporine in veterinary dermatology. Vet Clin North Am Small Anim Pract 2013;43:153–71.

119. Heinrich NA, McKeever PJ, Eisenschenk MC. Adverse events in 50 cats with allergic dermatitis receiving ciclosporin. Vet Dermatol 2011;22:511–20.

120. Roberts ES, Tapp T, Trimmer A, et al. Clinical efficacy and safety following dose tapering of ciclosporin in cats with hypersensitivity dermatitis. J Feline Med Surg 2016;18:898–905.

121. Riehl J, Bell CM, Constantaras ME, et al. Clinicopathologic characterization of oral pyogenic granuloma in 8 cats. J Vet Dent 2014;31:80–6.

122. Gracis M, Molinari E, Ferro S. Caudal mucogingival lesions secondary to traumatic dental occlusion in 27 cats: macroscopic and microscopic description, treatment and follow-up. J Feline Med Surg 2015;17:318–28.

123. Jafarzadeh H, Sanatkhani M, Mohtasham N. Oral pyogenic granuloma: a review. J Oral Sci 2006;48:167–75.

124. Kamal R, Dahiya P, Puri A. Oral pyogenic granuloma: various concepts of etiopathogenesis. J Oral Maxillofac Pathol 2012;16:79–82.

125. Tham HL, Linder KE, Olivry T. Deep pemphigus (pemphigus vulgaris, pemphigus vegetans and paraneoplastic pemphigus) in dogs, cats and horses: a comprehensive review. BMC Vet Res 2020;16(1):457.

126. Scott DW, Walton DK, Slater MR, et al. Immune-mediated dermatoses in domestic animals - 10 years after part 1. Comp Cont Educ Pract 1987;9:424–551.

127. Olivry T, Jackson HA. Diagnosing new autoimmune blistering skin diseases of dogs and cats. Clin Tech Small Anim Pract 2001;16:225–9.

128. Olivry T, Chan LS, Xu L, et al. Novel feline autoimmune blistering disease resembling bullous pemphigoid in humans: IgG autoantibodies target the NC16A ectodomain of type XVII collagen (BP180/BPAG2). Vet Pathol 1999;36:328–35.

129. Olivry T, Dunston SM, Zhang G, et al. Laminin-5 is targeted by autoantibodies in feline mucous membrane (cicatricial) pemphigoid. Vet Immunol Immunopathol 2002;88:123–9.

130. Buonavoglia A, Leone P, Dammacco R, et al. Pemphigus and mucous membrane pemphigoid: An update from diagnosis to therapy. Autoimmun Rev 2019;18:349–58.

# Update on Endodontic, Restorative, and Prosthodontic Therapy

Brian Hewitt, DVM[a],*, Curt Coffman, DVM[b]

## KEYWORDS

- Endodontic • Pulpitis • Pulp • Necrosis • Apex • Vital pulp therapy
- Root canal therapy • Prosthodontic • Restoration

## KEY POINTS

- Endodontic therapy can preserve the function of teeth with irreversible pulpitis or pulp necrosis
- Root canal therapy success depends on the tooth pathology, as well as the materials and procedures used.
- Mineral trioxide aggregate can increase the success rate of endodontic procedures.
- Vital pulp therapy preserves tooth vitality when appropriate timing and materials used.
- Crown preparation is critical for successful prosthodontic restoration.

## INTRODUCTION

Endodontics is the field of dentistry related to treating disorders of the pulp–dentin complex and periapical tissues. The goals of treatment include preservation (vital pulp therapy) or renewal (regenerative endodontics) of vital tissues within the tooth, or preservation of natural tooth structure as a comfortable and functional component of the oral/dental mechanism when vitality cannot be maintained. Endodontic therapies may include standard root canal therapy (for pulpitis and pulp necrosis), surgical root canal therapy (when standard root canal therapy fails), vital pulp therapy (with direct pulp capping), indirect pulp capping (for near pulp exposure), apexification (to close an open apex), and regenerative endodontics (to revitalize a nonvital tooth).

## ANTIBIOTIC USE IN ENDODONTICS

Although their use in endodontic therapy is controversial,[1] antibiotics are rarely indicated for endodontic procedures. There is an effort in the veterinary profession toward appropriate antimicrobial stewardship.[2] Furthermore, bacteria in endodontic and

[a] Cheyenne West Animal Hospital, 3650 N. Buffalo Drive, Las Vegas, NV 89129, USA; [b] Arizona Veterinary Dental Specialists, 7908 East Chaparral Road #108, Scottsdale, AZ 85250, USA
* Corresponding author.
E-mail address: DocBHew@aol.com

Vet Clin Small Anim 52 (2022) 185–220
https://doi.org/10.1016/j.cvsm.2021.09.003
0195-5616/22/© 2021 Elsevier Inc. All rights reserved.

periapical disease typically exist in biofilms[3,4] and exhibit antibiotic resistance.[5] Finally, many of the materials used in dentistry have antibacterial properties.[6–8] The judicious use of antibiotics is at the discretion of the veterinarian.

## ENDODONTIC ANATOMY

The tooth is divided into 3 anatomic areas, namely, the crown, neck, and root. The pulp contains the vital tissues within the tooth. It is located in the pulp chamber within the crown and the root canal within the root of the tooth, together making up the pulp cavity. The external surface of the crown is nonporous enamel. The external surface of the root is cementum, which is in direct communication with the periodontal ligament. Between the enamel or cementum and the pulp is dentin. Dentin is a porous structure that is permeated with tubules in a roughly conical shape. The dentinal tubules that approximate the pulp are larger in diameter and number than the tubules immediately deep to the pulp or cementum.[9] Immature permanent teeth in both dogs and cats have an open apex until approximately 10 to 11 months of age.[10,11] Multiple ramifications at the apex of the mature tooth exit the root canal, allowing passage of vessels and nerves to the neurovascular systems. This area is the apical delta. Cat canine teeth may have 7 to 22 ramifications,[12] and dog canine teeth may have up to 47 ramifications.[13] The apical delta typically encompasses the apical 3 mm of the root in both dogs and cats,[12,13] but this structure can extend more than 3 mm in the mandibular first molar tooth of the dog.[14] Roots may have lateral canals located at any part of the root, or have furcational canals.[14,15] Furcational and lateral canals in the cervical one-third of the root seem to be rare in dogs.[14] In cats, furcational canals have been shown to be present in 27.2% of maxillary fourth premolar and mandibular first molar teeth.[16] Furcational canals can cause failure of endodontic treatment. Furcational canals are difficult to obturate adequately and not only can harbor endodontic bacteria, but also can act as a conduit for oral bacteria to enter the endodontic system if there is compromise of the periodontal tissues.[16] Immature teeth have a relatively large diameter pulp cavity. After apexogenesis (development of the apex), there is progressive narrowing of the pulp cavity. In nonvital teeth, this narrowing ceases, as a result of the odontoblasts no longer producing dentin. Continued narrowing of the pulp cavity is an important sign when assessing the success of vital pulp therapy (ie, endodontic treatment of vital teeth).

## INDICATIONS AND CONTRAINDICATIONS

Endodontic therapy is indicated when there is compromise of the endodontic system, including:

- Dentoalveolar injuries, including maxillary and mandibular fractures
- Congenital disorders
- Inflammatory and infectious pathologies, including deep caries and periodontal–endodontic lesions
- Idiopathic and miscellaneous disorders

Contraindications to endodontic therapy can be divided into general contraindications and situational contraindications. One general contraindication is a lack of experience of the practitioner. Without appropriate training in the form of lecture and wet laboratory procedures, one should not attempt endodontic treatment on a patient. Another general contraindication is a lack of armamentarium. Without the proper equipment, it is not possible to perform endodontic therapy. Standard root canal therapy cannot be performed on a tooth with 45 mm working length if only 31 mm instruments are available. Situational contraindications occur when the endodontic therapy is not appropriate for the tooth. Comorbid pathology, such as periodontal disease, tooth resorption, or concurrent malignancy, may be a contraindication owing to the poor overall prognosis for the tooth. Another contraindication is endodontic disease of deciduous teeth. A final contraindication is cat teeth other than canines, owing to size, potential comorbid conditions, and potential furcational canals.

## DENTOALVEOLAR INJURIES

Dentoalveolar injuries can be divided into tooth fracture with pulp exposure, tooth fracture without pulp exposure, root fracture, subluxation, luxation, avulsion, concussive injury, thermal injury, alveolar bone fracture, and iatrogenic injury.

### Tooth Fracture with Pulp Exposure

Tooth fractures are relatively common in animals.[17] Tooth fractures that result in pulp exposure are referred to as complicated tooth fractures and may affect the crown only or the crown and root(s). Complicated fractures have a relatively rapid ingress of oral bacteria, resulting in irreversible pulpitis in mature teeth. Complicated fractures are treated by root canal therapy, vital pulp therapy (discussed elsewhere in this article), or extraction.

### Tooth Fracture without Pulp Exposure

Tooth fractures that do not expose the pulp directly are referred to as uncomplicated crown or crown–root fractures. However, endodontic compromise could still happen.[18] These fractures expose dentinal tubules, creating potential bacterial ingress into the pulp. Because the dentinal tubules have a larger diameter as they approximate the pulp chamber,[9] fractures that result in peripulpal dentin exposure are more likely to result in bacterial ingress. If an uncomplicated fracture has no endodontic compromise, it may be treated by indirect pulp capping, composite restoration,[19] or dentin bonding.[20] If a tooth with an uncomplicated fracture remains vital, the exposed dentinal tubules will mineralize and close naturally over several months.[20] Treated teeth should be monitored for signs of endodontic disease, which may take 2 to 3 months, or longer, to develop.[21]

### Root fracture

Root fractures may result from trauma or be secondary to external resorption. With root fractures above the alveolar margin, extraction is indicated. Root fractures in the coronal one-third of the root but below the alveolar margin often require additional stabilization.[22,23] Root fractures in the middle or apical one-third of the root are often stable and may have reversible pulpitis with eventual healing, or may develop endodontic disease of the coronal segment.[22] The tooth must be monitored for apical and periapical disease. Treatment of endodontically compromised teeth with root fractures has been documented using mineral trioxide aggregate (MTA).[24]

### Subluxation, Luxation, and Avulsion

Subluxation, luxation, and avulsion are injuries wherein there is damage of the periodontal ligament. Primary treatment of these injuries has been well-documented.[22,25,26] Subluxation results in loosening of the periodontal ligament without tooth displacement,[25] but may result in endodontic compromise. The affected tooth should be monitored for development of endodontic disease. Luxation is the partial displacement of a tooth within its alveolus. Luxation may be lateral, intrusive, or extrusive,[25] and often results in endodontic compromise. Endodontically compromised teeth should have root canal therapy or be extracted. Immature luxated teeth may be more resistant to endodontic compromise.[25] Avulsion is the complete displacement of the tooth from its alveolus.[25] Avulsed teeth are nonvital and require replantation, fixation, and endodontic treatment. Successful root canal therapy up to 40 days after replantation has been documented,[25] but it is typically recommended to be performed 7 to 14 days after replantation.[25]

### Concussive injury

A concussive injury may result in pulpal hemorrhage and pulp necrosis. The affected tooth may or may not become discolored. Transillumination of the tooth will often be abnormal. Pulp necrosis causes the normal narrowing of the pulp cavity to cease. This is identifiable on intraoral radiography when the injury occurs before complete maturation of the tooth (**Fig. 1**). However, radiography has limited accuracy in diagnosing a nonvital tooth. A study of intrinsically stained teeth revealed radiographic changes in 57.1% of affected teeth, yet 92.2% had pulp necrosis.[27] This finding was corroborated by a more recent study.[28] Pulp vitality testing may include specific testers made for human teeth[29] or pulse oximetry to detect pulpal blood flow.[30] The accuracy of these techniques in animal teeth is not consistently confirmed.

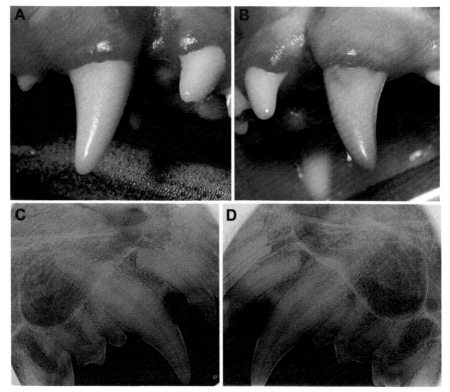

**Fig. 1.** (*A*) Clinical photograph of a vital tooth 104. (*B*) Clinical photograph of a nonvital tooth 204; note the intrinsic discoloration of its crown. (*C*) Intraoral radiography of tooth 104. (*D*) Intraoral radiography of the nonvital tooth 204; note its wider root canal and thinner dentinal walls compared with tooth 104.

## Thermal injury

Thermal injury can cause reversible or irreversible pulpitis and may occur as a result of electric shock or iatrogenic injury (discussed elsewhere in this article).

## Alveolar Bone Fracture

Dentoalveolar injuries may result in alveolar bone fracture. Alveolar fracture is also associated with maxillary or mandibular fracture.[31] Such fractures may damage the alveolus or disrupt the blood supply to teeth, resulting in pulp necrosis.

## Iatrogenic Tooth Injury

Prolonged contact time between a dental scaler or rubber polishing cup and the tooth surface can result in thermal injury.[32] Insufficient water cooling or excessive pressure during defect preparation can result in heating of the tooth surface. Thermal injury may result in reversible or irreversible pulpitis and pulp necrosis. Pulp necrosis is treated with root canal therapy or extraction. Iatrogenic tooth injury can result from inadvertent pulp exposure during preparation for a restoration. This type of injury is treated typically with direct pulp capping and restoration.

## CONGENITAL DISORDERS

A carnassial tooth malformation[33] may result in communication between the pulp and the oral cavity through furcational canals. Dens invaginatus[34] or enamel hypoplasia[19] create potential for endodontic compromise.

## INFLAMMATORY DENTAL DISEASES

Inflammatory or infectious causes may result in endodontic compromise of the teeth. Carious lesions that approximate the pulp may result in pulpal inflammation or infection. Fungal infections, osteomyelitis, and osteonecrosis may result in endodontic disease. Periodontal disease that reaches the apical delta (ie, a "perio-endo lesion") can result in bacteria entering the pulp through the apical delta. Bacterial ingress through exposed root dentin or lateral accessory, or furcational canals is possible, although uncommon,[1] except in the mandibular first molar tooth of the dog owing to the incidence of lateral canals.[14]

## IDIOPATHIC AND MISCELLANEOUS CONDITIONS

Vascular compromise of the teeth resulting from maxillectomy or mandibulectomy procedures may result in pulp necrosis. In the authors' experience, some brachycephalic breeds (eg, Pugs and French bulldogs), seem to have a predisposition to nonvital teeth with no apparent underlying pathology. A congenital disorder may be the underlying cause. Other miscellaneous causes include disruption of the blood supply owing to odontogenic cyst[35] or neoplasia.

## STANDARD (NONSURGICAL) ROOT CANAL THERAPY

The most common endodontic procedure performed in veterinary dentistry is standard root canal therapy. The instruments and materials required can be divided into 4 categories, based on the different steps of this procedure.

- Endodontic access
- Cleaning, shaping, and disinfecting the pulp cavity
- Obturation

- Restoration

Standard root canal therapy is indicated for the treatment of mature teeth (ie, teeth with a closed apex) and endodontic compromise owing to pulp exposure (traumatic or intentional crown reduction), irreversible pulpitis, or pulp necrosis. Contraindications include an open apex, concurrent disease (eg, periodontal disease or tooth resorption), complicating factors (eg, pulp stones, sclerotic root canal, carnassial tooth malformation), and deciduous teeth. The basic equipment and step-by-step hybrid procedure for root canal therapy are listed in **Boxes 1** and **2**.

---

**Box 1**
**Basic endodontic equipment**

*General*
Dental delivery system, with high and low-speed handpieces
Dental radiology generator and radiographic film or software
Dental dam or rubber glove

*Access*
Friction grip burs: #1, 1S, 2, 2S, 4, 4S, 333L
Right angle burs: #1, 1S, 2, 2S, 4, 4S
Mueller right angle burs #140 to 180
Peeso reamers: #1 to 6
Gates-Glidden #1 to 4

*Cleaning*
Barbed broaches
Endodontic irrigation needles
Irrigation solution
- 5.25% NaOCl (bleach)
- EDTA 15% to 17%
- Chlorhexidine gluconate 0.12% to 2.00%
Endodontic ruler
Endodontic files
- H-files, 21 to 60 mm
- K-files, 21 to 60 mm
- K-reamers (optional)
Rubber endo stops
File lubricant

*Obturation*
Absorbent points
Gutta percha points
Root canal sealer
Lentulo paste fillers
Pluggers/spreaders
Heat source

*Restoration*
Diamond bur
Acid etch
Curing light
Glass ionomer or Compomer
Bonding agent
Composite (flowable, hybrid, or both)
Composite finishing system
Liquid polish/sealer

**Box 2**
**Root canal therapy (step by step)**

*Preparation*
- Clean/polish tooth (glycerin and fluoride-free paste)
- Radiograph
- Disinfect with 0.12% to 2.00% chlorhexidine
- Apply rubber dam

*Access*
- Initial access: #1 to 4 friction grip round bur
- Continued access with friction grip or right angle round bur
- Achieve straight-line access
  - Hand files
  - Peeso reamer
- Coronal widening
  - Gates Glidden
  - Peeso reamer

*Cleaning and shaping*

Remove pulp with barbed broach
- Measure the working length
- Radiograph to confirm working length
- Cleaning/shaping canal
  - Hand files
  - Engine driven system
  - Lubrication (aqueous or gel)
- Frequent irrigation
  - 5.25% NaOCl (bleach)/15% to 17% EDTA (alternating)
  - Chlorhexidine 0.12% to 2.00% (alternative to bleach)
- Reciprocate with master file

*Obturation*
- Dry canal with absorbent points
- Choose master gutta percha point (slight tug-back)
- Radiograph to confirm fit
- Place root canal sealer (technique depends on sealer)
- Place master gutta percha point
- Place accessory gutta percha, if needed (lateral/vertical compaction)
- Radiograph to confirm fill

*Restoration (composite)*
- Remove damaged enamel/dentin from fracture site
- Bevel enamel at access site (on nonocclusal sites)
- Clean debris from access/fracture site (spoon excavator or bur)
- Acid etch
- Place intermediate layer (glass ionomer)
- Apply dentin bonding agent
- Place composite restoration
  - Flowable composite
  - Hybrid composite
  - Thin layer flowable, followed by hybrid
  - Shape/finish restoration surface
  - Apply liquid polish
  - Radiograph

## ENDODONTIC ACCESS

A dental dam is advised for endodontic treatment.[1,36] Endodontic access may be achieved through a coronal fracture site in some canine and all incisor teeth in the dog and all canine teeth in the cat.[1] Typical access sites have been described.[37-40]

Access is achieved using a standard or surgical length round bur, size 1, 2, or 4. For larger canine teeth, an extended-length round bur (Mueller bur) is used. The bur is initially positioned perpendicular to the enamel. After the enamel is breached (1–2 mm), the bur is angled within dentin toward the apex of the tooth. Access to the root canal is confirmed with a small file (size 10 or Pathfinder).

### Tips

- More control can be achieved if a high-speed friction grip bur is used to penetrate the enamel, followed by a low-speed right angle bur of a similar size to enter the pulp chamber.
- If the bur does not enter the pulp chamber, remove the bur from the handpiece, place it in the access site, and take a 2-view radiograph to assess the accuracy and proximity of the approach (**Fig. 2**).

After access is confirmed, the opening is widened and a straight-line access to the apex achieved. The term "straight-line" is a misnomer because a true straight line from access to apex is not feasible. Near straight-line access decreases potential complications such as perforation, zipping, ledging, or instrument separation.[26,41] The coronal root canal is widened to allow access of endodontic instruments without binding. Straight-line access and access widening are performed concurrently using hand files, Gates–Glidden reamers, Peeso reamers, or rotary access widening files.

In stenotic or calcified coronal aspects of the root canal, diamond-coated ultrasonic tips may improve access. If a small (06–08) endodontic file can access the root canal, filing with lubricant will allow progressively larger files to be used. If the root canal cannot be accessed by the measures described elsewhere in this article, treatment options are s follows.

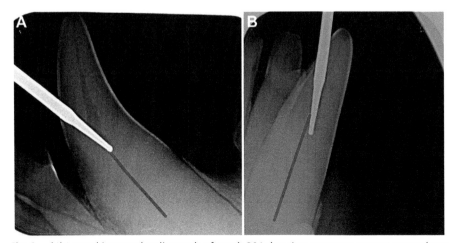

**Fig. 2.** . (*A*) Lateral intraoral radiograph of tooth 304 showing apparent correct access (root canal marked in red). (*B*) Occlusal intraoral radiograph of same tooth 304 showing missed root canal access, indicating the importance of multiple views.

- Surgical root canal therapy.
- Multirooted tooth: Amputate the obstructed root and continue root canal therapy on the remaining roots.
- Extraction.
- If the root canal seems to be completely obstructed and apical pathology is absent, restore the fracture and access sites and monitor for future periapical pathology. If preexisting periapical pathology is present, one of the options described elsewhere in this article is required.

## INSTRUMENTATION

The root canal is then cleaned of debris and tissue. A barbed broach is used to remove any residual pulp. The root canal is cleaned and shaped by one of several methods. These can be divided into hand instrumentation, engine-driven systems, or a combination of these.

### Hand Instrumentation

The basic technique for cleaning is instrumentation with hand files. All operators must become proficient in hand-filing before using any other cleaning system. Hand-filing is required for wide root canals, when engine-driven systems cannot engage the root canal walls, or in the event of equipment failure of other systems.

Hand files are divided into 3 types: Hedstrom (H) files, Kerr (K) files, and K-Reamers. They are made in standardized ISO sizes from size 06 to size 140. The ISO size indicates the tip diameter of the file. A size 10 file is 0.1 mm diameter at the tip, size 40 file is 0.4 mm diameter at the tip, and so on. Standard files come in 21 mm, 25 mm, and 31 mm lengths. Veterinary-length files are made in 40 mm, 60 mm, 120 mm, and 180 mm lengths. Files may be made of stainless steel or nickel–titanium alloy.

### Hedstrom files

H-files have an aggressive cutting edge on a smaller central core.[1] They are used with a push–pull action, with no rotation. H-files have aggressive cutting with rapid removal of dentin. However, the smaller core increases risk for separation. If an H-file is rotated in the root canal, it can become lodged in the dentin, with a risk of separation.

### Kerr files

K-files are made by twisting a triangular, square, or rhomboidal tapered metal blank. Triangular files are more flexible but have less strength than square or rhomboidal files.[1] They are used in a push–pull action or one-quarter turn followed by pull. K-files are less likely to break or become lodged in the dentin than H-files, are more flexible that K-reamers, and have greater contact with the dentinal surface than K-reamers owing to the increased number of flutes.[1] K-files have less effective cutting and debris removal than H-files, and more than K-reamers.

### K-reamers

K-reamers are prepared similar to K-files, but with fewer twists.[1] They have less dentin contact, are stiffer than K-files, and are used in a rotational "watch-winding" action. K-reamers are stronger than other file types. However, they have less effective cutting and removal of dentinal debris.

Once the root canal working length has been determined, rubber endo stops are set to the working length on all instruments. In the step–down or crown–down techniques, larger files are used to enlarge the coronal aspect of the root canal, followed by progressively smaller instruments, until the working length is reached. In the step–back technique, the smallest file that will reach working length is used, followed by progressively larger files, until the largest file (master file) that can be passed to the working length is reached.[1,26,42] A hybrid technique combines initial enlargement and flaring of the coronal aspect of the root canal, reducing midshaft binding of files, followed by a step–back technique. File-binding can lead to the erroneous tactile sensation that a file has reached the apex when it has not.

### Engine-driven Instruments

Engine-driven instruments come in 2 basic types: rotary or reciprocating. Rotary instruments operate with continuous rotation. Reciprocating instruments operate in an automated push–pull action or with alternating forward and reverse rotation. Engine-driven instruments can increase the speed of performing root canal procedures.[43] The nickel–titanium alloy used for these instruments is flexible, allowing instruments to navigate curved canals better than rigid instruments.[44] Engine-driven instruments have a higher operating cost, the need for specialized equipment, and difficulty retrieving separated instruments from curved canals.[41,45] Each system has advantages and disadvantages. All engine-driven systems should be used with copious irrigation.[1] Appropriate training in the use of any engine-driven instrument is necessary to avoid procedure complications.

### Lubrication

During the cleaning and shaping of canals, lubrication is necessary. Lubricants help the instruments to negotiate the root canal, dissolve organic and mineral components of the root canal, and decrease friction and file binding. Lubricants may be aqueous or in paste form. For hand-files, a paste lubricant is acceptable. Aqueous lubricants are preferred for rotary instruments, with EDTA being preferred over NaOCl (bleach).[46]

### Irrigation

During the cleaning of the canal, irrigation is essential. The purpose of irrigation is disinfection, lubrication, dissolution of organic and/or mineral material, disruption of biofilms, removal of debris, and removal of the smear layer.[1,47,48] Irrigants include bleach, chlorhexidine, EDTA, and MTAD.

#### Sodium hypochlorite (NaOCl, bleach)
Bleach has antimicrobial, lubricant, and tissue-dissolving properties. It is able to dissolve the organic components of the smear layer.[49] Strengths between 1% and 6% are used. The strength does not significantly impact the antibacterial efficacy.[50,51] Full-strength (5.25%) bleach is recommended. One study indicated that only higher strength bleach had the ability to disrupt biofilms.[49] The use of higher strength bleach may result in increased potential for complications and pain in humans.[52,53] Bleach effectiveness can be enhanced by warming, increased volume, longer contact time, and ultrasonic agitation.[47]

#### Chlorhexidine gluconate
Chlorhexidine gluconate is antimicrobial and has less tissue toxicity than bleach. It has no tissue dissolution properties, nor any effect on the smear layer or biofilms. However, clinical success using chlorhexidine as an irrigant is comparable with that of bleach.[7,54,55] Chlorhexidine gluconate should not be used concurrently with bleach owing to the potential for the formation of the insoluble, toxic compound parachloroaniline.[47]

*Ethylenediamine tetra-acetic acid*
During cleaning of the root canal both organic and mineral debris become lodged in the dentinal tubules. This debris is called the smear layer. There is disagreement as to whether there is benefit from leaving or removing the smear layer in endodontic therapy.[48] Removal of the smear layer is generally recommended. Bleach dissolves the organic components of the smear layer, but not mineral components. EDTA is a chelator that dissolves the mineral components of the smear layer. EDTA has no anti-microbial activity and does not disrupt biofilms.[47] EDTA and bleach used in alternating irrigation cycles is a very effective combination.[47]

*Mixture of tetracycline, detergent, and acid*
MTAD is a combination irrigant that has been promoted for final canal irrigation.[42] MTAD has antimicrobial properties, the ability to remove the smear layer, and is less toxic to tissues than bleach.[42] However, 5.25% bleach is more effective than MTAD at disrupting biofilms.[3,47]

*Irrigant Delivery*

Irrigants can be delivered by positive pressure, using a side-vented endodontic needle, with or without ultrasonic agitation, or with a negative-pressure system. Ultrasonic agitation in addition to positive-pressure irrigation has been promoted, but the effect on the clinical outcome is variable.[56] Positive-pressure irrigation may increase potential for complications from extrusion in humans,[57] which is exacerbated by ultrasonic agitation.[58] Negative-pressure irrigation systems provide for larger volumes of irrigant delivery and less chance of extrusion.[47]

## OBTURATION

Obturation is the 3-dimensional filling of the root canal, with the goal of blocking all apical and nonapical ramifications (apical delta, secondary, lateral, and furcational canals). Obturation is accomplished by the use of a root canal sealer with gutta percha (GP) in some form.

*Root Canal Sealers*

Root canal sealers help to prevent apical leakage, prevent bacterial ingress into the root canal, and entomb any residual bacteria in the root canal.[59] Common types include zinc oxide-eugenol, calcium hydroxide (CaOH), resin, soft bonded resin, silicone, and MTA-based sealers. Sealer examples are listed in **Table 1**. Bleach as the final irrigant may interfere with resin-based sealers.[47] Guttaflow 2, AH Plus, and MTA Fillapex have generally performed well, and are logical choices.[8,59–64]

*Obturation Techniques*

Obturation material is typically GP or resilon, although studies have shown GP to be more reliable than resilon.[65,66] With most techniques, a master GP cone is used (typically corresponding with the master file used), which should be trial fit in the root canal, and a radiograph is obtained. The master cone must reach the apical stop (apical end of the prepared root canal). A slight "tug-back" when the cone is removed is desirable, indicating a snug fit. A cone that has slight tug-back, but does not reach the apical end of the root canal is not appropriate.

Tip: When the appropriate fit of the master GP cone is confirmed, the cone should be marked at the level it enters the tooth with a marker or a slight nick in the surface of the cone, so that when the final placement is made, the operator is certain that the cone is fully inserted.

**Table 1**
**Root canal sealers**

| Product | Manufacturer | Sealer Type |
|---|---|---|
| TubliSeal | Kerr Endodontics – Brea, CA | Zinc oxide-eugenol |
| Sealapex | Kerr Endodontics – Brea, CA | Calcium hydroxide-based |
| AH Plus | Dentsply Sirona USA - New York, NY | Resin-based |
| Epiphany | Kerr Endodontics – Brea, CA | Soft bonded resin |
| Guttaflow 2 | Coltene/Whaledent - Cuyahoga Falls, OH | Silicone-based |
| MTA Fillapex | Angelus - Londrina-PR, Brazil | MTA-based |
| Neosealer Flo | Avalon Biomed - Bradenton, FL | MTA-based |
| Endoseal | Maruchi, Inc. - Gangwon-do, South Korea | MTA-based |
| Endosequence BC sealer | Brassler USA - Savannah, GA | MTA-based |
| BioRoot RCS | Septodont - Saint Maur des Fosses, France | MTA-based |

When using a root canal sealer that has a longer setting time (eg, AH Plus = 8 hours[59] or MTA Fillapex = 130 minutes[61]), the canal should be filled with accessory GP cones. Guttaflow 2 is a combination of silicone-based sealer with powdered GP and nano silver particles[59] and has a curing time of 25 to 30 minutes. The fast-setting version of Guttaflow 2 has a curing time of 8 to 10 minutes.[59] Guttaflow 2 is used with a single GP master cone.

### Gutta Percha Placement Techniques

1. Cold lateral condensation: The master GP cone is coated with sealer and placed to working length. Spreaders are used to adapt the GP to the walls of the root canal. Accessory GP cones are subsequently placed and adapted with spreaders until the root canal is filled.
2. Warm vertical condensation: After placement of the master GP cone, the GP is warmed with a heated instrument (eg, Kerr Touch N Heat or Sybron Endo System B), and pluggers are used to vertically compact the warmed GP and accessory cones to fill the root canal.
3. Thermoplastic technique: In this technique, the accessory GP cones are heated before placement manually or with a carrier-based system, followed by manual compaction. Some techniques are less effective or have a higher rate of complications.[43,67]
4. Thermomechanical technique (McSpadden): A rotational condensation instrument on a low-speed handpiece warms the GP via friction and mechanically compacts the GP. Although the condenser is rotating, accessory GP cones are fed in to the root canal until it has been completely obturated.[1,68,69]

Mechanical compaction of the GP may increase the risk of complications, such as extrusion of the sealer or GP, or fracture of a compromised root.[67,70]

### Guttaflow 2

The Guttaflow 2 has ease of use, a rapid setting time, and slight expansion on setting, resulting in improved adaptation to the root canal. The root canal is filled with Guttaflow 2 using mixing tips with a lentulo paste filler, veterinary-length tips (45 mm × 17G, 45 mm × 20G, or flexible 11 cm × 0.5 mm diameter), 20G to 22G intravenous catheter, or a 3.5F polypropylene urinary catheter for placement. After root canal filling, the master GP cone is placed and the Guttaflow 2 allowed to cure before restoration.

## RESTORATION

The final step in root canal therapy is restoration, which is covered in detail elsewhere in this article.

## SUCCESS RATE OF STANDARD ROOT CANAL THERAPY

Standard root canal therapy in dogs has a high success rate. One study indicated a 94% rate of success or no evidence of failure,[71] with periapical lucency or root resorption being a negative prognostic indicator. A study in cats indicated an 81% rate of success or no evidence of failure,[72] with external root resorption or cats 5 years of age or older being negative prognostic indicators. Success is determined by subsequent imaging of the treated tooth (intraoral radiography or a cone beam computed tomography scan [CBCT]). Periapical pathology may take 6 months to develop after a failed procedure.[47] Post-treatment imaging at 6 months, followed by additional imaging annually, is reasonable.

## IMAGING IN ENDODONTICS

Traditionally, intraoral radiography has been used for imaging dental pathology. With the advent of CBCT scans, options have expanded. Traditional CT scanners (64-Multi-detector Row Computed Tomography) are of limited benefit in veterinary dentistry.[73] If a traditional CT scan is used, a slice size of 0.5 to 1.0 mm is ncessary.[74] A CBCT scan is equal to or superior to intraoral radiography in detecting dental pathology and determining procedure success.[75,76] A CBCT scan is more cost effective, faster, and has less radiation exposure than traditional CT scanners.

## ROOT CANAL THERAPY COMPLICATIONS

Complications include damage caused by instruments, anatomic or endodontic-related complications, extrusion of materials, inadequate obturation, and instrument separation.

### Damage Caused by Instruments

An inappropriate angle or depth of access preparation can result in a missed root canal and tooth damage, including perforation of the lateral wall or furcation of the tooth. Minor perforations may be repaired by routine obturation, whereas others should be repaired with MTA.[77] Inadequate straight-line access can result in underinstrumentation or overinstrumentation of the root canal with hand files, resulting in ledging, transportation, or zipping.[1]

### Anatomic or Endodontic Pathology

Anatomic complications, such as sclerosis, diffuse pulpal mineralization, pulp stones, or enamel pearls, can make root canals inaccessible. Congenital defects (eg, carnassial tooth malformation) may cause an inability to seal all routes of bacterial ingress and extraction is often warranted. Roots with chronic endodontic pathology or endodontic disease that developed during apexogenesis may have a thin apex that is easily perforated by instruments. Apex perforation is treated by means of an apexification procedure. Another complication is persistent bleeding from the root canal. Persistent bleeding may be related to an incomplete cleaning of the root canal or may originate from larger ramifications in the apical delta or other locations (lateral canals). Persistent bleeding can be treated by the following methods.

- Two-step treatment: The root canal is filled with a CaOH paste, a sterile cotton pellet, and a temporary restoration. The CaOH is left for 2 weeks to 2 months, then removed, and root canal therapy is completed in the normal manner after stimulated closure of the open apex.[47,78,79]
- One-step treatment: An apical plug of MTA is placed. A small amount of powdered MTA can initially be placed, followed by layers of MTA in a putty-like consistency to an apical fill of 3 to 5 mm.
- One-step treatment, option 2: A bleach-moistened paper point can be placed in the canal until bleeding halts, then root canal therapy can be performed using an MTA-based root canal sealer.[61]

### Extrusion of Materials

Extrusion of GP, sealer,[59] irrigant, or MTA may occur. Extrusion of GP and some sealers does not create significant reactions.[21] Extrusion of bleach has been associated with pathology in humans.[52,53] Guttaflow and MTA have good biocompatibility.[63,80] However, there is at least 1 documented case of paresthesia associated with the extrusion of MTA.[81] The extrusion of materials is unlikely in cats with intact apices owing to small diameter ramifications.[12]

### Inadequate Obturation

Voids in the obturation on final radiographs are not uncommon. If the apical one-third of the root canal is free of voids, success is more likely. However, owing to the possibility of lateral canals or residual contaminants contributing to treatment failure, repeat cleaning and obturation is advised when voids are present.

### Instrument Separation

The separation of instruments during endodontic procedures can occur.[42,46] Separation may happen with files, broaches, and rotary instruments. Instrument separation commonly occurs owing to user error. Broaches can separate if they are too large and engage the root canal walls. Separation can happen with dull or damaged hand files. Burs, Gates Glidden, and Peeso reamers can separate if they are overused (dull), are used with too much apical force (binding), or are passed into a root canal such that angular stress is applied to the shaft. Nickel–titanium alloy rotary instruments can separate if dull or excessive apical force results in binding. If an instrument separates, a radiograph should be obtained to determine the location of the instrument. Instruments deeper in the root canal are difficult to retrieve. Retrieval techniques have been addressed in detail in other publications.[1,41] If the instrument cannot be removed and adequate apical cleaning and obturation can be performed around the instrument, the instrument is included in the obturation. If the separated instrument obstructs apical cleaning, then surgical root canal therapy or extraction should be considered. If an instrument is left in a root canal, the tooth is monitored for failure in the future. To reduce potential for instrument separation, follow these guidelines.[41]

- Use appropriately sized instruments
- Achieve straight-line access to decrease bending
- Use appropriate lubrication (never instrument a dry root canal)
- Flare the coronal aspect of the root canal to prevent shaft binding
- Do not overuse instruments; change files and rotary instruments as directed by the manufacturer (most human files are single use)

- Do not rotate H-files in root canal
- Use caution with prebent files because prebending weakens them
- Never use excessive force on an instrument in a root canal

### Air Embolism

Although rare, human death by air embolism during root canal therapy has been reported. The presumed cause is from blowing high-pressure air into the root canal orifice. An animal study confirmed that this can be a fatal complication in dogs.[82]

## MINERAL TRIOXIDE AGGREGATE AND OTHER CALCIUM SILICATE CEMENTS

Certain endodontic procedures require the use of a bioactive cement. Previously, the standard material used was CaOH. The use of MTA, rather than CaOH, results in higher success rates and has certain procedural advantages over the use of CaOH. Some specific calcium silicate cements are listed in **Table 2**. Some MTA products can be used in a thinner consistency as a root canal sealer.[83]

## ENDODONTIC PROCEDURES OF VITAL PULP TISSUE

Procedures for vital pulp tissues are indirect pulp capping and vital pulp therapy. Vital pulp therapy is commonly used.

### Indirect Pulp Capping

Indirect pulp capping is performed when there is near-pulp exposure owing to fracture, carious lesion, or preparation for restoration. If the dentin is 5 mm or more thick, direct composite restoration may be performed.[26] If the dentin is thinner, a layer of CaOH or MTA is placed over the area, followed by glass ionomer and composite restoration.[84]

### Vital Pulp Therapy

Vital pulp therapy is indicated when there is pulp exposure of an immature tooth, recent (ideally <48 hours)[85] complicated fracture of a mature tooth, or secondary to a crown reduction procedure. The procedure involves partial pulpectomy, direct pulp capping, and restoration. Direct pulp capping may also be performed when there is iatrogenic pulp exposure during preparation for the placement of a composite restoration on a vital tooth. A thin layer of MTA is placed,[86,87] followed by glass ionomer and composite restoration.

Tip: In most patients, mature teeth with closed apices and complicated fractures of any duration are best treated by root canal therapy, owing to higher success rate and fewer required follow-up procedures.

Contraindications for vital pulp therapy include complicated tooth fractures of uncertain duration of pulp exposure, complicated fractures of mature teeth with greater than 48 hours duration of pulp exposure, teeth with suspected irreversible pulpitis, nonvital teeth, and teeth with periapical pathology. Some complicated fractures of immature teeth of 7 to 14 days or longer duration of pulp exposure may be successfully treated by vital pulp therapy. If vital pulp therapy is not successful in these teeth, it may allow the pulp to remain vital long enough for apexogenesis to occur before failure, allowing root canal therapy to be performed later. Additional equipment and step-by-step procedure are listed in **Boxes 3** and **4**.

### Success Rate and Complications of Vital Pulp Therapy

The success of vital pulp therapy depends on the duration of pulp exposure and the materials used. Radiographic follow-up should initially be performed at 3 to 6 months

**Table 2**
**Calcium silicate cements**

| Product | Manufacturer | Setting Time[a] | Advantages | Dis-advantages |
|---------|--------------|-----------------|------------|----------------|
| ProRoot MTA | Dentsply Sirona USA - New York, NY | 2.5–4.0 hours[b] | Most research performed | Long setting time |
| Biodentine | Septodont - Saint Maur des Fosses, France | 10–12 min | Excellent performance, increased calcium release | Unit dose[c] capsules |
| MTA Angelus | Angelus - Londrina-PR, Brazil | 15 min | Multidose vials | |
| MTA Repair HP | Angelus - Londrina-PR, Brazil | 15 min | Improved handling | Unit dose[c] |
| NeoMTA 2 | Avalon Biomed - Bradenton, FL | 14 min (putty), 70 min (sealer consistency) | 3-y shelf life, mix to variable consistency | |
| NeoPUTTY | Avalon Biomed - Bradenton, FL | 4 hours[b] | Easy handling, 3-y shelf life | |
| MTA Flow | Ultradent Products Inc. - South Jordan, UT | 15 min | 2-y shelf life, mix to variable consistency with specific mixing instructions | |
| Endocem ZR | Maruchi, Inc. - Gangwon-do, South Korea | 4 min | Rapid setting | Unit dose,[c] limited working time |
| Endosequence BC RRM regular set putty | Brassler USA - Savannah, GA | 2 h | Easy handling | |
| Endosequence BC RRM fast set putty | Brassler USA - Savannah, GA | 20 min | Easy handling, rapid setting | |
| Theracal PT, dual cure | Bisco Inc. - Shaumburg, IL | 5 min or 10 s Light cure | Light cure, syringe delivery | |

[a] Per manufacturer data.
[b] MTA is amenable to placement of a glass ionomer directly over MTA before complete set, compensating for long setting time.
[c] Unit-dose products allow fewer uses per package, limited flexibility of use, and more product waste.

after vital pulp therapy, followed by intraoral radiography at 6- to 12-month intervals for a minimum of 2 years. The formation of a radiopaque dentin bridge is a positive finding, but does not indicate success. The primary indicators of vital pulp therapy success are:

- Apical closure
- Progressive thickening of dentin and narrowing of the root canal
- Lack of apical (ie, root resorption) and periapical pathology (ie, radiolucency)

---

**Box 3**
**Vital pulp therapy – additional equipment**

Cold LRS or saline solution

MTA or CaOH powder and cement

Mixing surface (glass slab, poly pad, dappen dish)

Wax spatula

MTA carrier (various types)

Medium or coarse round diamond burs

---

Previously, CaOH was recommended for vital pulp therapy. However, success using MTA has surpassed CaOH in multiple studies.[86–89] One study documented an overall vital pulp therapy success rate of 85%. However, the success rate using MTA (92%) was higher than for CaOH (58%).[88] The duration of pulp exposure is also a factor. One study showed a 100% success rate for vital pulp therapy after

---

**Box 4**
**Vital pulp therapy (with MTA), step-by-step procedure**

- Disinfect tooth to be treated
- Isolate tooth with dental dam or rubber glove
- Reduce crown with 699 or 701L bur (if ortho)
- Smooth fracture or resection margins (fine diamond bur)
- Remove pulp to a depth of 5 to 8 mm
  - Medium or coarse round or round-end cylinder diamond bur
  - Copious irrigation with cold, sterile LRS or saline
- Place moistened sterile absorbent paper points until bleeding stops
  - Chilled sterile LRS[a] or saline
  - Wait 5 minutes
  - If persistent bleeding, use cold NaOCl-soaked sterile points
- Optional: Place thin layer powder MTA over pulp
- Mix MTA to appropriate thickness (putty-like)
- Place approximately 2 mm thick layer of MTA over pulp, and allow to set
- Clean walls of residual blood or MTA (important)
- ???Etch???
- Place intermediate layer of glass ionomer (or compomer)
- Etch
- Place bonding agent
- With or without a thin layer flowable composite
- Hybrid composite
- Shaping to low-profile restoration
- Seal restoration margins with unfilled resin

[a] LRS is less toxic to fibroblasts than saline.[101]

---

crown reduction, and 0% success rate in teeth with complicated fractures more than 7 days old.[90] Another study showed a success rate of 88.2% in fractured teeth with a pulp exposure of less than 48 hours of duration, 41.4% if the duration was 2 to 7 days, and 23.5% if the duration was 1 to 3 weeks.[85] Both studies were performed using CaOH, rather than MTA, potentially impacting success rate.

## APEXIFICATION

Apexification is a procedure intended to induce apical closure in a nonvital tooth. This includes immature teeth with pulp necrosis or mature teeth with apical resorption owing to chronic apical periodontitis. Previously, this procedure was performed using CaOH. After cleaning and disinfecting of the canal, CaOH was mixed into a paste and placed in the canal, followed by a temporary restoration. This procedure was repeated every 1 to 2 months until the apical closure is accomplished and root canal therapy can be performed. This process often needed to be repeated multiple times before apical closure was obvious. With MTA, the procedure is simplified. MTA previously had an extended setting time (ProRoot approximately 4 hours; see **Box 3**). Apexification with this product was performed in a 2-step procedure, to allow the MTA to set.[91] Newer MTA products have a shorter setting time, allowing apexification in a single procedure. If the tooth has significant periapical disease, as indicated by a large periapical radiolucency or a fistulous tract, there may be a decreased success rate.[84] In this case, the following alternatives can be considered.

- Filling of the root canal with CaOH and temporary restoration, followed by MTA apical fill and root canal therapy in 2 to 4 weeks
- Surgical root canal therapy (apicoectomy and retrograde filling)

Additional equipment and the step-by-step procedure are listed in **Boxes 5** and **6**. Radiographic follow-up is performed in 3 to 6 months, and at 6- to 12-month intervals thereafter until healing is confirmed.

## SURGICAL ROOT CANAL

Surgical root canal therapy (apicoectomy and retrograde filling) is indicated when a tooth is nonvital or has irreversible pulpitis or necrosis and a standard root canal procedure cannot be performed owing to obstruction of the canal (eg, separated instrument, enamel pearls, diffuse calcification/sclerosis of the root canal, or pulp stones) or has periapical destruction that is not amenable to apexification. Surgical root canal therapy is also indicated in patients when periapical lesions have failed to resolve or have enlarged after treatment. In these patients, root canal therapy may be repeated or an apicoectomy can be performed. In multirooted teeth, only the affected root(s) are treated. The alternative to surgical root canal therapy is extraction. Additional equipment and procedure steps are listed in **Boxes 7** and **8**.

---

**Box 5**
**Apexification – additional equipment**

MTA or CaOH paste and sterile cotton pellets

Mixing surface (glass slab, poly pad, dappen dish)

Wax spatula

MTA carrier (various types)

---

**Box 6**
**Apexification step-by-step procedure**

*Single-visit apexification*
- Initial steps are similar to standard root canal therapy
  - ○ Avoid passing instruments beyond radiographic apical stop
  - ○ Avoid excessive positive-pressure irrigation with NaOCl (risk of extrusion)
  - ○ Use negative-pressure system or irrigation with chlorhexidine gluconate
  - ○ Instrument to the level of the radiographic apical stop
- Radiograph frequently to avoid insufficient or excessive apical instrumentation
- Mix MTA to appropriate, putty-like, consistency
- Place base layer of MTA over apical tissues (avoid extensive compaction to prevent extrusion)
- Place additional layers of MTA until apical fill of 4 to 5 mm
- Allow time for MTA to set (see **Table 2**)
- Obturate remainder of the root canal, avoiding excessive apical pressure
- Restoration as for standard root canal therapy

*Two-visit apexification*
- Initial steps are similar to standard root canal therapy
  - ○ Avoid passing instruments beyond the radiographic apical stop
  - ○ Avoid excessive positive-pressure irrigation with NaOCl (risk of extrusion)
  - ○ Use negative-pressure system or irrigation with chlorhexidine gluconate
  - ○ Instrument to the level of radiographic apical stop
- Mix CaOH powder into a thick slurry and place in the root canal with lentulo paste filler
- Place sterile cotton pellet
- Place temporary restorative material
- 2 weeks later, remove restorative, cotton and CaOH
- Mix MTA to appropriate, putty-like, consistency
- Place base layer of MTA over apical tissues (avoid extensive compaction to prevent extrusion)
- Place additional layers of MTA until apical fill of 4 to 5 mm
- Allow time for MTA to set (see **Table 2**)
- Obturate remainder of root canal, avoiding excessive apical pressure
- Restoration as for standard root canal therapy

---

## Access

Access sites have been described (alveolar mucosa for the maxillary canine, maxillary fourth premolar, and mandibular first molar teeth; skin for the mandibular canine tooth).[92] If there is difficulty locating the access site, two 25G hypodermic needles are placed in the tissue and a radiograph is obtained to identify the correct site (**Fig. 3**). After flap creation, alveolar bone over the root apex is removed. Bone removal is performed to expose the apical 3 to 4 mm of the root without damaging neurovascular tissue (infraorbital bundle for the maxillary fourth premolar tooth and inferior alveolar bundle for the mandibular first molar tooth) or perforating the thin palatal/lingual bony wall.

Tip: When creating mucosal flaps for this procedure, leave at least 2 to 3 mm of mucosa adjacent to the mucogingival line, to have accessible tissue for suturing the flap.

### Maxillary Fourth Premolar Tooth

When the mesiopalatal root of the maxillary fourth premolar tooth is affected, hemisection and extraction of the affected root has been recommended.[93] Anecdotally, a buccal approach to the palatal root has been performed.[94]

### Mandibular First Molar Tooth

The main concern when approaching the roots of this tooth is the location of the mandibular canal, often obstructing access to the root apex. Access is made at the

**Box 7**
**Apicoectomy – additional equipment**

Fine diamond bur, rounded end

MTA or other retrofilling material

Mixing surface (glass slab, poly pad, dappen dish)

MTA carrier (various types)

3 to 4 mm angled ultrasonic tip

Small bone curette

Spoon excavator, angled

Amalgam plugger, angled

Surgical pack
- Scalpel handle/blade
- Periosteal elevator
- Tissue forceps
- Needle holders
- Suture

dorsal aspect of the mandibular canal, being cautious not to damage the inferior alveolar neurovascular bundle.

## Apicoectomy

After apical exposure, 3 to 4 mm of the root is resected, or the root is resected flush with the wall of the periapical lesion, whichever is greater. Roots of the mandibular first molar tooth should have approximately 6 mm of the root resected owing to the potential for lateral canals.[14] To prevent perforation of the palatal/lingual bony wall, the apex is removed with light strokes using a round or straight fissure bur until it is easily fractured with a root elevator. Using the bur to transect the root completely increases potential for perforation. The root surface is smoothed with a fine diamond bur.

## Apical Cleaning and Filling

GP/sealer are removed from the apical 3 to 4 mm of the root canal. This procedure can be performed with the combination of an extended-length round bur and a small, angled spoon excavator. Cleaning in this manner is difficult owing to limited access. Amputation of the apex at a 45° angle improves access, but runs the risk of not removing enough of the apical delta at the palatal/lingual aspect.[95] The preferred method of cleaning the apical root canal is with an ultrasonic scaler using an angled tip intended for this purpose.[95,96] Radiographs are obtained to confirm the depth of cleaning and removal of all obturation material. The apical root canal is filled with an appropriate filling material. Common materials include MTA, Super EBA, and IRM (both reinforced zinc oxide-eugenol cements), and glass ionomer cements. MTA has been shown to have advantages over these materials and is preferred.[95–98]

## Closure

Residual bony debris and GP are removed. The mucosal flap is sutured in a simple interrupted or cruciate pattern using a 4-0 or 5-0 absorbable suture material. The skin is closed in at least 2 layers. Bone grafting material is not necessary for the defect.

**Box 8**
**Apicoectomy step-by-step procedure**

- Perform standard root canal therapy, if indicated
- Place 25G needles, and radiograph to assist in access location
- Incise alveolar mucosa or skin (mandibular canine tooth only)
- Elevate with periosteal elevator
- Remove alveolar bone with #2 or #4 round bur to expose the root apex
- Remove periapical bone to expose 3 to 4 mm of the root (6 mm for the mandibular first molar tooth)
- Amputate 3 to 4 mm of the apex with straight fissure or round bur
  - Avoid perforation of palatal/lingual bone surface
  - Amputate perpendicular to root
- Leave a thin wall of tooth at the palatal/lingual aspect
- Fracture apical root with a root elevator
- Smooth remaining tooth margins with fine diamond bur
- Curette granulation and or epithelial tissue from apical defect
  - Caution when in proximity of neurovascular bundles or thin alveolar walls
  - Control hemorrhage
- Remove 3 to 4 mm of obturation material and sealer
- Measure to confirm depth of 3 to 4 mm removal
- Radiograph to confirm complete obturation material removal
- Mix MTA into a thick, putty-like consistency
- Place MTA with an MTA carrier and gently compact
- Clean periapical defect of any residual contaminants
- With or without placement of a barrier membrane over the defect (make tacking sutures)
- Suture mucosal flap or subcutaneous tissue and skin (for the mandibular canine tooth)

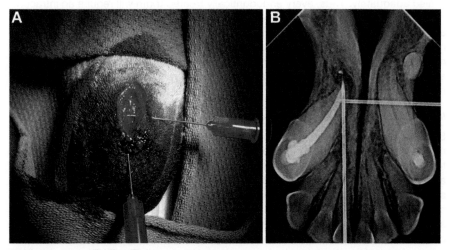

**Fig. 3.** (A) Hypodermic needles are used to locate the surgical root canal therapy site through skin of tooth 304. (B) Intraoral radiography showing needle placement.

One study showed improved healing in cats when a barrier membrane was used (with or without a bone graft), compared with closure with a bone graft alone or with no graft/membrane.[99] With large periapical defects, a membrane may be considered.

### Success Rates and Follow-up

Surgical root canal procedures are highly successful.[100] Follow-up imaging should be performed at 3 to 6 months, and then at intervals determined by the extent and progression of the healing apical defect.

## REGENERATIVE ENDODONTIC TREATMENT

Regenerative endodontics aims to use the concepts of tissue engineering to restore the root canals to a healthy state, allowing for continued development of the tooth and surrounding tissue. Published reports in humans have described various methods for the treatment of immature permanent teeth with infected root canal systems, with the goal of converting a nonvital tooth into a vital one and retaining the natural dentition. Currently, published reports of these techniques in veterinary patients are limited. However, continued evolution in this area of endodontics is moving closer to the successful regeneration of a functional pulp-dentin complex.[101,102]

## RESTORATION AFTER ENDODONTIC TREATMENT

Restoration of an endodontically treated tooth follows cleaning and obturation of the root canal. The quality of the restorative dentistry performed after root canal treatment directly impacts the prognosis of the endodontically treated tooth.[103] Two types of final restorations are commonly used in veterinary patients after endodontic treatment, namely, direct composite restoration and prosthodontic crown restoration.

The goal of restoring the tooth is to provide optimal sealing of the obturated root canal. This seal is vital to the long-term success of endodontically treated teeth because contamination of the root canal system by saliva, often referred to as "coronal microleakage," is a potential cause of endodontic failure.[104] Even if a tooth is planned to receive a prosthodontic crown restoration, the root canal access site must still be sealed adequately. Thus, every endodontically treated tooth will require an intracoronal restoration of the access site even if it will eventually receive prosthodontic therapy. If prosthodontic therapy is not planned, the intracoronal access restoration must also protect against recurrent fractures, abrasions, or decay that may lead to recontamination of the root canal system. These restorations must withstand repeated exposure to physical insult, chemical stressors, and micro-organisms in the oral environment to maintain a hermetically sealed root canal system.

### Intracoronal Direct Composite Restoration

Both the endodontic access site and any other traumatized areas of the tooth are restored in conjunction with endodontic treatment. After the completion of endodontic treatment, obturation material should be condensed or removed from the fracture and access sites. Restoration is begun by removing any unsupported enamel using a high-speed handpiece and an appropriately sized carbide or diamond bur (**Fig. 4**) and compaction of GP (**Fig. 5**). To allow for a better resin adaptation, all internal line angles should be rounded and cavity walls should be smoothed. The cavosurface margins on occlusal surfaces should not be beveled (**Fig. 6**). Any beveling should be restricted to the gingival and proximal margins where enamel is present (**Fig. 7**). The site should be rinsed well and gently dried to ensure all debris is removed.[105–107]

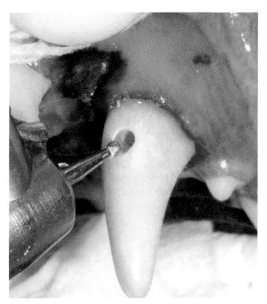

**Fig. 4.** A round diamond bur is used to removed excess gutta percha from the access site.

An initial restorative layer is typically placed in the deep part of the preparation. Low viscosity materials such as glass ionomer, resin-modified glass ionomer, or flowable composite will adapt well to the deep confines of the preparation. If a eugenol-based sealer was used for obturation, a glass ionomer or resin modified glass ionomer should be placed over the GP to prevent any remaining eugenol from affecting the composite setting. With the current, commonly used obturation techniques using resin-based sealers and endodontic obturation materials, flowable composite resin

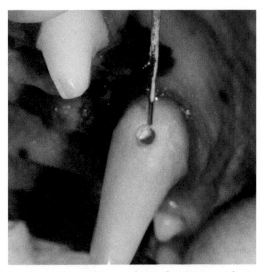

**Fig. 5.** An endodontic plugger is used to condense the gutta percha into the access site.

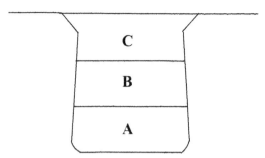

**Fig. 6.** Nonocclusal restorative layers. The prepared site requires an initial restorative layer of flowable composite, resin modified glass ionomer or glass ionomer (A) and incremental layers of packable composite (B, C). Note the beveling at the occlusal surface to allow for increased surface contact of composite with enamel.

may also be considered as an initial base.[107–109] Each restorative material should be placed and cured according to the manufacturer's directions.

### Adhesive Bonding

Whenever composite resin is placed, an adhesive bonding agent is used to adhere the composite to the prepared tooth surfaces. Adhesive bonding agents continue to evolve. There are 2 main types, the self-etch and the total-etch. Total-etch requires a separate phosphoric acid step to etch the enamel and dentin, a subsequent rinse, and application of the adhesive bonding agent. Self-etch systems have an acidic resin that etches, primes, and bonds in one step with the application of the agent without the need for separate etching and rinsing.

When using total-etch adhesive bonding agents, the prepared dentin and enamel is etched for 10 to 20 seconds with 37% phosphoric acid, rinsed, and gently air dried, but left moist. This etching and rinsing step is omitted with self-etch systems. The adhesive bonding agent is then applied and light-cured according to manufacturer's directions.[110,111]

### Composite Placement

A layer of flowable composite is deposited over the cured adhesive bonding agent as the syringe tip is slowly retracted. This thin layer of composite (1–2 mm thick) is placed on the floor of the cavity and light cured according to manufacturer's directions.

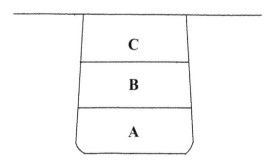

**Fig. 7.** Occlusal restorative layers. The prepared site requires an initial restorative layer of flowable composite, resin modified glass ionomer or glass ionomer (A) and incremental layers of flowable composite (B, C). Beveling of the enamel is not performed.

Incremental layers of composite of approximately 2 mm thickness should be placed and cured to completely fill the prepared cavity (see **Figs. 6 and 7**). For occlusal surfaces, a higher viscosity composite with improved strength and wear characteristics should be considered for the final restoration layer.[111] With higher viscosity, packable composites, each layer is condensed gently with a clean, nonsticking composite condenser or filling instrument to ensure complete adaptation to the underlying resin and the prepared walls of the cavity. Each composite layer (curing light only penetrates about 2 mm) is light cured according to the manufacturer's directions.

### Contouring and Finishing

There are numerous methods for finishing the restoration to shape and smooth the composite to ensure no rough or sharp edges are present. If the intracoronal restoration will be the final restoration, excess composite bulk should also be removed using medium or fine diamond burs, so that the composite is confined within the prepared enamel and dentin and no overfill of unsupported composite exists. Fine diamond burs, fine polishing points, discs, or polishing pastes are used for finishing the restoration.[111]

### Materials for Occlusal versus Nonocclusal Restorations

The type of composite used for the final restoration depends on the anticipated stresses that will be placed on the restored tooth during normal use.[109,111] For restorations on occlusal surfaces that will be placed under continuous chewing forces, a universal microhybrid composite or other packable composite would be appropriate choices. For restoration on a nonocclusal surface (such as the mesiolabial access site of a maxillary canine tooth), a lower viscosity (flowable) composite with less filler can be used.[109] Recently, nanofilled composites have become available that offer both mechanical strength and high polishability.[111] to provide an optimal restoration for commonly used endodontic access sites, the clinician should have access to different types of composites and an understanding of the indication of use for each.

### Subgingival Restoration

The maxillary fourth premolar tooth in dogs can present as a sagittal fracture ("slab fracture"), where a buccal portion of the crown or crown and root are separated from the tooth. This separation can lead to a periodontal defect at the injured site. A technique for composite restoration of this type of defect using a periodontal flap to allow open debridement and composite restoration of the fracture has been described.[112] If the fracture extends significantly into the root and below the gingival attachment, extraction may be the treatment of choice.

## PROSTHODONTIC THERAPY
### Indications

Endodontically treated teeth are structurally different from unrestored vital teeth owing to a number of factors. It was originally thought that endodontic treatment weakened teeth by desiccating the dentin, thus making them brittle.[113,114] Several previous studies supported this fact; however, recent studies have contradicted this line of thinking. Although some mechanical properties of pulpless teeth are different from normal vital teeth, the compressive and tensile strength of dentin from endodontically treated teeth was not significantly different than dentin from vital teeth.[115] In veterinary patients, coronal fractures are a common reason for endodontic treatment, and this traumatic loss of coronal structure will contribute to a weakened tooth. Access made for endodontic treatment also alters the structural integrity of the tooth. The access combined with an original coronal fracture can lead to greater cuspal flexion of the tooth under normal use.[116] Ultimately, the diminished volume of tooth structure from the combined effects of prior fracture, disease, and endodontic therapy all affect the strength of nonvital teeth. When possible, restorations for endodontically treated teeth should be designed to compensate for these effects.

If the cause of tooth trauma or disease can be determined, steps should be taken to resolve the cause of the problem. The long-term success of the planned restorative treatment may be compromised if the cause of the initial trauma cannot be identified and resolved. Good success rates for retention of full crowns in dogs have been reported by multiple sources.[117–120] The selection of the type, material, and design of the restoration should be based on multiple factors.

- The amount of remaining sound tooth structure
- The anatomic position of the tooth
- Forces on the tooth (pet's behavior or working requirements)
- Financial considerations
- Esthetics

Various combinations of these factors will help the clinician to decide if a prosthodontic crown or an intracoronal restoration is selected as the final restoration. If the degree of tooth destruction from the original injury requires the restoration to add strength and protection to the remaining tooth structure or risk factors for refracture cannot be eliminated, a full crown may be indicated in addition to a direct composite resin restoration of the fracture and access sites. When planning for prosthodontic therapy, preparation for a full or partial crown coverage, margin design, the need for additional retentive features and tooth preservation must all be considered.

### Contraindications

Several situations may lead to a decision not to perform prosthodontic crown restoration. If the pet owner is unable to alter the behavior of the pet or prevent the actions that caused the original tooth trauma, the prognosis for successful long-term outcome of prosthodontic therapy may be decreased. The patient's overall periodontal health status as well as the tooth requiring treatment must be in good condition when planning prosthodontic therapy. If the pet has active periodontitis or significant attachment loss, and the pet owner is not able to commit to regular home oral hygiene and in-office follow-up, then the tooth may not be a good candidate for treatment.

Ultimately, not having adequate sound tooth structure remaining may lead the clinician to decide against prosthodontic therapy. There is no single measurement or number to follow when evaluating the remaining tooth structure for prosthodontic therapy. The remaining tooth structure must be evaluated for its ability to sustain normal occlusal load and stress as well as its retentive qualities and the esthetic requirements of the restoration. In general, greater amounts of remaining, sound tooth structure result in a more retentive and resistant crown restoration. Multiple factors, including the shape, height, diameter, and surface area play a role in the strength of the restored tooth.[118,121,122] If the amount of remaining tooth structure is deemed insufficient, a post-and-core buildup or crown lengthening procedure (gingivectomy or crown lengthening procedure) can be performed, or an alternative to prosthodontic therapy should be considered.

### Partial and Full Crowns

For veterinary patients, the material used for the crown is commonly chosen based on the need for strength and protection. As a result, full metal crowns are by far the most commonly used prosthodontic restorations reported in the literature.[117–120] If esthetics are the primary concern, then other materials such as ceramic or porcelain fused to metal can be considered. However, there are limited reports of the long-term clinical success of these materials in veterinary patients.

In some dogs that are "cage biters" (abrasive loss of enamel and dentin on the distal crown surfaces of canine teeth without pulp exposure), reduction of less coronal structure for placement of a three-quarter crown onlay may help to prevent further abrasion.[123] Full crowns (covering all sides of the crown) are generally accepted to be the most retentive restorations when compared with three-quarter crowns and other types of partial coverage crowns.[118] Studies have shown that full crowns are generally more retentive than partial crowns.[124,125]

### Tooth Preparation and Types of Preparation Margins

Crown restorations should be designed to replace lost tooth structure and at the same time preserve and protect remaining healthy tooth structure. A balance between removing sound tooth structure to allow enough room for the prosthodontic crown and preserving sound tooth structure must be made. For the restoration to accomplish its purpose, it must stay in place. The size and shape of the tooth preparation, along with the adhesive properties of the cement used, provide retention and resistance to the restoration.

The common preparation margins used in veterinary patients include chamfer, shoulder, and deep chamfer. Shoulder and deep chamfer may be provided with a bevel that is an oblique cut into the external angle of the recess.[126] The potential benefit to adding a bevel is that it will decrease the thickness of the cement interface at the restoration margin. Occult finish lines such as a feather margin may leave a stronger tooth structure to support the crown, but it also results in an oversized restoration. Additionally, these finish lines are clinically more difficult to prepare and reproduce in the dental laboratory.[127] Although subgingival finish lines may increase clinical crown height, there are many disadvantages to their use in regard to periodontal health.[128] Because esthetic preferences are less important in companion animals, supragingival finish lines are generally chosen to maintain periodontal health and preserve as much healthy tooth structure as possible (**Fig. 8**).

In the past decade, significant additions to the veterinary literature have added to the body of knowledge available to help with decision-making regarding the tooth preparation in veterinary patients.[129] The height, diameter, surface area, and shape of the clinical crown and the preparation all play a role in the retention, resistance, strength, and long-term success of prosthodontic therapy of the endodontically treated tooth.[118,122] Additionally, it was demonstrated that the addition of axial grooves in the crown preparation of canine teeth with otherwise poor retention/resistance form (low crown height/mesiodistal diameter, high convergence angle) significantly increased the force required for canine tooth crown dislodgment.[130]

The equipment, materials, and clinical steps used for preparing a tooth for full crown restoration have been described in detail.[126,131] Ultimately, the equipment and techniques used are personal preference, and an optimal outcome can be achieved if the principles of preparation summarized elsewhere in this article are followed.

### Crown Manufacturing

Impression techniques, typically with polyvinylsiloxane, are used to produce a negative form of the teeth, thus allowing a positive reproduction or cast (model) to be made. This exact duplicate of the prepared tooth should include enough area around the preparation to allow the dental laboratory technician to be certain of the

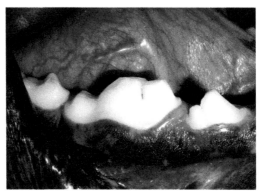

**Fig. 8.** A mandibular first molar tooth is prepared for a full prosthodontic crown with a supragingival, chamfer margin.

configuration and location of the restoration margin on the prepared tooth. This indirect technique allows the prosthodontic crown to be made away from the patient at the dental laboratory.[126] Recently, it was shown that computer-aided design/computer-aided manufacturing technology can be a useful tool for making accurate prosthodontic crowns in veterinary patients.[120] Moreover, computer-aided design/computer-aided manufacturing enables the production of prosthodontic crowns in a very short clinical time, although the number of anesthetic procedures required for prosthodontic therapy remains the same as with traditional techniques. As computer-aided design and manufacturing continues to evolve, its availability and ultimately its use in veterinary prosthodontics will become more common.

### Temporary (Provisional) Crowns

Provisional restorations are used in people between tooth preparation and cementing a definitive (permanent) prosthodontic crown. They are used to cover freshly cut dentin in the vital tooth or prepared dentin in the nonvital tooth, prevent tooth movement, and maintain esthetics.[132] A clinical review of the techniques used for chairside manufacture and placement of temporary crowns in dogs has been reported.[133] However, there are no data in the scientific literature reporting how they may affect the long-term success of the endodontic treatment or the permanent crown restoration in veterinary patients.

### Prosthodontic Crown Placement and Cementing

When the prosthodontic crown is received from the dental laboratory, it should be examined closely to ensure it has been cast accurately and verified to fit, has appropriate contour, and maintains occlusion. A dental explorer can be used to evaluate marginal integrity of the prosthodontic crown and ensure that the margins are closed when it is properly seated (**Fig. 9**). If the prosthodontic crown does not seat onto the preparation properly, minor adjustments to the prosthodontic (not natural) crown can be made. A spray articulation marking material can be used on the inside of the prosthodontic crown to indicate areas of minor adjustments. However, if the prosthodontic crown does not seat properly, or the shape and contour are incorrect, the tooth preparation should be corrected and a new impression obtained to allow a new prosthodontic crown to be cast.[134]

When the clinician is satisfied that the crown is properly adapted to the preparation, the tooth surface should be cleaned with pumice and water to remove any plaque and

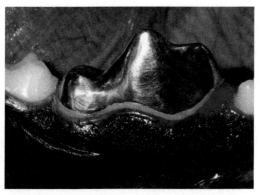

**Fig. 9.** The mandibular first molar tooth after crown cementation.

debris. Resin-based cements provide a strong bond and are advised for animals.[135] Careful adherence to the manufacturer's directions will yield optimal results. Newer preparations of resin-based cements have decreased number of steps and often use auto-mixing tips, which help to limit operator error in mixing and application. Specific directions vary between different brands of resin cement.

### Follow-up and Maintenance of Crowns

Daily tooth brushing with a pet-approved dentifrice should be performed. However, calculus will form on crown restorations as plaque mineralizes. Regular care of prosthodontic restorations is important to prevent the degradation of the restorative margin, reduce the adherence of plaque, reduce corrosion, and maintain periodontal health. Polishing materials and techniques for metal crowns have been described.[136] A professional dental cleaning with the pet under general anesthesia is necessary to maintain the prosthodontic crowns and ensure the health of the restored tooth. Hand scaling should be performed on the affected tooth, because power scaling could cause failure of the adhesive/cohesive bond between the prosthodontic crown and the tooth.

### DISCLOSURE

The authors have nothing to disclose.

### REFERENCES

1. Boyd R. Basic endodontic therapy. In: Lobprise HB, Dodd JR, editors. Wiggs' veterinary dentistry: principles and practice. 2nd edition. Hoboken: John Wiley & Sons; 2019. p. 311–34.
2. Smith DR, Gaunt PS, Plummer PJ, et al. The AVMA's definitions of antimicrobial uses for prevention, control, and treatment of disease. J Am Vet Med Assoc 2019;254:792–7.
3. Giardino L, Ambu E, Savoldi E, et al. Comparative evaluation of antimicrobial efficacy of sodium hypochlorite, MTAD, and tetraclean against enterococcus faecalis biofilm. J Endod 2007;33:852–5.
4. Ricucci D, Siqueira JF. Biofilms and apical periodontitis: study of prevalence and association with clinical and histopathologic findings. J Endod 2010;36: 1277–88.

5. Al-Ahmad A, Ameen H, Pelz K, et al. Antibiotic resistance and capacity for biofilm formation of different bacteria isolated from endodontic infections associated with root-filled teeth. J Endod 2014;40:223–30.
6. Kapralos V, Rukke HV, Ørstavik D, et al. Antimicrobial and physicochemical characterization of endodontic sealers after exposure to chlorhexidine digluconate. Dent Mater 2021;37:249–63.
7. Ruksakiet K, Hanák L, Farkas N, et al. Antimicrobial efficacy of chlorhexidine and sodium hypochlorite in root canal disinfection: a systematic review and meta-analysis of randomized controlled trials. J Endod 2020;46:1032–41.
8. Almeida LHS, Moraes RP, Morgental RD, et al. Are premixed calcium silicate-based sealers comparable to conventional materials? A systematic review of in vitro studies. J Endod 2017;43:527–35.
9. Hernández SZ, Negro VB, Paulero RH, et al. Scanning electron microscopy of pulp cavity dentin in dogs. J Vet Dent 2010;27:7–11.
10. Gracis M. Dental anatomy and physiology. In: Reiter AM, Gracis M, editors. BSAVA manual of canine and feline dentistry and oral surgery. 4th edition. Gloucester: BSAVA; 2018. p. 6–32.
11. Wilson G. Timing of apical closure of the maxillary canine and mandibular first molar teeth of cats. J Vet Dent 1999;16:19–21.
12. Hennet PR, Harvey CE. Apical root canal anatomy of canine teeth in cats. Am J Vet Res 1996;57:1545–8.
13. Hernandez SZ, Negro VB, de Puch G, et al. Scanning electron microscopic evaluation of tooth root apices in the dog. J Vet Dent 2014;31:148–52.
14. Hernández SZ, Negro VB, Maresca BM. Morphologic features of the root canal system of the maxillary fourth premolar and the mandibular first molar in dogs. J Vet Dent 2001;18:9–13.
15. Gioso MA, Knobl T, Venturini MA, et al. Non-apical root canal ramifications in the teeth of dogs. J Vet Dent 1997;14(3):89–90.
16. Negro VB, Hernández SZ, Maresca BM, et al. Furcation canals of the maxillary fourth premolar and the mandibular first molar teeth in cats. J Vet Dent 2004; 21:10–4.
17. Soukup JW, Hetzel S, Paul A. Classification and epidemiology of traumatic dentoalveolar injuries in dogs and cats: 959 injuries in 660 patient visits (2004-2012). J Vet Dent 2015;32:6–14.
18. Goodman AE, Niemiec BA, Carmichael DT, et al. The incidence of radiographic lesions of endodontic origin associated with uncomplicated crown fractures of the maxillary fourth premolar in canine patients. J Vet Dent 2020;37:71–6.
19. Greenfield BA. Enamel defect restoration of the left mandibular first molar tooth. J Vet Dent 2012;29:36–43.
20. Theuns P, Niemiec BA. Bonded sealants for uncomplicated crown fractures. J Vet Dent 2011;28:130–2.
21. Barker BC, Lockett BC. Utilization of the mandibular premolars of the dog for endodontic research. Aust Dent J 1971;16(5):280–6.
22. Soukup J. Traumatic dentoalveolar injuries. In: Lobprise HB, Dodd JR, editors. Wiggs' veterinary dentistry: principles and practice. 2nd edition. Hoboken: John Wiley & Sons; 2019. p. 109–30.
23. Abbott PV. Diagnosis and management of transverse root fractures. J Endod 2019;45(12s):s13–27.
24. Kim D, Yue W, Yoon TC, et al. Healing of horizontal intra-alveolar root fractures after endodontic treatment with mineral trioxide aggregate. J Endod 2016;42: 230–5.

25. Gracis M. Management of periodontal trauma. In: Verstraete FJM, Lommer MJ, Arzi B, editors. Oral and Maxillofacial Surgery in dogs and cats. 2nd edition. St. Louis: Elsevier; 2020. p. 218–34.
26. Reiter AM, Gracis M. Management of dental and oral trauma. In: Reiter AM, Gracis M, editors. BSAVA manual of canine and Feline dentistry and oral Surgery. 4th edition. Gloucester: BSAVA; 2018. p. 196–227.
27. Hale FA. Localized intrinsic staining of teeth due to pulpitis and pulp necrosis in dogs. J Vet Dent 2001;18:14–20.
28. Feigin K. Fifty shades of grey: contemporary understanding of intrinsically stained dog teeth. In: Proceedings of the 33rd Annual Veterinary Dental Forum 2019;235.
29. Remeeus P, Verbeek M. Use of the dental pulp tester in veterinary dentistry. J Vet Dent 1997;14(1):23–8.
30. Riehl J, Hetzel SJ, Snyder CJ, et al. Detection of pulpal blood flow in vivo with pulse oximetry in dogs. Front Vet Sci 2016;3:36. https://doi.org/10.3389/fvets.2016.00036.
31. Soukup JW, Mulherin BL, Snyder CJ. Prevalence and nature of dentoalveolar injuries among patients with maxillofacial fractures. J Small Anim Pract 2013; 54:9–14.
32. Stepaniuk K. Periodontology. In: Lobprise HB, Dodd JR, editors. Wiggs' Veterinary dentistry: principles and practice. 2nd edition. Hoboken: John Wiley & Sons; 2019. p. 81–108.
33. Ng KK, Rine S, Choi E, et al. Mandibular carnassial tooth malformations in 6 dogs-micro-computed tomography and histology findings. Front Vet Sci 2019; 6:464. https://doi.org/10.3389/fvets.2019.00464.
34. Coffman CR, Visser CJ, Visser L. Endodontic treatment of dens invaginatus in a dog. J Vet Dent 2009;26:220–5.
35. MacGee S. Endodontic therapy of a mandibular canine tooth with irreversible pulpitis secondary to dentigerous cyst. J Vet Dent 2014;31:30–9.
36. LeVan LM, Russell DA, Galburt RB, et al. Use of the dental dam in endodontic procedures in dogs. J Vet Dent 1994;11(2):49–53.
37. Visser CJ. Coronal access of the canine dentition. J Vet Dent 1991;8(4):12–5.
38. Marretta SM, Golab G, Anthony JM, et al. Ideal coronal endodontic access points for the canine dentition. J Vet Dent 1993;10(4):12–5.
39. Eisner ER. Transcoronal approach to the palatal root of the maxillary fourth premolar in the dog. J Vet Dent 1990;7(2):14–5.
40. Matelski J, Rendahl A, Goldschmidt S. Effect of alternative palatal root access technique on fracture resistance of root canal treated maxillary fourth premolar teeth in dogs. Front Vet Sci 2020;7:600145. https://doi.org/10.3389/fvets.2020.600145.
41. McCoy T. Managing endodontic instrument separation. J Vet Dent 2015;32:262–5.
42. Hiscox L. Cleaning and shaping the canal. In: Niemiec BA, editor. Veterinary endodontics. San Diego: Practical Veterinary Publishing; 2011. p. 101–11.
43. Stein KE, Marretta SM, Siegel A, et al. Comparison of hand-instrumented, heated gutta-percha and engine-driven, cold gutta-percha endodontic techniques. J Vet Dent 2004;21:136–45.
44. Beckman BW. Engine driven rotary instrumentation for endodontic therapy in a cat. J Vet Dent 2004;21:88–92.
45. Terauchi Y, O'Leary L, Suda H. Removal of separated files from root canals with a new file-removal system: case reports. J Endod 2006;32:789–97.

46. Boessler C, Peters OA, Zehnder M. Impact of lubricant parameters on rotary instrument torque and force. J Endod 2007;33:280–3.
47. Sasser L. Endodontic disinfection for orthograde root canal treatment in veterinary dentistry. J Vet Dent 2020;37:35–40.
48. Violich DR, Chandler NP. The smear layer in endodontics - a review. Int Endod J 2010;43:2–15.
49. Zehnder M. Root canal irrigants. J Endod 2006;32:389–98.
50. Clegg MS, Vertucci FJ, Walker C, et al. The effect of exposure to irrigant solutions on apical dentin biofilms in vitro. J Endod 2006;32:434–7.
51. Verma N, Sangwan P, Tewari S, et al. Effect of different concentrations of sodium hypochlorite on outcome of primary root canal treatment: a randomized controlled trial. J Endod 2019;45:357–63.
52. MEHAA Mostafa, El-Shrief YAI, Anous WIO, et al. Postoperative pain following endodontic irrigation using 1.3% versus 5.25% sodium hypochlorite in mandibular molars with necrotic pulps: a randomized double-blind clinical trial. Int Endod J 2020;53:154–66.
53. Swanljung O, Vehkalahti MM. root canal irrigants and medicaments in endodontic malpractice cases: a nationwide longitudinal observation. J Endod 2018;44:559–64.
54. Ferguson DB, Marley JT, Hartwell GR. The effect of chlorhexidine gluconate as an endodontic irrigant on the apical seal: long-term results. J Endod 2003;29:91–4.
55. Zandi H, Petronijevic N, Mdala I, et al. Outcome of endodontic retreatment using 2 root canal irrigants and influence of infection on healing as determined by a molecular method: a randomized clinical trial. J Endod 2019;45:1089–98.
56. Căpută PE, Retsas A, Kuijk L, et al. Ultrasonic irrigant activation during root canal treatment: a systematic review. J Endod 2019;45:31–44.
57. Topçuoğlu HS, Topçuoğlu G, Arslan H. The effect of apical positive and negative pressure irrigation methods on postoperative pain in mandibular molar teeth with symptomatic irreversible pulpitis: a randomized clinical trial. J Endod 2018;44:1210–5.
58. Dos Reis S, Cruz VM, Hungaro Duarte MA, et al. Volumetric analysis of irrigant extrusion in immature teeth after different final agitation techniques. J Endod 2020;46:682–7.
59. Lothamer CW, Anderson A, Hetzel SJ, et al. Apical microleakage in root canals obturated with 2 different endodontic sealer systems in canine teeth of dogs. J Vet Dent 2017;34:86–91.
60. Krug W, Marretta SM, Thomas MW, et al. Comparison of cold GP/sealer and resin bonded obturation techniques in canine teeth in dogs. J Vet Dent 2008;25:10–4.
61. Gomes-Filho JE, Watanabe S, Cintra LT, et al. Effect of MTA-based sealer on the healing of periapical lesions. J Appl Oral Sci 2013;21:235–42.
62. Lee BN, Hong JU, Kim SM, et al. Anti-inflammatory and osteogenic effects of calcium silicate-based root canal sealers. J Endod 2019;45:73–8.
63. Mandal P, Zhao J, Sah SK, et al. In vitro cytotoxicity of guttaflow 2 on human gingival fibroblasts. J Endod 2014;40:1156–9.
64. Thorne S, Johnston N, Adams VJ. Successful Use of MTA fillapex as a sealant for feline root canal therapy of 50 canines in 37 cats. J Vet Dent 2020;37:77–87.
65. Strange KA, Tawil PZ, Phillips C, et al. Long-term outcomes of endodontic treatment performed with resilon/epiphany. J Endod 2019;45:507–12.

66. Payne LA, Tawil PZ, Phillips C, et al. Resilon: assessment of degraded filling material in nonhealed cases. J Endod 2019;45:691–5.
67. Mendoza KA, Manfra Marretta S, Siegel AM, et al. Comparison of two heated gutta percha and sealer obturation techniques in canine teeth of dogs. J Vet Dent 2000;17:69–74.
68. Wiggs RB. Use of the McSpadden compactor for root canal obturation in dogs and macaques. J Vet Dent 1988;5(3):9–10.
69. Gawor J. Obturation of the properly prepared root canal. In: Niemiec BA, editor. Veterinary endodontics. San Diego: Practical Veterinary Publishing; 2011. p. 112–35.
70. Flake NM, Johnson JD. Obturation and temporization. In: Torabinejad M, Fouad AF, Shabahang S, editors. Endodontics: principles and practice. 6th edition. London: Elsevier; 2020. p. 327–49.
71. Kuntsi-Vaattovaara H, Verstraete F, Kass P. Results of root canal treatment in dogs: 127 cases (1995-2000). J Am Vet Med Assoc 2002;220:775–80.
72. Strøm PC, Arzi B, Lommer MJ, et al. Radiographic outcome of root canal treatment of canine teeth in cats: 32 cases (1998-2016). J Am Vet Med Assoc 2018; 252:572–80.
73. Soukup JW, Drees R, Koenig LJ, et al. Comparison of the diagnostic image quality of the canine maxillary dentoalveolar structures obtained by cone beam computed tomography and 64-multidetector row computed tomography. J Vet Dent 2015;32:80–6.
74. Campbell RD, Peralta S, Fiani N, et al. Comparing intraoral radiography and computed tomography for detecting radiographic signs of periodontitis and endodontic disease in dogs: an agreement study. Front Vet Sci 2016;3:68.
75. Garcia de Paula-Silva FW, Hassan B, Bezerra da Silva LA, et al. Outcome of root canal treatment in dogs determined by periapical radiography and cone-beam computed tomography scans. J Endod 2009;35:724–6.
76. Roza MR, Silva LA, Barriviera M, et al. Cone beam computed tomography and intraoral radiography for diagnosis of dental abnormalities in dogs and cats. J Vet Sci 2011;12:387–92.
77. Bogen G, Kuttler S. Mineral trioxide aggregate obturation: a review and case series. J Endod 2009;35:777–90.
78. Holland R, Otoboni Filho JA, de Souza V, et al. A comparison of one versus two appointment endodontic therapy in dogs' teeth with apical periodontitis. J Endod 2003;29:121–4.
79. Leonardo MR, Hernandez ME, Silva LA, et al. Effect of a calcium hydroxide-based root canal dressing on periapical repair in dogs: a histological study. Oral Surg Oral Med Oral Pathol Oral Radiol Endod 2006;102:680–5.
80. Katsamakis S, Slot DE, Van der Sluis LW, et al. Histological responses of the periodontium to MTA: a systematic review. J Clin Periodontol 2013;40:334–44.
81. Alves FRF, Dias MCC, Mansa MGCB, et al. Permanent labiomandibular paresthesia after bioceramic sealer extrusion: a case report. J Endod 2020;46:301–6.
82. Rickles NH, Joshi BA. A possible case in a human and an investigation in dogs of death from air embolism during root canal therapy. J Am Dent Assoc 1963;67: 397–404.
83. McMichael GE, Primus CM, Opperman LA. Dentinal tubule penetration of tricalcium silicate sealers. J Endod 2016;42:632–6.
84. Diogenes A, Botero T, Kang M. Management of the vital pulp and of immature teeth. In: Torabinejad M, Fouad AF, Shabahang S, editors. Endodontics: principles and practice. 6th edition. London: Elsevier; 2020. p. 176–95.

85. Clarke DE. Vital pulp therapy for complicated crown fracture of permanent canine teeth in dogs: a three-year retrospective study. J Vet Dent 2001;18: 117–21.
86. Suhag K, Duhan J, Tewari S, et al. Success of direct pulp capping using mineral trioxide aggregate and calcium hydroxide in mature permanent molars with pulps exposed during carious tissue removal: 1-year follow-up. J Endod 2019;45:840–7.
87. Zaen El-Din AM, Hamama HH, Abo El-Elaa MA, et al. The effect of four materials on direct pulp capping: an animal study. Aust Endod J 2020;46:249–56.
88. Luotonen N, Kuntsi-Vaattovaara H, Sarkiala-Kessel E, et al. Vital pulp therapy in dogs: 190 cases (2001-2011). J Am Vet Med Assoc 2014;244:449–59.
89. Meschi N, Patel B, Ruparel NB. Material pulp cells and tissue interactions. J Endod 2020;46(9S):S150–60.
90. Niemiec BA. Assessment of vital pulp therapy for nine complicated crown fractures and fifty-four crown reductions in dogs and cats. J Vet Dent 2001;18: 122–5.
91. Juriga S, Maretta SM, Weeks SM. Endodontic treatment of a non-vital permanent tooth with an open root apex using mineral trioxide aggregate. J Vet Dent 2008; 25:189–95.
92. Marretta SM, Eurell JA, Klippert L. Development of a teaching model for surgical endodontic access sites in the dog. J Vet Dent 1994;11(3):89–93.
93. Reiter AM, Lewis JR, Rawlinson JE, et al. Hemisection and partial retention of carnassial teeth in client-owned dogs. J Vet Dent 2005;22:216–26.
94. Personal communication: John F Huff III, BS, DVM, FAVD, DAVDC; Castle Pines, CO, USA.
95. Hennet P, Girard N. Surgical endodontics in dogs: a review. J Vet Dent 2005;22: 148–56.
96. Rubinstein R, Fayad MI, Torabinejad M. Apical microsurgery. In: Torabinejad M, Fouad AF, Shabahang S, editors. Endodontics: principles and practice. 6th edition. London: Elsevier; 2020. p. 428–41.
97. Bernabe PF, Gomes-Filho JE, Rocha WC, et al. Histological evaluation of MTA as a root-end filling material. Int Endod J 2007;40:758–65.
98. Baek SH, Plenk H Jr, Kim S. Periapical tissue responses and cementum regeneration with amalgam, SuperEBA, and MTA as root-end filling materials. J Endod 2005;31:444–9.
99. Artzi Z, Wasersprung N, Weinreb M, et al. Effect of guided tissue regeneration on newly formed bone and cementum in periapical tissue healing after endodontic surgery: an in vivo study in the cat. J Endod 2012;38:163–9.
100. Fulton AJ, Fiani N, Arzi B, et al. Outcome of surgical endodontic treatment in dogs: 15 cases (1995-2011). J Am Vet Med Assoc 2012;241(12):1633–8.
101. Feigin K, Shope B. Regenerative endodontics. J Vet Dent 2017;34:161–78.
102. Peak M, Lobprise HB. Advanced endodontic therapy. In: Lobprise HB, Dodd JR, editors. Wiggs' veterinary dentistry: principles and practice. 2nd edition. Hoboken: John Wiley & Sons; 2019. p. 335–55.
103. Ray HA, Trope M. Periapical status of endodontically treated teeth in relation to the technical quality of the root filling and the coronal restoration. Int Endod J 1995;28(1):12–8.
104. Saunders WP, Saunders EM. Coronal leakage as a cause of failure in root-canal therapy: a review. Endod Dent Traumatol 1994;10(3):105–8.
105. Small BW. Direct posterior composite restorations – state of the art 1998. Gen Dent 1998;46:26–32.

106. Leinfelder KF. Using composite resin as a posterior restorative material. J Am Dent Assoc 1991;122:65–70.
107. Roberson TM, Heyman HO, Ritter AV. Introduction to composite restorations, . Sturdevants Art and science of operative dentistry. 4th edition. St. Louis: Mosby; 2002. p. 488–92.
108. Wagnild G, Mueller K. Restoration of endodontically treated teeth. In: Cohen S, Hargreaves KM, editors. Pathways of the pulp. 9th edition. St Louis: Mosby; 2006. p. 786–821.
109. Mannocci F, Cowie J. Restoration of endodontically treated teeth. Br Dent J 2014;216:341–6.
110. Kugel G, Ferrari M. The Science of bonding: from first to sixth generation. J Am Dent Assoc 2000;131:20S–5S.
111. Caifa A, Visser L. Restorative dentistry. In: Lobprise HB, Dodd JR, editors. Wiggs' *veterinary dentistry: principles and practice*. 2nd edition. Hoboken: John Wiley & Sons; 2019. p. 357–86.
112. Reiter AM, Lewis JR. Dental bulge restoration and gingival collar expansion after endodontic treatment of a complicated maxillary fourth premolar crown-root fracture in a dog. J Vet Dent 2008;25:34–45.
113. Carter JM, Sorensen SE, Johnson RR, et al. Punch shear testing of extracted vital and endodontically treated teeth. J Biomech 1983;16(10):841–8.
114. Helfer AR, Melnick S, Schilder H. Determination of moisture content of vital and pulpless teeth. Oral Surg Oral Med Oral Pathol 1972;34:661–70.
115. Huang TJ, Schilder H, Nathanson D. Effects of moisture content and endodontic treatment on some mechanical properties of human dentin. J Endod 1992;18(5): 209–15.
116. Panitvisai P, Messer HH. Cuspal deflection in molars in relation to endodontic and restorative procedures. J Endod 1995;21(2):57–61.
117. Van Foreest A, Roeters J. Evaluation of the clinical performance and effectiveness of adhesively-bonded metal crowns on damaged canine teeth of working dogs over a two- to 52-month period. J Vet Dent 1998;15:13–20.
118. Soukup JW, Snyder CJ, Karls TL, et al. Achievable convergence angle and the effect of preparation design on the clinical outcome of full veneer crowns in dogs. J Vet Dent 2011;28:72–82.
119. Fink L, Reiter A. Assessment of 68 prosthodontic crowns in 41 pet and working dogs (2000-2012). J Vet Dent 2015;32:148–54.
120. Mestrinho LA, Gordo I, Gawor J, et al. Retrospective study of 18 titanium alloy crowns produced by computer-aided design and manufacturing in dogs. Front Vet Sci 2019;6:97.
121. Zimmerman C, Soukup JW. Evaluation of the natural crown convergence angle of dog carnassial teeth. J Vet Dent 2015;32:222–5.
122. Riehl J, Soukup JW, Collins C, et al. Effect of preparation surface area on the clinical outcome of full veneer crowns in dogs. J Vet Dent 2014;31:22–5.
123. Luskin IR. Three-quarter crown preparation. J Vet Dent 2001;18:102–5.
124. Lorey RE, Myers GE. The retentive qualities of bridge retainers. J Am Dent Assoc 1968;76:568–72.
125. Potts RG, Shillingburg HT, Duncanson MG. Retention and resistance of preparations for cast restorations. J Prosthet Dent 1980;43:303–8.
126. Coffman C, Visser C, Soukup J, et al. Crowns and prosthodontics. In: Lobprise HB, Dodd JR, editors. Wiggs' Veterinary dentistry: principles and practice. 2nd edition. Hoboken: John Wiley & Sons; 2019. p. 387–410.

127. Shillingburg HT, Sumiya H, Whitsett LD, et al. Principles of tooth preparation, . Fundamentals of fixed prosthodontics. 3rd edition. Batavia: Quintessence Publishing Inc.; 1997. p. 119–37.

128. Sarandha DL. Effects of location of gingival finish lines on periodontal integrity. J Nepal Dent Assoc 2013;13:74–7.

129. Soukup JW. Crown preparation design: an evidence-based review. J Vet Dent 2013;30:214–9.

130. Goldschmidt S, Collins CJ, Hetzel S, et al. The influence of axial grooves on dislodgment resistance of prosthetic metal crowns in canine teeth of dogs. J Vet Dent 2016;33:146–50.

131. Coffman CR, Visser L, Visser CJ. Tooth preparation and impression for full metal crown restoration. J Vet Dent 2007;24:59–65.

132. Wassell R, George G, et al. Crowns and other extra-coronal restorations: provisional restorations. Br Dent J 2002;192:619–30.

133. Carle D, Shope B, Ogrodnick D. Temporary crowns. J Vet Dent 2013;30:34–8.

134. Wingo K. Cementation of full coverage metal crowns in dogs. J Vet Dent 2018; 35:46–53.

135. Wingo K. A review of dental cements. J Vet Dent 2018;35:18–27.

136. Crowder SE. Care of metal crown restorations. J Vet Dent 2010;27:191–6.

# Virtual Surgical Planning and 3D Printing in Veterinary Dentistry and Oromaxillofacial Surgery

Graham P. Thatcher, DVM, Jason W. Soukup, DVM*

## KEYWORDS

- Virtual surgical planning (VSP) • Computer-aided surgical planning
- Computer-aided design (CAD) • Computer-aided manufacturing (CAM) • 3D printing
- Additive manufacturing • Stereolithography (SLA)

## KEY POINTS

- Three-dimensional printing was invented in the early 1980's with the first paten for stereolithography being awarded to Charles Hull in 1987.
- The human oral and maxillofacial surgical field has been a driving force in the field of 3DP and VSP due to the complex anatomy of the midface and mandibles.
- Imaging data from Computed Tomography, Magnetic Resonance Imaging, and 3D Laser Scanners is required by the VSP and 3DP software.
- VSP has a steep learning curve and requires the operator to import the DICOM file into a software designed to create a 3D object, which can be manipulated and saved as an STL (Standard Tesselation Language) file.
- Most 3D printers will have proprietary software that converts the STL file into a language recognized by that printer.

## INTRODUCTION

The specialized field of veterinary dentistry and oromaxillofacial surgery (OMFS) has been evolving at a rapid rate. Advancements in the technology of three-dimensional (3D) printing and surgical planning software have also become more accessible and affordable in the past 3 decades. In the human surgical fields, computer-aided surgical planning and additive manufacturing have revolutionized the surgeon's ability to create patient-specific models, design and fabricate surgical guides, and customize surgical implants.[1,2] *Virtual surgical planning* (VSP) has become a common practice

University of Wisconsin-Madison, School of Veterinary Medicine, 2015 Linden Drive, Madison, WI 53706, USA
* Corresponding author.
*E-mail address:* jason.soukup@wisc.edu

Vet Clin Small Anim 52 (2022) 221–234
https://doi.org/10.1016/j.cvsm.2021.09.009
0195-5616/22/© 2021 Elsevier Inc. All rights reserved.

in human craniomaxillofacial surgery with benefits of improved patient outcomes as a result of increased precision, shorter operating room times and a decrease in complications. VSP comes with an increased preoperative planning time and a steep learning curve if the operator is performing the surgical simulations without the help of an experienced biomedical engineering team. In veterinary medicine, the use of VSP and 3D printing has grown to include anatomic models for teaching and surgical rehearsal, surgical applications of patient-specific cutting guides and reconstruction implants.

## HISTORY OF THREE-DIMENSIONAL PRINTING TECHNOLOGY

A Japanese engineer, named Hideo Kodama at the Nagoya Municipal Industrial Research Institute, pioneered and published his work on a rapid prototyping technique using a laser beam to cure successive layers of photopolymer in 1981.[3] Kodama was unsuccessful in securing a patent for this invention. In 1984, an American physics engineer named Charles Hull further refined the *stereolithography* (SLA) process first reported by Kodama. Later that same year, Hull cofounded 3D Systems Inc, which has been widely used by the automotive, aerospace, and medical industries.[4] Hull received a patent for stereolithography in 1986, thereby crowning him as the inventor of 3D printing. Hull described the process of using ultraviolet light to solidify liquid polymers in cross-sections of a 3D model. 3D Systems produced the world's first commercial SLA printer in 1988.[4]

Also, in 1984 an undergraduate student from the University of Texas named Carl Deckard along with his mentor, Joe Beaman, developed similar 3D printing technology. This new method of 3D printing used a laser beam to selectively sinter or melt powdered materials such as metal, plastic, ceramic, or glass.[5] This technology, known as *selective laser sintering* (SLS), was refined by a company called Desktop Manufacturing Corporation (DTM Corp) founded by Deckard. DTM produced the first SLS printers in 1992 before being acquired by 3D Systems.[4]

In 1989, Scott and Lisa Crum developed a new form of rapid prototyping called *fused deposition modeling* (FDM) and founded Stratasys Inc. Stratasys patented the FDM technology that heated a plastic filament or metal wire that was extruded through a nozzle. The thin strands of material are deposited on a printing platform, controlled by a computer based on a digital model (computer-aided design [CAD]/computer-aided manufacturing [CAM]).

In 2005, after the expiration of the patent for Stratasys' FDM technology, a professor of mechanical engineering named Adrian Bower started a self-replicating rapid-prototyper project known as RepRap. Bower's first open-source printer, called Darwin, was the first self-replicating printer created in 2008. This design was refined in 2009 in the Czech Republic by Josef Prusa, which led to the release of the Prusa Mendel; this was a simplified version of Darwin, which rapidly improved the printer models and eventually the release of commercial kits, including one in the same year known as the Makerbot Cupcake CNC, followed by the Makerbot Thing-O-Matic in 2010.[4,6] Stratasys acquired Makerbot in 2013.

Medical fields have been a driving force for the improvement in 3D printing technologies. VSP and patient-specific anatomic models, guides, and implants for orthopedic patients were among the first applications of this technology in practice.[7,8] Starting as early as 2005, patient-specific radiographic models, based on computed tomography (CT) scans have been used to 3D print hydroxyapatite scaffolds as medium for live cell growth following implantation.[9] In recent years, 3D printing has been used extensively by the human oral and maxillofacial surgical field to improve surgical times as well as functional and cosmetic outcomes due to the complex anatomy of the head with extensive networks of vital structures.[10] It is only natural that the veterinary oral and maxillofacial teams will follow suit, as the technologies become more mainstream along with the expectations of the clients.

## IMAGE ACQUISITION, COMPUTER MODELING, AND VIRTUAL SURGICAL PLANNING

VSP is a preoperative process that uses computer software to simulate a surgical procedure virtually in 3D or with 3D models. The major steps required to perform VSP include acquisition of appropriate images, patient work-up, the virtual planning session including image segmentation, and finally the surgical execution.[11] To create an accurate anatomic 3D model, medical imaging technologies including CT, cone-beam computed tomography (CBCT), MRI, and intraoral scanners have been used. Because of the complex nature of the oral and maxillofacial regions of our veterinary patients, high-resolution CT scans are typically used. Depending on the nature of the case, various algorithms will be needed to appropriately capture the imaging data required for the surgical plan. Bone algorithms with thin slices are required for osseous segmentation in most oral and maxillofacial trauma and neoplasia cases. However, soft-tissue algorithms may also be required to properly segment and isolate the margins of a tumor and therefore assist in the surgical plan in oncologic surgery.

Spatial resolution and contrast resolution need to be considered when deciding on the imaging modality that is most appropriate for the tissues involved in the surgical plan.[12] *Spatial resolution* is the ability of an imaging modality to differentiate between two adjacent objects or structures. An example of spatial resolution would be the ability to differentiate a tooth root from the surrounding periodontal ligament space. *Contrast resolution* refers to the ability of an imaging modality to distinguish between differences in intensity of an image.[12] An example of contrast resolution is the ability to visualize the variable image intensities in an area of contrast medium (iohexol) uptake in a tumor. Good spatial resolution is important for hard tissue interventions such as osseous trauma repair. However, good contrast resolution is required for planning and evaluation of soft tissue margins in oncologic surgery. Conventional CT scans have good spatial but limited contrast resolution. This limited contrast resolution is improved with the application of contrast imaging studies to evaluate lymph nodes and tumors and other oral and maxillofacial structures with increased vascularity. CT is the imaging modality of choice for oral and maxillofacial patients because of the involvement of variable osseous and soft tissue structures such as teeth, bone, muscle, lymph nodes, and so forth. CBCT has gained popularity in dentistry and oral surgery practices due to their portability, lower cost, ease of use, and decreased radiation exposure. CBCT has good spatial resolution, making it a good imaging modality for osseous lesions and craniomaxillofacial trauma. The contrast resolution of CBCT is poor, making it a poor choice for evaluation of soft tissue such as in the surgical planning of oral and maxillofacial neoplasia cases.[13] MRI technology is the most appropriate imaging modality for soft tissue structures not involving bone due to their superior contrast resolution. However, this is not typically applicable to most oral and maxillofacial cases due to the proximity of the bones of the skull.[14] Most recently gaining popularity in dentistry and oral surgery practices is the use of 3D laser scanners to achieve high resolution of surface structures such as the dentition, for the creation of surgical cutting guides in orthognathic surgery as well as planning for orthodontic aligners.[15]

Successful surgical planning requires the team to acquire a dataset that can accurately reproduce the anatomic detail within the modeling and editing software.[11] The imaging data are universally stored in digital imaging and communications in medicine

(DICOM) format for ease of use with multiple software applications. VSP requires the operator to import the DICOM file into a software designed to create a 3D object, which can be manipulated and saved as an STL (Standard *Tesselation Language* or *Stereolithographic*) file. Mimics (Materialise, Leuven, Belgium) is a commonly used software in research and clinical practice for VSP. Importation of a DICOM file into the software allows the surgical team to manipulate data to create 3D computer models of any tissues or regions of interest (ROI) within the dataset. The process of digitally isolating the ROI from surrounding structures and tissue is known as *segmentation*. *Thresholding* is a semiautomated segmentation tool within the software in which a range of Hounsfield units (HU) is selected to represent the tissues of interest. Additional desirable structures that may fall within the selected HU range can be added from the ROI by various region growing functions within the software. Undesirable structures falling within the selected HU range can also be removed, using various software trimming functions. The 3D image that results from the completion of segmentation, trimming, and region growing results in a 3D computer model that can be used with additional software tools to create a virtual surgical environment, allowing the surgeon to rehearse the surgery (approach, osteotomy, tumor resection, graft harvesting and placing, and so forth) within the software (**Fig. 1**). In addition, the exported STL files can be printed as anatomically accurate 3D models that can be used for a similar surgical rehearsal. Lastly, the STL file can be uploaded into a software with design functions for additional virtual planning, including creation of cutting guides or patient-specific implants, which can then also be printed and sterilized for surgical use. To optimize surgical outcome, the anatomic accuracy of the imaging dataset and fidelity to the patient of the resultant models, surgical guides, and implants must be maintained. Any loss of anatomic accuracy during the virtual surgical plan, such as selection of an inadequate HU range for thresholding, can lead to loss of anatomic fidelity to the patient, and this can result in inappropriate surgical margins, poorly fitting surgical guides and patient-specific implants a negative surgical outcome.

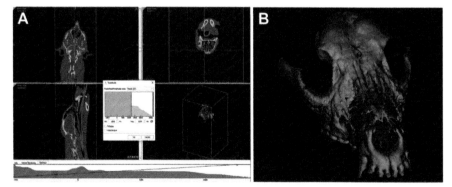

**Fig. 1.** Screenshot of Materialise Mimics image processing software (*A*) in which a thresholding process (centrally located histogram) with an HU range of 1200 to 3006 has been used to complete the segmentation of a patient's skull. The osseous structures of the head can be seen highlighted in a green color in the dorsal, transverse, and sagittal CT slices in the top and bottom left windows. The 3D computer model of the skull can be seen in purple in bottom right window of 1A and in 1B. In this case, a large osseous defect can be seen on the patient's right, which was a result of a thermal or chemical burn. In this case VSP was used to perform a virtual ostectomy of necrotic bone before printing a 3D model of the maxilla, which was then used to contour a titanium mesh implant.

VSP and 3D printing has become widely used in OMFS in part due to the anatomic complexity of the region. Surgical resection of large tumors involving the orbitozygomaticomaxillary complex is challenging and often requires osteotomies with poor direct visualization of the tumor in addition to vital structures in the region such as the maxillary artery, branches of the facial nerve, sinuses, cribriform plate, tympanic bullae, and calvarium. Surgical rehearsal using the software and 3D printed models and guides enhances the ability of the surgeon to improve precision, accuracy, and confidence. Recent studies have demonstrated an improved ability of the surgeon to achieve tumor-free surgical margins with the use of VSP.[16,17] In addition, it has been demonstrated that the use of 3D printed surgical models and cutting guides can increase surgical speed and decrease complications associated with extended surgical times such as wound dehiscence and infection.[18,19]

VSP is not without limitations outside of the control of the surgical team, notwithstanding the improved outcomes for these complex oromaxillofacial surgeries. These limitations include, but are not limited to, time delays, a steep learning curve with planning and design software, and human error with communications between the operator and the design engineer. Many surgical facilities have in-house VSP software and printing capabilities. However, even with strong knowledge of the planning tool there can often be delays of more than 24 hours from the time of medical imaging to completing a virtual plan and printing models, guides, or implants based on the experience of the authors. Many hospitals in veterinary and human medicine will use the services of a third-party surgical planning and design wing of larger surgical instrument companies such as DePuy Synthes, Materialise, and KLS Martin. Although this takes away the need for the surgeon to be intimately aware of the software, the communication between the surgeon and the design team is of paramount importance. Typically, a rough sketch is drawn up by the surgeon followed by planning sessions between the design engineers and the surgeon to create the model, implants, and guides. The time from imaging to delivery of custom, patient-specific implant has been reported to take 14 to 17 days due to planning time, printing, processing, and delivery of the parts.[11]

## THREE-DIMENSIONAL PRINTING TECHNIQUES

Before printing a model or part in 3 dimensions, a high-quality DICOM file is required. In veterinary medicine and particularly OMFS, the most appropriate imaging modality is the CT scan with thin slices in order to provide the most anatomic detail possible. The next step is to import the DICOM compliant files into the 3D software package. There are several commercial software companies available, including, but not limited to, Mimics (Materialize, Plymouth, MI), Geomagic (3D Systems, Wilsonville, OR), ScanIP (Simpleware, Ashburn, VA), Solidworks (Dassault Systems, Waltham, MA).[20] In addition, there are several open-source (freeware) software packages available, including Meshmixer, InVesalius, ITK SNAP, and 3D Slicer. The commercial products come with customer support and have powerful engineering capabilities in comparison to the open-source products. However, there is generally a steeper learning curve with the commercial products. If simple planning tasks are required before printing, such as segmentation and mirroring, then it is the authors' opinion that freeware such as Meshmixer will suffice. Within the 3D modeling/planning software, the ROI must be isolated by thresholding and segmentation techniques to isolate the pixels within an operator-determined HU range and to remove nonessential anatomy or objects such as the endotracheal tube. The resulting surface details of the ROI will be represented in 3D as a continuous mesh made up of 30,000 to millions of polygons depending on the complexity of the file.[20,21] The particularly highly detailed anatomy of the oromaxillofacial structures often results in large data files, which can lead to delayed processing and printing. Once the model is complete, the part is exported as an STL file, which is a universally recognized CAD file.[20] At this stage, if no further parts design or refinements are required, the STL file is uploaded into a printing software. This software is commonly a proprietary software that is bound to the printer to be used. However, there are commercial (3D Systems, Wilsonville, OR) and open-source (Replicator G) software programs that are compatible with multiple printers. In addition to recoding the data to be recognized by the printer to be used, these software packages function to optimize orientation of the part to be printed (in order to minimize material and time) and provide adequate scaffold supports to avoid unsupported minima. Remote printing services are becoming a common alternative to in-house printing and can be found at public libraries and makerspace settings. A complete step-by-step guideline of how to create 3D printed anatomic models has been described, which demonstrates the accessibility of high-resolution 3D prints from digital files.[22] A simplified schematic process of 3D printing from start to finish is shown in **Fig. 2**.

## VIRTUAL SURGICAL PLANNING AND THREE-DIMENSIONAL PRINTING APPLICATIONS

Although it is still relatively uncommon in veterinary medicine, 3D printing applications have been reported in orthopedics as far back as 2 decades for management of limb deformities and more recently for the management of oromaxillofacial trauma and tumor management.[23–26] The oromaxillofacial structures have complex anatomy including, but not limited to, the dentoalveolar arches, dense network of craniofacial neurovascular structures, masticatory apparatus, temporomandibular joints (TMJ), orbitozygomaticomaxillary complex, and the calvarium. These structures contribute to several vital functions including breathing, nutrient, and fluid intake, communication, vision, and defense to name a few. Patient-specific anatomic complexities have, in part, led veterinary oromaxillofacial surgeons to use the technologies of VSP and 3D printing in academic centers and in private practice. Our human counterparts in craniomaxillofacial surgery have been ground breakers in the development and use of 3D printing since the advent of CAD/CAM, which has paved the way for veterinarians to provide similar advanced services to our patients.

The most common uses of 3D printing in veterinary OMFS are very similar to the usage in human craniomaxillofacial surgeries and can be described in 4 categories including anatomic models for implant contouring, surgical guides, splints, and patient-specific implants.[27] In the authors' experience, the most common usage of 3D printing is for contour models. These anatomic models used for implant contouring are positive-space models with the 3D print maintaining patient-specific anatomic fidelity.[28] This fidelity allows the surgeon to precontour standard implants such as titanium mandibular reconstruction plates, adaptation plates, and titanium mesh implants for traumatic bone injuries and tumor excisions without the surgical field being obscured by blood and soft tissues (**Fig. 3**). This decreases the time in the operating room in addition to increasing the likelihood of returning the patient to a pretrauma anatomic form. To achieve a model representative of pretrauma or pretumor anatomy, VSP including mirroring of unaffected bones is often performed. In addition to these

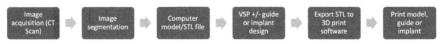

**Fig. 2.** A typical workflow from image acquisition to 3D printing. Note that VSP and implant design may be an optional step depending on the goals and complexity of the case.

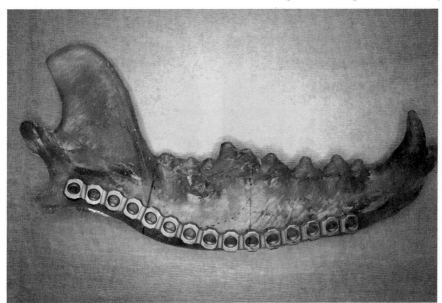

**Fig. 3.** A 3D printed mandible with a precontoured mandibular reconstruction plate. The printed model reflects a canine acanthomatous ameloblastoma at the distal aspect of the right mandibular first molar tooth as well as a 1 cm margin (*dashed line*) and planned osteotomy locations (*solid lines*). In this case, the mandible was reconstructed immediately at the time of tumor excision.

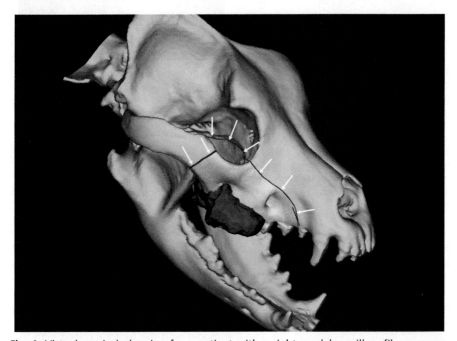

**Fig. 4.** Virtual surgical planning for a patient with a right caudal maxillary fibrosarcoma. This 3D computer model was created in Materialise Mimics from a helical CT study. VSP included separate segmentation of the skull (*blue*), contrast-enhancing soft tissue tumor (*red*), and planned surgical excision (*yellow*). Osteotomies (*white arrows*) were performed virtually within the software, and both the complete preoperative skull and the skull after virtual excision were printed for use as anatomic guides in the operating room.

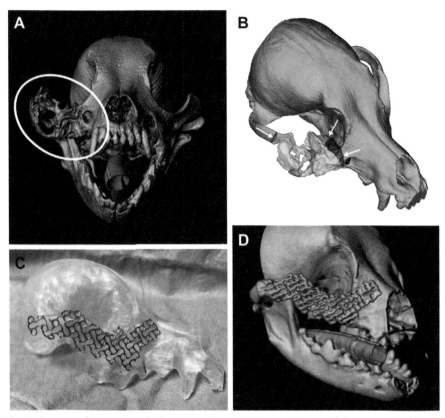

**Fig. 5.** Images of a case in which an invasive odontogenic lesion of the ventral orbit and rostral zygomatic arch was surgically excised. The preoperative CT (*A*) reveals an invasive multilocular lesion (*white ellipse*). The helical CT study DICOM file was imported into the image processing software (*B*). Subsequently, the maxilla was segmented (*green*), the infraorbital neurovascular bundle was segmented (*red*), and osteotomies were performed virtually (*white arrows*). The resultant computer model with the excised lesion (translucent blue) was then used to design a 3D printed cutting guide (not shown) in a design software. A mirror image of the segmented skull was also created and printed, which allowed for precontouring of a titanium mesh implant to reconstruct the ventral orbit and zygomatic arch (*C*). Fig. 5D shows a postoperative volumetric rendering of the excision and reconstructed orbit/zygoma.

models being used preoperatively to contour implants, they are frequently sterilized and brought into the operating room for anatomic reference and teaching during surgery.

For many oromaxillofacial tumor cases, VSP offers the opportunity to plan and create the osteotomy planes within the software, followed by virtual surgical excision of the tumor (**Fig. 4**); this allows the operator to print not only the pretumor contouring model for implant preparation but also the model with the tumor excised with the desired margins and osteotomies that will be replicated on the patient in the operating room (**Fig. 5**).

The second most common use of 3D printing in the authors' OMFS caseload is the application of surgical cutting guides. These guides are designed to attach to the

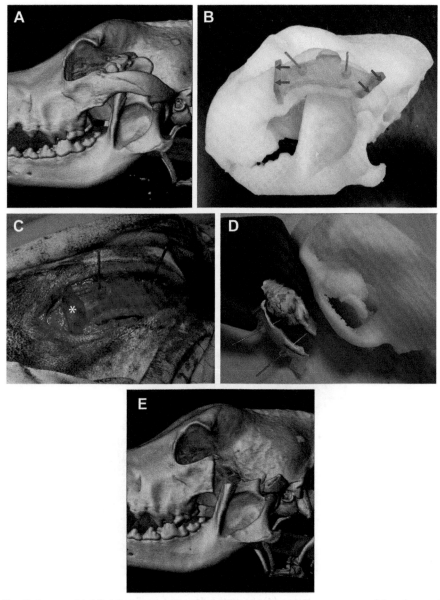

**Fig. 6.** Images highlighting a case in which VSP and 3D printing were used to plan and execute a gap arthroplasty to treat an extraarticular TMJ ankylosis. A preoperative CT (*A*) revealed osseous union of the coronoid process of the left mandibular ramus and the medial aspect of the left zygomatic arch likely secondary to previous trauma. Design software was used to create a surgical cutting guide, which is shown in (*B*) attached to a 3D printed skull with 2 Steinmann pins. The rostral and caudal aspects of the surgical cutting guide are designed with flat edges (red *arrows*) that provide a flat surface to guide the surgical saw. This flat edge (white *asterisk*) can be better appreciated in (*C*), which shows the surgical cutting guide in place intraoperatively. (*D*) shows the surgical cutting guide affixed to the resected zygomatic arch and coronoid process adjacent to the 3D printed skull for purposes of comparison. The surgical outcome can be appreciated in the postoperative CT (*E*).

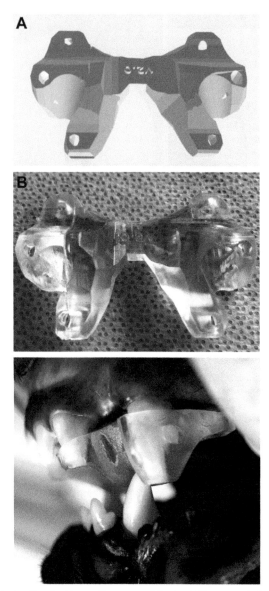

**Fig. 7.** A 3D printed orthodontic appliance used to treat linguoverted mandibular canine teeth in a dog. An STL file image (A) shows the designed appliance, which can be seen in the 3D printed form (B) to be an exact duplicate. Note that strategically placed holes were designed as locations in which bis-acryl composite could be placed as a means of securing the appliance to the maxillary dentition (C).

patient in only one orientation, which provides precision osteotomies with appropriate surgical margins, all while avoiding vital structures. Oncologic resections and TMJ ankylosis are examples of the use of surgical cutting guides in veterinary OMFS. In the human field, there has been documentation of improved surgical times and precision in addition to aesthetic and clinical outcomes with the use of surgical cutting

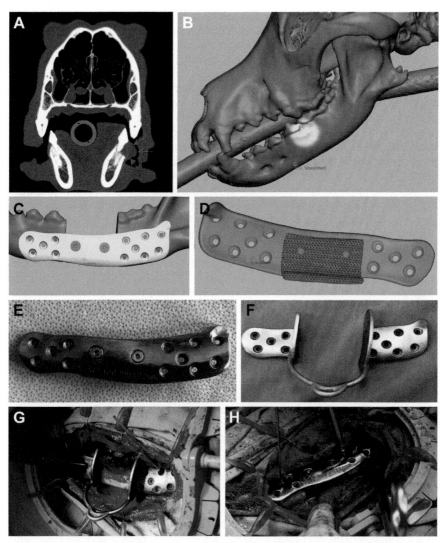

**Fig. 8.** A series of images of a case in which VSP, 3D models, and patient-specific implants were used to excise a canine acanthomatous ameloblastoma and reconstruct the left mandible. The tumor can be appreciated (*red arrows*) in the preoperative CT (*A*). A third-party medical implant design company (Voxelmed, Germersheim, Germany) was used to create a patient-specific implant for mandibular reconstruction. The helical CT DICOM study of the skull (*blue*) was segmented and the location of the tumor (*yellow*) identified (*B*). Subsequently, the implant (*C, yellow*) and a corresponding cutting guide (*F*) were designed, and the osteotomies performed virtually in order to mimic the surgical procedure (*C*). In (*D*), the lingual aspect of the implant (now in *blue*) can be seen to incorporate a mesh basket to receive a graft. The implant (*E*) and cutting guide (*F*) were printed in a titanium SLS printer. The cutting guide (*G*) and the implant (*H*) can be seen held in place by Steinmann pins during the surgical procedure.

guides for dental implants, maxillary obturators, orthognathic surgery, and mandibular reconstruction (**Fig. 6**).[29] While providing for better patient outcomes and shorter surgery times, the creation of these guides require a strong operating knowledge of the design software, which generally has steep learning curves and requires substantial preoperative planning.

Patient-specific 3D printed splints are not commonly used in veterinary OMFS. However, the authors have used this modality to create orthodontic appliances to correct traumatic malocclusion in a dog (**Fig. 7**). Splints are negative space models with enhanced detail due to the complex dental anatomy. In order to closely match the anatomic contours of the oromaxillofacial region, high-resolution imaging is required. Optimizing the use of 3D printed splints in veterinary patients for orthodontic management may require the use of intraoral scanners and adaptation of human dental software designed for these functions. In addition, 3D printed splints have been proposed as a novel method of mandibular and maxillary fracture fixation in place of the commonly applied bis-acryl composite splints, which use the negative space around to the teeth. The use of 3D printed splints may hold great promise for the future management of veterinary patients.

Although most implants used in veterinary OMFS are standard commercially produced titanium plates and screws, patient-specific 3D printed implants are also being used in practice.[30] These implants are commonly designed to maintain normal maxillomandibular occlusion as well as a scaffold for fibrous or osseous integration (**Fig. 8**). Implants used for veterinary OMFS are currently using SLS printers to print in titanium, as this is considered biocompatible due to the formation of a corrosion resistant oxide layer.[31] This protective oxide layer persists in environments with a pH of a human body, which is similar to the common veterinary patients.[32] More recently in human OMFS, bioresorbable implants composed of polymers such as poly-L-lactic acid and poly-lactic-co-glycolic acid and ceramics composed of hydroxyapatite or tricalcium phosphates have been used for bone reconstruction particularly in non–weight-bearing regions and in pediatric patients.[29,33] The authors consider bioresorbable 3D printed, patient-specific implants to be an exciting opportunity for management of oromaxillofacial trauma in veterinary patients in the near future.

## SUMMARY

Advances in VSP and 3D printing are being led by craniomaxillofacial surgeons in human medicine. Because medical information is becoming more mainstream, there is and will continue to be increasing expectations for similar patient-specific treatments in our veterinary patients. Improved patient outcomes can be achieved when VSP and 3D printing are integrated into the surgeon's armamentarium. There are costs and time considerations in addition to steep learning curves with respect to the design aspects of VSP and 3D printing. However, third-party consultants can be integrated into the team. Veterinary OMFS teams are among those pushing the boundaries of these tools, which will no doubt become a bigger component of other subspecialties within veterinary surgery.

## CLINICS CARE POINTS

- The most common uses of 3D printing in veterinary OMFS can be described in 4 categories including anatomic models for implant contouring, surgical guides, splints, and patient-specific implants.

- Conventional helical CT scan is required for VSP of oncologic cases, whereas cone beam CT scan is adequate for VSP of trauma and orthodontic cases.
- There are third party vendors available to assist the clinician with VSP and 3DP, which creates a delay from the time of clinical imaging to use of the virtual plan and 3D print in the surgical patient.

## DISCLOSURE

The authors have no commercial or financial interests that would constitute a conflict of interest regarding this article.

## REFERENCES

1. Doi K. Computer-aided diagnosis in medical imaging: historical review, current status and future potential. Comput Med Imaging Graph 2007;31(4–5):198–211.
2. Efanov JI, Roy AA, Huang KN, et al. Virtual surgical planning: the pearls and pitfalls. Plast Reconstr Surg Glob Open 2018;6(1):e1443.
3. Kodama H. Automatic method of fabricating a three-dimensional plastic model with photo-hardening polymer. Rev Sci Instrum 1981;52:1770–3.
4. Su A, Al'Aref SJ. History of 3D Printing. *3D Printing Applications in Cardiovascular Medicine*. Available at: https://doi/10.1016/B978-0-12-803917-5.00001-8. Accessed July 22, 2021.
5. McGurk M, Amis A, Potamianos P, et al. Rapid prototyping techniques for anatomical modelling in medicine. Ann R Coll Surg Eng 1997;79(3):169–74.
6. The Official History of the RepRap Project. All about 3D printing 2016. Available at: https://all3dp.com/history-of-the-reprap-project/. Accessed July 22, 2021.
7. Robiony M, Salvo, Costa F, et al. Virtual reality surgical planning for maxillofacial distraction osteogenesis: the role of reverse engineering rapid prototyping and cooperative work. J Oral Maxillofac Surg 2007;65:1198–208.
8. Mazzoli A. Selective laser sintering in biomedical engineering. Med Biol Eng Comput 2013;51:245–56.
9. Leuker B, Gulkan H, Irsen S, et al. Hydroxyapatite scaffolds for bone tissue engineering made by 3D printing. J Mater Sci Mater Med 2005;16:1121–4.
10. Serrano C, van den Brink H, Pineay J, et al. Benefits of 3D printing applications in jaw reconstruction: A systematic review and meta-analysis. J Cran Max Fac Surg 2019;47:1387–97.
11. Hua J, Aziz S, Shum JW. Virtual surgical planning in oral and maxillofacial surgery. Oral Maxillofacial Surg Clin N Am 2019;31:519–30.
12. Allisy-Roberts P, Williams J. Farr's physics for medical imaging. New York: W.B. Saunders Company; 2007.
13. Pauwels R, Beinsberger J, Stamatakis H, et al. Comparison of spatial and contrast resolution for cone-beam computed tomography scanners. Oral Surg Oral Med Oral Pathol Oral Radiol 2012;114:127–35.
14. Lin E, Alessio A. What are the basic concepts of temporal, contrast and spatial resolution in cardiac CT? J Cardiovasc Comput Tomogr 2009;3:403–8.
15. Kusnoto B, Evans CA. Reliability of a 3D surface laser scanner for orthodontic applications. Am J Orthod Dentofacial Orthop 2002;122:342–8.
16. Tarsitano A, Ricotta F, Baldino G, et al. Navigation-guided resection of maxillary tumours: the accuracy of computer-assisted surgery in terms of control of resection margins – a feasibility study. J Craniomaxillofac Surg 2017;45:2109–14.

17. Ricotta F, Cercenelli L, Battaglia S, et al. Navigation-guided resection of maxillary tumours: can a new volumetric virtual planning method improve outcomes in terms of control of resection margins? J Craniomaxillofac Surg 2018;46:2240–7.
18. Bernardino MM, Chiodo MV, Patel PA. Customized "in-office" three-dimensional printing for virtual surgical planning in craniofacial surgery. J Craniofac Surg 2015;26:1584–6.
19. Mazzoni S, Marchetti C, Sgarzani R, et al. Prosthetically guided maxillofacial surgery: evaluation of the accuracy of a surgical guide and custom-made bone plate in oncology patients after mandibular reconstruction. Plast Reconstr Surg 2013; 131:1376–85.
20. Hespel AM, Wilhite R, Hudson J. Invited review – Application for 3D printers in veterinary medicine. Vet Radiol Ultrasound 2014;55:347–58.
21. Baker T, Earwaker W, Lisle D. Accuracy of stereolithographic models of human anatomy. Australas Radiol 1994;38:106–11.
22. Doney E, Krumdick L, Diener J, et al. 3D printing of preclinical X-ray computed tomographic data sets. J Vis Exp 2013;73:e50250. https://doi.org/10.3791/50250.
23. Harrysson OL, Cormier DR, Marcellin-Little DJ, et al. Rapid prototyping for treatment of canine angular limb deformities. Rapid Prototyping J 2003;9:37–42.
24. Dismukes DI, Fox DB, Tomlinson JL, et al. Use of radiographic measures and three-dimensional computed tomographic imaging in surgical correction of an antebrachial deformity in a dog. J Am Vet Med Assoc 2008;232:68–73.
25. Radke A, Morello S, Muir P, et al. Application of computed tomography and stereolithography to correct a complex angular and torsional limb deformity in a donkey. Vet Surg 2017;46:1131–8.
26. Winer JN, Verstraete FJM, Cissell DD, et al. The application of 3-dimensional printing for preoperative planning in oral and maxillofacial surgery in dogs and cats. Vet Surg 2017;46:942–51.
27. Jacobs CA, Lin AY. A new classification of three-dimensional printing technologies: systematic review of three-dimensional printing for patient-specific craniomaxillofacial surgery. Plast Reconstr Surg 2017;19:1211–20.
28. Ghai S, Sharma Y, Jain N, et al. Use of 3-D printing technologies in craniomaxillofacial surgery: a review. Oral Maxillofac Surg 2018;22:249–59.
29. Tack P, Victor J, Gemmel P, et al. 3D-printing techniques in a medical setting: a systematic literature review. Biomed Eng Online 2016;15(1):115.
30. Liptak JM, Thatcher GP, Bray JP. Reconstruction of a mandibular defect with a customize 3-dimensional-printed titanium prosthesis in a cat with a mandibular osteosarcoma. J Am Vet Med Assoc 2017;250:900–8.
31. Sidambe AT. Biocompatibility of advanced manufactured titanium implants – A review. Materials 2014;7:8168–88.
32. Schiff N, Grosgogeat B, Lissac M, et al. Influence of fluoride content and pH on the corrosion resistance of titanium and its alloys. Biomaterials 2002;23:1995–2002.
33. Grün NG, Holweg PL, Donohue N, et al. Resorbable implants in pediatric fracture treatment. Innov Surg Sci 2018;3(2):119–25.

# Oral and Maxillofacial Tumor Management - From Biopsy to Surgical Removal

Ana C. Castejón-González, DVM, PhD,
Alexander M. Reiter, Dr Med Vet, FF-AVDC-OMFS*

## KEYWORDS

- Oral tumor • Staging • Oral biopsy • Mandibulectomy • Maxillectomy
- Glossectomy • Lip/cheek resection

## KEY POINTS

- Despite the advances in medical oncology and radiation therapy, surgical excision remains the best treatment to achieve the local control of OMF tumors.
- Determination of the type of tumor, as well as the local, regional and distal extension of the disease (staging), is necessary to appropriately manage the disease.
- Dogs respond better to radical OMF surgeries than cats.

## INTRODUCTION

The incidence of OMF tumors is 0.5% for dogs and cats.[1] OMF neoplasms account for 6% of all tumors in dogs. A variety of tumor and tumor-like lesions can be encountered in the oral cavity of dogs and cats. A recent study suggests that 61% of tumor-like (ie, neoplastic, hyperplastic, and inflammatory) oral lesions in dogs and 27% of such lesions in cats were, indeed, neoplastic in nature.[2] In dogs, the distribution of malignant and benign OMF tumors is about the same, while malignant tumors are far more frequent in cats (**Table 1**).[2–4]

Despite the advances in other treatment modalities, surgical excision is still the treatment of choice for OMF tumors to get local control, regardless of whether the tumor is benign or malignant. The surgeon might decide the best course of action based on the possibility of removing the tumor with clean surgical margins whereas maintaining oral function and preventing complications that will affect the quality of life of the patient. The presence of regional and distant metastasis might also have an impact on pursuing surgery or the need for additional therapy such as lymph node removal,

Both authors declare to have no conflict of interest. The authors wish to retain the copyright for any image material used in this article (©2021 Ana C. Castejon and Alexander M. Reiter). Department of Clinical Sciences and Advanced Medicine, School of Veterinary Medicine, University of Pennsylvania, 3900 Delancey Street, Philadelphia, PA 19104, USA
* Corresponding author.
*E-mail address:* reiter@vet.upenn.edu

**Table 1**
OMF tumors in dogs and cats

| Tumor | Frequent Location | Surgical Margins | Metastasis | Comments |
|---|---|---|---|---|
| Papillary SCC | Rostral maxilla or mandible | >1 cm | Not reported | Surgery is curative; definitive RT ≥ complete response in 8/9 cases |
| Tonsillar SCC | Tonsil | Difficult to obtain margins due to location | Yes | Poor prognosis when surgery only is used (MST = 137 d), local (MST = 75 d) or distant metastasis (MST = 134 d) is present, or with bilateral involvement; MST for unilateral tonsillar SCC is 637 d; better outcome with multimodal treatment (surgery, radiation, chemotherapy) |
| Non-tonsillar SCC | Gingiva, oral mucosa, palate, tongue | >1 cm | Yes; rare at diagnosis; 20%–30% at late diagnosis | Curative, local control possible; long survival times (mean ST >4.5 y, MST not reached) with clean surgical margins and no metastasis at diagnosis; postoperative RT after incomplete resection (MST = 2051 d) |
| FS | Mandible > maxilla | Wide and radical; >2 cm | Yes; late in the disease (20%–24%) | Curative or local control; MST = 557–743 d; recurrence high; longer survival time with clean surgical margins |
| OS | Maxilla > mandible | Wide and radical; >2 cm | Yes; rare at diagnosis, late in the disease (up to 58%) | Local control; local recurrence >51%; long-term ST (525 d) with surgery and clean surgical margins; grade and MI > 40 are negative prognostic indicators |
| MM | Mandibular gingiva > maxillary gingiva > oral mucosa of lip and tongue > palate > tonsils | Wide and radical; >2 cm | Yes; metastasis at diagnosis is more frequent than for other tumors; metastasis diagnosed after treatment in about 45% of dogs. | Curative or local control with surgery; long MST (326–723 d) with curative intent surgery and smaller size and no metastasis; the more advanced the disease, the worse the prognosis; adjuvant therapy might help. Long ST with RT (758 d for stage I; 80 for stage IV); presence of gross disease a negative prognostic factor for RT outcome |

| Tumor | Location | Surgical margin | Metastasis | Prognosis/outcome |
|---|---|---|---|---|
| Well-differentiated melanoma | Mucosa of the oral cavity and lips | <1 cm | Low | Favorable prognosis; curative or local control with marginal excision; good prognosis if MI <3 and smaller size (<1 cm) |
| CAA | Mandibular gingiva > maxillary gingiva | 1 cm; smaller margins might be appropriate | No | Surgery is curative; responsive to RT |
| Conventional ameloblastoma | Maxilla > mandible | Wide; >1 cm | No | Surgery is curative; responsive to RT |
| POF | Maxillary gingiva > mandibular gingiva | Marginal (>0.5 cm) | No | Curative |
| APOT | Maxillary and mandibular gingiva | >1 cm | Low potential for metastasis (reported in one case) | Curative or local control; responsive to RT |
| FIOT | Maxillary canine region; young cats <18 mo | Marginal; enucleation may be sufficient to have local control | No | Curative |
| Feline SCC | Mandibular and maxillary gingiva, oral mucosa, tongue, and sublingual region | Wide or radical; limited by the size of tumor, adjacent structures, and oral function | Yes | Favorable outcome possible if local control is achieved with surgery; MST = 217 d |

*Abbreviations:* APOT, amyloid producing odontogenic tumor; FS, fibrosarcoma; MM, malignant melanoma; MI, mitotic index; MST, median survival time; OS, osteosarcoma; POF, peripheral odontogenic fibroma; SCC squamous cell carcinoma; ST, survival time; RT, radiation therapy.
*Data from references*[5,6,8–11,16,17,50,71,82–89]

radiation therapy (RT), chemotherapy, or immunotherapy. Metastasis also affects the prognosis, influencing the progression of the disease and shortening survival times.[5,6] Survival times are very variable depending on the tumor, but long-term survival is still achievable with good local control for malignant tumors.[5–9] Survival times longer than 1.5 years were achieved for oral malignant melanoma (MM) smaller than 3 cm, with no metastasis at diagnosis when treated with surgery alone or with surgery and RT.[5,10] Patients with squamous cell carcinoma (SCC) may live more than 4.5 years after local control and those with fibrosarcoma (FS) more than 3 years.[6,8,11]

A thorough physical examination, complete blood count, serum chemistry panel, and urinalysis should be performed to assess general health and to determine if the OMF tumor patient is a good candidate for anesthesia. Thoracic radiographs and abdominal ultrasound can be conducted at an initial stage as part of the general assessment, but also as part of staging.[12]

## STAGING

Staging of a tumor refers to the TNM system (T for primary tumor size and extent, N for regional lymph node involvement, and M for presence of distant metastasis) of the World Health Organization (**Tables 2** and **3**).[13] Several variables measured during the staging process have been associated with the outcome of patients with malignant OMF tumors. Negative prognostic factors for OMM are higher stage, size greater than 2 cm, metastatic disease present at diagnosis, caudal location, nuclear atypia, mitotic index (MI), degree of pigmentation, and lymphatic invasion.[5,10,11,14,15] OMM shows lymphatic invasion when the tumor is > 24.5 mm in size and can be ruled out when less than 6.5 mm.[15] For osteosarcoma (OS), MI >40, higher grade, and calvarial versus

**Table 2**
**TNM staging scheme by WHO for tumors in the *oral cavity* of domestic animals.[13]**

| T: Primary tumor | Tis | Pre-invasive carcinoma (carcinoma *in situ*) | |
|---|---|---|---|
| | T0 | No evidence of tumor | |
| | T1 | <2 cm | a: NO bone invasion |
| | T2 | 2–4 cm | b: Bone invasion |
| | T3 | >4 cm | |
| | Add "m" to T category for multiple tumors | | |
| N: Regional lymph nodes (LN) | N0 | No evidence of LN involvement | |
| | N1 | Movable ipsilateral nodes | a: Nodes NOT considered to contain growth |
| | N2 | Movable contralateral or bilateral nodes | b: Nodes considered to contain growth |
| | N3 | Fixed nodes | |
| M: Distant metastasis | M0 | No evidence of distance metastasis | |
| | M1 | Distant metastasis | |
| Stage grouping | | | |
| I | T1 | N0, N1a or N2a | M0 |
| II | T2 | N0, N1a or N2a | M0 |
| III | T3 | N0, N1a or N2a | M0 |
| IV | Any T | N1b | M0 |
| | Any T | Any N2b or N3 | M1 |
| | Any T | Any N | |

**Table 3**
**TNM staging scheme by WHO for oral tumors in the *oropharynx* (mainly tonsillar carcinoma) of domestic animals.[13]**

| | | | |
|---|---|---|---|
| T: Primary Tumor | Tis | Pre-invasive Carcinoma (Carcinoma *in situ*) | |
| | T0 | No evidence of tumor | |
| | T1 | Tumor superficial or exophytic | a: NO systemic signs |
| | T2 | Tumor with the invasion of tonsil only | b: Systemic signs |
| | T3 | Tumor with the invasion of surrounding tissue | |
| | Add "m" to T category for multiple tumors | | |
| N: Regional lymph nodes (LN) | N0 | No evidence of LN involvement | |
| | N1 | Movable ipsilateral nodes | a: Nodes NOT considered to contain growth |
| | N2 | Movable contralateral or bilateral nodes | b: Nodes considered to contain growth |
| | N3 | Fixed nodes | |
| M: Distant metastasis | M0 | No evidence of distance metastasis | |
| | M1 | Distant metastasis | |
| No stage grouping | | | |

mandibular or maxillary location are negative prognostic factors.[9,16] Location, tumor size, grade, stage, and type of surgery performed influence the outcome of patients with FS.[8,17]

## CYTOLOGIC AND HISTOLOGIC EVALUATION

Presentation, signalment, macroscopic appearance, and diagnostic imaging may be suggestive of one type of tumor or another, but ultimately the final diagnosis requires cytology or histology. Cytology may be diagnostic in highly exfoliative tumors such as MM or SCC. The biopsy of tumors in the oral cavity should not be performed without anesthesia to avoid injury of the veterinarian or patient and to protect the airway in case of bleeding or airway obstruction. During the same anesthetic episode, the following information can be retrieved:

- Size of the tumor in all directions. Pedunculated tumors might appear larger than they really are at the base. A periodontal probe can be placed between the tumor and the pedicle to identify the attached area, as it can affect the extent of the resection. Areas of inflammation next to the tumor with no clear mass effect might be considered part of the tumor. Photographic images of the mass in different views (eg, lateral and occlusal) are important to help pathologists and surgeons to evaluate changes between the time the biopsy is performed and the time of the final procedure. This is of most importance if the biopsy is not performed by the same clinician who performs the surgery.
- Invasion and attachment to deeper tissues such as bone, mandibular canal, infraorbital canal, palate, nasal cavity, and orbit. Advanced diagnostic imaging is necessary.
- Record of other dental or oral pathology that can affect the surgical planning or worsen with RT or chemotherapy. Dental treatment may be performed during the same anesthesia to avoid trauma to flaps or upper lips (ie, crown reduction and vital pulp therapy or extraction of mandibular canine teeth in cases of rostral

maxillectomy or segmental or total mandibulectomy). Tooth extraction or flap creation next to the tumor or in the margins of the tumor is contraindicated because it may increase the size of the excision (an exception is a flap made to obtain a deeper tissue sample during biopsy). Scaling and polishing of the teeth can be performed before surgery to improve overall oral health following surgery.

## Cytology

Accuracy of cytologic examination by fine-needle aspiration (FNA), fine-needle insertion (FNI), and impression smear (IS) of OMF lesions in dogs and cats have recently been reported.[18] FNA, FNI, and IS showed almost perfect (more than 90%) agreement with histologic examination. However, none of these techniques provide any information about the architecture of the tissue which can affect prognosis and treatment plan.[12,18]

FNA and FNI are techniques with high sensitivity (98%) and specificity (100%).[18] Because an inconclusive diagnosis may be obtained if the cellularity of sampled tissue is poor or the sample is hemodiluted and samples from the mouth should be taken under sedation or anesthesia, the authors use cytologic techniques for lymph node diagnostics but rarely use them for the sampling of the primary OMF tumor. IS can be useful as a first noninvasive approach during an awake oral examination in calm and cooperative patients with MM or SCC by taking a sample with a Q-tip applicator and smear the sample on a glass slide, although many times this is unrewarding (**Box 1**).

## Histology

Samples taken from the OMF mass should be large enough to facilitate the pathologists' work. Multiple samples from areas without necrosis or ulceration and representative of the tissue should be taken. The biopsy should be performed safely without compromising the surgical margins, that is, the biopsy should ideally not involve

---

**Box 1**
**Cytologic techniques[12]**

Rinse the mouth with chlorhexidine 0.12% to 0.2%.
Fine-needle aspiration (FNA)
- Use a 22G or 25G[a] needle attached to a 3 to 10 mL syringe.
- Insert a needle in the lesion and retract and release the plunger multiple times, changing the position of the needle within the lesion.
- Withdraw the needle and syringe attached to the lesion.
- Detach the syringe from the needle, and fill the syringe with air.
- The syringe is then attached to the needle again, the opening of the needle should face the glass side, and the plunger is pushed, delivering the cells onto the slide.
- A second glass slide is used to spread the cells.
Fine-needle insertion (FNI)
- Hold a 22G or 25G needle with the dominant hand.
- Insert the needle into the lesion in different directions (do not exit the lesion when doing so).
- Retrieve the needle from the lesion.
- Attach a 3 to 10 mL syringe filled with air and proceed to create the smear as described above.

[a] Larger needles increase blood contamination. Smaller needles cause more cellular damage to the sampled cells (Arai et al 2019).

normal tissue because that would increase the lesion and the extension of the resected area during definitive treatment.[12,19]

A 4 to 8 mm biopsy punch or a #15 scalpel blade is used to obtain multiple samples from representative areas of the OMF lesion. When using a scalpel blade, a stay suture (5–0 suture material) can be placed through the sampling site to secure the tissue, facilitate manipulation, and minimize crushing artifacts with tissue forceps. The stay suture is removed from the sample before placing it in 10% buffered formalin. The sample should be completely submerged in formalin in a ratio of 10 times the volume of the sample. This ensures adequate fixation. Once the sample is removed, a few absorbable stitches can be used to close the defect and control any bleeding. If the tissue is too friable, hemostasis is achieved with pressure, hemostatic agents, or cautery. Electrosurgery or laser should not be used to take the sample because associated heat will destroy the cells, potentially making the sample nondiagnostic.

Samples of OMF tumors that cause expansile lesions within bone, or without obvious alteration of the mucosa, should be taken after the elevation of a mucosal or mucoperiosteal flap and exposure of the deeper tissues. The flap is located over the lesion without extending laterally to avoid seeding tumoral cells in nonaffected mucosa. Computed tomography (CT) can help to determine the area to be sampled when large areas of necrosis are encapsulated. Biopsies of osseous lesions can be obtained with rongeurs (**Fig. 1**).

Incisional biopsies are usually preferred to excisional biopsies because the lesion is still visible at the time of treatment that helps establish margins. Excisional biopsies are only indicated for benign small tumors, pedunculated lesions that cause airway obstruction or bleed spontaneously, and lymph nodes. Whatever technique is used, the clinician should have in mind the possible treatment plan to avoid spreading the tumor locally (ie, avoid flaps or extraction of teeth in the periphery of the lesion).[12,19,20]

## EVALUATION OF REGIONAL LYMPH NODES

A recent study in dogs showed that treatment (RT or surgical removal) of locoregional lymph nodes in patients with high-grade mast cell tumors improved the outcome of these patients.[21] However, there is no clear evidence of how treatment of regional

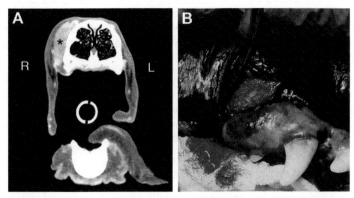

**Fig. 1.** Open biopsy. (*A*) Transverse post-contrast CT image of a dog with right maxillary fibrosarcoma (*). R, right; L, left. The mass is centrally located on the lateral aspect of the right maxilla. (*B*) The mass was accessed by elevating a mucosal flap apical to the mucogingival junction of the canine tooth. (© 2021 Ana C. Castejon-Gonzalez and Alexander M. Reiter.)

lymph nodes of the head and neck affect the outcome in patients with OMF tumors. The diagnostic and treatment approaches are variable and dependent on the clinician, as real guidelines have not been published.[22] Extension of the disease to lymph nodes may change treatment recommendations, prognosis, and owner expectations. Lymph node involvement can be challenging due to several factors:

- The only palpable lymph nodes of the head are the mandibular lymph nodes. The medial retropharyngeal lymph node is located too deep to be palpated, and the parotid lymph node can only be palpated if it is enlarged. The medial retropharyngeal lymph node is located deep in the neck, medial, and slightly caudal to the mandibular salivary gland. Severe enlargement of this node causes lateral and cranial displacement of the salivary gland misleading one to aspirate a normal salivary gland. Aspiration of the medial retropharyngeal lymph node may be facilitated by ultrasound or CT-guidance.
- The size of the lymph node does not rule out metastatic disease. Therefore, cytology or histology should be performed to detect lymph node involvement.[23] Cytology correlates with histopathology in 80% to 90% cases.[24,25]
- The drainage of the oral cavity and head is complex. Evaluation only of the mandibular lymph node may not be representative of true lymph node involvement. Metastatic disease in medial retropharyngeal lymph nodes without the involvement of the mandibular lymph nodes is possible (~40%). Based on this, some clinicians may choose to remove all lymph centers, mandibular and medial retropharyngeal lymph nodes only, or enlarged lymph nodes only with cytologic evidence of metastasis in the presence of a known malignant tumor.[22,24,26–28]
- Surgical removal of lymph nodes may be performed through a lateral incision in the upper neck to reach the 3 lymph centers or through a ventral midline approach in the upper neck to reach the mandibular and medial retropharyngeal lymph nodes.[24,27–30] Recently, studies have been published to determine the sentinel lymph nodes of head and neck tumors in dogs.[30–35] Detection of the first lymph node to which the tumor drains and histologic examination of that lymph node to rule out metastasis would avoid further dissection of more lymph nodes and decrease the time of anesthesia and postoperative morbidity (pain, swelling, infection) associated with the dissection. In a recent study, the sentinel lymph node could be determined in 94% of dogs by CT lymphangiography with iohexol medium. In most OMF tumor cases it was the ipsilateral mandibular lymph node; however, in some tumors located close to midline the sentinel lymph node was on the other side.[35]

Diagnostic imaging of the lymph node may also suggest metastatic disease. Lymph nodes can be evaluated with CT regarding size, contrast enhancement, attenuation, and margins. For OMF tumors the technique showed low sensitivity, but a severely enlarged, heterogeneously attenuated, and contrast- enhanced medial retropharyngeal lymph node may be indicative of tonsillar or pharyngeal tumors.[36–38]

## EVALUATION OF DISTANT METASTATIC DISEASE

Thorax evaluation in search of lesions and nodules consistent with metastasis is one of the first steps. Lungs are a predilection organ whereby many of the malignant tumors spread, but osseous, cutaneous, and abdominal metastases can occur. Mast cell tumors rarely affect the lungs. A 3-view thoracic study is initially performed as a screening, although a negative result does not exclude the presence of metastasis.

Sensitivity for the detection of nodules is higher for CT scan than conventional radiography. In patients with MM, we tend to do an evaluation with conventional radiography because it is the tumor with higher rates of metastasis at diagnosis, and the presence of metastasis is a negative prognostic indicator. Usually, in the absence of respiratory clinical signs and if the patient can be sedated or anesthetized for imaging, we tend to recommend CT of the thorax and head at the same time. Nodules larger than 3 mm can be identified on radiography and as small as 1 mm on CT.[39,40] CT allows for the identification of smaller nodules, a higher number of nodules, and its lobar location, and reduce the superimposition of structures.[40,41] Abdominal ultrasound is indicated to look for evaluation and sampling of nodules in the liver or spleen.

## DIAGNOSTIC IMAGING OF THE ORAL AND MAXILLOFACIAL TUMOR

CT is the gold standard for imaging OMF masses. It has shown advantages regarding the invasion of adjacent structures such as the orbit or nasal cavity compared to conventional radiography, and it allows for the evaluation of soft tissue.[42] Pre and postcontrast multi-planar reconstructions in the 3 planes (transverse, dorsal, and sagittal) should be evaluated for surgical planning (**Fig. 2**). In some exceptions, surgical planning can be safely performed in cases of small tumors in the gingiva with minimal or no bone invasion by evaluating them only with dental radiography, but a combination of dental radiography and CT images provides more information regarding bone, soft tissue, and teeth. Conventional radiography is discouraged due to the excessive superimposition of structures and not being as good for the evaluation of soft tissue. Bony lysis is visible with dental radiography when the bone has lost 30% of its mineral content.[43] Therefore, if only evaluated with dental radiography, larger margins for surgical planning should be considered. Cone-beam computed tomography (CBCT) is a relatively new tool in veterinary medicine focused on the evaluation of bone and teeth. Adequate postcontrast soft tissue algorithm is not yet possible with CBCT. Therefore, soft tissue involvement and surgical margins cannot be accurately assessed with this technique.

Frequent diagnostic imaging findings of OMF tumors include a soft tissue mass, alveolar bone lysis extending into the bone and causing cortical lysis, bone expansion, tooth displacement, cortical bone thinning, heterogeneous or rim contrast enhancement, and presence of cystic structures.[43–47] Locally aggressive tumors can invade other structures such as the mandibular canal, infraorbital canal, nasal cavity, orbit, intermandibular space, and sublingual area.[43,44] Failure in identifying the true tumor extension causes suboptimal surgical planning, leaving tumor tissue behind, and increasing the risk of recurrence and progression of the disease.

## ORAL ONCOLOGIC SURGERY

Overall, benign tumors, including those that are locally aggressive, have a good to excellent prognosis when the tumor is removed with clean margins, and that would be the main goal of surgery. Small malignant tumors have a better prognosis than larger tumors because the surgical excision of smaller tumors provides the best chance for complete removal with suitable margins. Malignant tumors have worste prognosis; however, long-term survival with good quality of life can be obtained if treatment is performed at earlier stages, but in many cases, if local control fails, the patient will succumb to local disease instead of metastatic disease.

The goals of the OMF surgeon should be to create an adequate environment to facilitate healing, remove the tumor with curative-intent or to achieve local control, and maintain masticatory function that keeps the good quality of life of the patient.

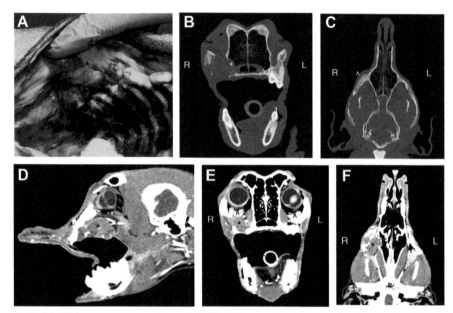

**Fig. 2.** Multiplanar reconstructions with CT. (*A*) Intraoral photograph of an oral malignant melanoma distal to the right maxillary third premolar tooth (#107). The fourth premolar and first molar teeth are missing. The second molar tooth (#110) is still present. Sutures are visible resulting from a previous biopsy. (*B*) Transverse CT image in bone algorithm. There is osteolysis of the zygomatic arch, maxilla, and orbit. The mass invades the right maxillary recess (*). (*C*) Dorsal CT image in the bone algorithm. Periosteal reaction and thickened zygomatic arch (ˆ). (*D*) Postcontrast sagittal CT image in soft tissue algorithm. The tumor extends caudally into the orbit (*), ventral to the globe. The maxillary artery and the descending palatine artery are visible caudal to the tumor (+). (*E*) Postcontrast transverse CT image in soft tissue algorithm. The mass (*) displaces the right zygomatic salivary gland dorsocaudally (ˆ). (*F*) Postcontrast dorsal CT image in soft tissue algorithm. The mass (*) expands laterally and medially. R, right; L, left. (© 2021 Ana C. Castejon-Gonzalez and Alexander M. Reiter.)

Debulking is usually unrewarding. It is performed for exceptional cases if the mass is obstructing the airway or the patient can be treated with adjuvant therapies such as RT. Better results are obtained with RT in the presence of microscopic disease than if the gross lesion is left behind after surgery. Palliative surgery is indicated with the intention of improving pain management, masticatory function, and quality of life.[12,48,49] The main aspects to consider during the surgical procedure are:[12,48,49]

- Preserve the vascularization of the tissues by adequate surgical planning of the incisions and atraumatic surgical technique. The use of stay sutures to retract and gentle manipulation of the tissue are of utmost importance. To avoid electrocautery in the oral mucosa and skin, and if used in deeper tissues, it should be used consciously.
- Reconstruct the facial structures with tension-free closures.
- Avoid infection of the surgical site. Infection of maxillectomy and mandibulectomy sites is unlikely due to the excellent vascularization of the oral cavity if the principles of surgical techniques are followed. Broad-spectrum antibiotics are recommended during the procedure and in the immediate postoperative

period. The oral cavity should be rinsed with 0.12% chlorhexidine, and scaling and polishing of the teeth after induction should be performed. The skin is prepared routinely for aseptic surgery.

- Decrease the risk of bleeding and seeding of neoplastic cells by the ligation of the arteries and veins as early as possible and limiting the manipulation of the tumor (retracting with stay sutures, wrapping the tumor with bandage material) and abundant rinsing with sterile Ringer's lactate solution. Drapes, surgical instruments, and surgical gloves should be changed between tumor excision and reconstruction.

The ideal surgical margin for OMF tumors in dogs and cats is not described. Wide (removing the tumor, reactive zone around it, and normal tissue in all planes) or radical excision is recommended for most OMF tumors. Overall, at least 1 cm margin is acceptable for odontogenic tumors and SCC, 1 to 2 cm for MM, greater than 2 cm for sarcomas.[12] However, the surgical margin is usually limited by the size of the patient, the tissue available to close the resulting defect or the presence of important structures next to the tumor. Therefore, the excision is based on the proportion of the lesion and size of the tissues around. We tend to do surgery with curative intention or to achieve local control of the disease by the removal of the whole tumor and obtaining clean margins.

A recent study showed that surgical margins for canine acanthomatous ameloblastoma (CAA) smaller than 1 cm might be curative.[50] Benign noninvasive tumors, such as peripheral odontogenic fibromas or odontomas, can be controlled with marginal excision or enucleation, though still wide removal is recommended to avoid recurrence. The tumor with the bone, soft tissue, and teeth should be removed *en bloc*. The roots of the affected teeth should be included with the resection, as the tumor can track along the periodontal ligament. Any root remnants of sectioned teeth are elevated and extracted before wound closure and after radiographic confirmation that all root remnants were removed.[12,48]

## MANDIBULECTOMY

The American College of Veterinary Dentistry (AVDC) classifies resections of the lower jaw as partial and total mandibulectomy.[51] Partial mandibulectomy could be unilateral or bilateral, rostral, segmental, dorsal marginal, or caudal. Total mandibulectomy would entail removal of one entire mandible. Partial and total mandibulectomy can be combined if needed (ie, removal of one mandible and parts of the other mandible). Other classifications have been published in various sources (**Table 4**).[52–54]

### Unilateral Rostral Mandibulectomy

This partial mandibulectomy includes removal of the tumor, bone, and soft tissues from the mandibular symphysis up to the second premolar tooth.[53] This technique can be extended to the premolar and molar teeth as needed. The surgical technique is similar for all situations with differences regarding the location of the osteotomy and ligation of the mental and inferior alveolar neurovascular bundles. The patient is positioned in lateral or dorsal recumbency, and the technique can be conducted by an intra- or extraoral approach. An intraoral approach facilitates the visualization of the intraoral margins. A sterile surgical pen is used to draw the intended margins in the oral mucosa and skin. If margins allow, the mucosa of the lateral lip frenulum can be preserved to reconstruct the oral vestibule.

An incision is made in the oral mucosa with a #15 blade, the soft tissues are elevated away from the surgical margin and the tumor by blunt and sharp dissection until

**Table 4**
**Mandibulectomy and maxillectomy procedures**

| | Extent | Location | Description |
|---|---|---|---|
| Mandibulectomy | Partial (removal of part of one or both mandibles and surrounding soft tissues) | Unilateral rostral | Removal of the rostral portion of one mandible (usually up to the second premolar tooth); can be extended caudally if needed |
| | | Extended subtotal | Removal of one mandibular body including the whole mandibular canal |
| | | Caudal | Removal of the caudal portion of one mandible (i.e., mandibular ramus) |
| | | Segmental | Removal of a full dorsoventral segment of one mandible |
| | | Dorsal marginal (also called mandibular rim excision) | Removal of the dorsal portion of one mandible with maintenance of the ventral border |
| | | Bilateral rostral | Removal of the rostral portion of both mandibles; can be extended caudally if needed |
| | Total | Removal of one mandible and surrounding soft tissues | |
| Maxillectomy | Partial (removal of part of one or both maxillae[a] and surrounding soft tissues) | Unilateral rostral | Removal of the rostral aspect of one maxilla (incisivectomy: removal of the incisive bone) |
| | | Central | Removal of the mid-portion of one maxilla |
| | | Caudal | Removal of the caudal portion of one maxilla |
| | | Palatectomy | Removal of part of the palate |
| | | Bilateral rostral | Removal of the rostral portion of both maxillae; can be extended caudally if needed |
| | Total | Removal of one maxilla and surrounding soft tissues (usually an extensive maxillectomy with the removal of all tooth-bearing parts with osteotomies reaching the midline and extending dorsally into nasal and caudally into zygomatic bones) | |

[a] Maxilla (plural: maxillae) is used for maxilla and other facial bones (incisive, vomer, nasal, nasal turbinates, palatine, and/or zygomatic).

exposing the bone (**Fig. 3**). The papillae of the sublingual and mandibular salivary glands can often be preserved in the mucosa caudal to the mandibular symphysis. For tumors localized on the incisor teeth, excision of the mandible rostral to the middle mental foramen may be enough to obtain margins. In this situation, the neurovascular bundles at the rostral and middle mental foramina are ligated and transected with 3-0

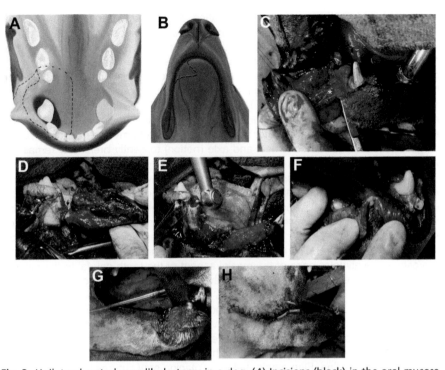

**Fig. 3.** Unilateral rostral mandibulectomy in a dog. (*A*) Incisions (black) in the oral mucosa for a tumor located at the mandibular canine tooth. If the tumor is larger, removal of skin will be necessary (purple). (*B*) V-shaped incision in the skin of the lower lip. The lines connect with the intraoral incision in (*A*). (*C*) Exposure of the middle mental neurovascular bundle (*), which is ligated. No attempt is made to separate the nerves from the vascular structures. (*D*) Ligation of the inferior alveolar neurovascular bundle (*black arrow*) after osteotomy should be made through a tooth (or in the interproximal bone between teeth if there is enough space to avoid damage to the teeth). Sutures were used (*white arrows*) to retract the soft tissue and avoid soft tissue injury during osteotomy. (*E*) Following the extraction of tooth segments or root remnants, osteoplasty is performed with a large round diamond bur under sterile Ringer's lactate cooling. Depending on the extent of unilateral rostral mandibulectomy, wound closure can be (*F*) without and (*G*) with prior skin incisions or (*H*) with commissuroplasty with tension-relieving sutures. (© 2021 Ana C. Castejon-Gonzalez and Alexander M. Reiter.)

to 4-0 polydioxanone or poliglecaprone 25 suture material. Further dissection is continued until the bone is exposed and freed of soft tissue. The mandibular symphysis is separated with an osteotome and mallet. In small patients, an incision into the soft intermandibular synchondrosis with a #15 scalpel blade and separation of the 2 mandibles with a dental or periosteal elevator may be sufficient. The separation of the symphysis facilitates access to the sublingual area and the intermandibular musculature.

Dental radiographs or CT images can be used to plan the osteotomy line which may be curved, abiding by the shape of the tumor and leaving more length in the ventral border of the mandible than in the alveolar margin to provide some osseous support for the gingiva and alveolar mucosa following wound closure. The osteotomy in the body of the mandible is made with a sterile 700L-702S bur in a sterile dental handpiece and sterile cold irrigation to prevent overheating, avoiding any trauma in the soft tissue. Alternatively, a sagittal saw or piezotome is used for the osteotomy. If the tumor is larger and the osteotomy is made caudal to the second premolar tooth, then the middle mental foramen with its neurovascular bundle will be removed together with the tumor. In that case, the osteotomy would involve the mandibular canal. A full-thickness cut is made dorsal (through teeth) and ventral (through the ventral mandibular cortex) to the mandibular canal. The bony cortices at the labial and lingual aspect of the mandible are cut without penetrating the mandibular canal. Then, a dental elevator or Seldin periosteal elevator is placed in the osteotomy site near the alveolar margin and carefully twisted (wheel and axle motion) to gently break any remaining bony connections.

The inferior alveolar neurovascular vessels are ligated with 3-0 to 4-0 polydioxanone or poliglecaprone 25 suture material, then it is transected, and the tumor is removed en block. If the ligature fails and the neurovascular vessels retract into the mandibular canal, access to it might be impossible without removing more bone. Bone wax or other hemostatic agents can be applied to control bleeding (bone wax should be removed before closure). The authors usually perform the osteotomy through a tooth to preserve the alveolar bone of the mesial aspect of the tooth caudal to the osteotomy. Tooth fragments are extracted. The alveolar bone of the extracted mesial root can be shaped to slightly slope downward, thus allowing reliable closure of gingiva and alveolar mucosa. The remaining mandibular bone is smoothed (osteoplasty) with a #23 to 29 round diamond bur to remove any sharp edges which may contribute to ischemic necrosis and wound dehiscence.

Tension-free closure and gentle tissue handling are mandatory to avoid dehiscence at the suture line. Flap manipulation by placing stay sutures in the connective tissue of the mucosal flap prevents the crushing trauma that usually occurs with tissue forceps and facilitates stretching the tissues and testing their correct positioning. Releasing of the periosteum in the caudal, labial and rostral aspects along with the elevation of the mucosal flap sometimes near to the mucocutaneous junction allows the apposition of the tissue and reconstruction of an oral vestibule. A mucosal releasing incision extending caudally, 1 to 2 mm ventral to the mucogingival junction may be necessary. Soft tissue closure is performed in layers with 3-0 (large and giant breed dogs) or 4-0 poliglecaprone 25 suture material covering the rostroventral aspect of the remaining mandible with connective tissue from labial and lingual. Small holes can be made with a #½ or 1 carbide bur 1 to 2 mm away from the bony edge to anchor the connective tissue attachments to the mandibular body. Furthermore, the remaining fibrocartilaginous tissue of the mandibular symphysis can be used to suture the connective tissue of the lip to the opposite mandible. A two-layer closure of the oral mucosa (connective tissue/submucosa first, mucosa second) with an absorbable suture material is made, carefully avoiding the accidental ligation of the mandibular and sublingual salivary ducts and trauma to the sublingual caruncles.

The skin should not be sutured to sublingual mucosa. For small tumors not requiring skin excision, labial advancement flaps from the mucosa may be sufficient. However, skin excision is usually necessary to remove the tumor, bone, teeth, and sufficient normal tissue en block or to remove excess skin that would be in the way of achieving cosmetic appearance. The oral mucosa is advanced from the margins of the resection to the center, closing the defect in a T-shape, or a wedge resection of centered skin may be necessary for the closure and reconstruction of the oral vestibule with closure in a T-shape. The skin is apposed routinely, ensuring that mucocutaneous junctions are accurately apposed if skin was incised.

*Extended Subtotal Mandibulectomy*

The extended subtotal mandibulectomy was recently described.[52] This type of mandibulectomy is indicated for tumors affecting the body of the mandible and extending caudally within the mandibular canal, but not yet involving the mandibular ramus. A commissurotomy may improve the visualization of the caudal OMF tissues. A ventral approach can be made instead to facilitate the approach to the mandibular foramen. The initial steps of the procedure are the same as described above.

As this technique exposes the ventral and caudal parts of the mandibular body and the angular process, the digastricus muscle is transected or elevated with a periosteal elevator from the mandible. The facial artery and vein may be visualized during the commissurotomy or the ventral approach to the caudal part of the mandible. The maxillary artery courses caudomedial to the angular process. The medial pterygoid muscle attaches to the ventromedial aspect of the mandibular ramus covering the neurovascular bundle ventrally, and insertions of the temporal muscle are just dorsal to it.[55] Blunt and careful elevation of the muscle insertions are needed to visualize the neurovascular bundle. Ligation and transection of the bundle should be made rostral to the lingual nerve just before it enters the mandibular foramen using 3-0 or 4-0 polydioxanone or poliglecaprone 25.

The caudal osteotomy is oblique from the dorsal transition between the mandibular body and ramus to the angular process. A Cawood-Minnesota retractor or Seldin periosteal elevator is placed medial to the mandibular ramus to protect adjacent soft tissue. The osteotomy is performed with a piezoelectric surgical unit, a 700L-702S dental bur, or an oscillating saw. An osteotome and mallet can be combined with powered cutting tools if access to the medial aspect of the mandible is difficult. The soft tissue is apposed routinely as described earlier. The lip commissure is reconstructed by closing the initial incision in three layers (oral mucosal, muscular, and cutaneous). Tension-relieving sutures are placed through plastic tubes at the rostral end of the rostrally advanced lip commissure. The new commissure can be extended forward up to the level of the second premolar tooth to provide some support to the tongue, preserve an oral vestibule, decrease drooling, and reduce the instability of the mandible.

*Bilateral Rostral Mandibulectomy*

Bilateral rostral mandibulectomy is the excision of the right and left rostral mandible. Depending on the location and extension of the tumor, the procedure may spare the caudal aspect of the mandibular symphysis preserving the stability of the mandibles and temporomandibular joints (TMJ) and causing minimal functional and cosmetic changes. Procedures extending beyond the second premolar tooth cause independent movement of the mandibles and some TMJ instability.[56] The further caudal the osteotomies are made, the more likely will this affect masticatory function.

The patient is positioned in dorsal recumbency (or lateral with the head rotated 45°). Bilateral labial mucosal incisions are made along the rostral aspect of the lateral lip frenula, coursing rostrally toward the mucocutaneous junction at the level of the canine teeth, from where they continue in a V-shaped form into skin (**Fig. 4**). If the margins and size of the patient allow, the caudal part of the mandibular symphysis can be spared. If the osteotomy goes through the mandibular canine teeth, then their roots must be elevated after excision of the tumor and before wound closure. The attachment of the genioglossus muscle to the caudal aspect of the mandibular symphysis and sublingual mucosa might be included in the resection if the tumor extends caudal to the symphysis. If the excision occurs caudal to the sublingual caruncles, bilateral

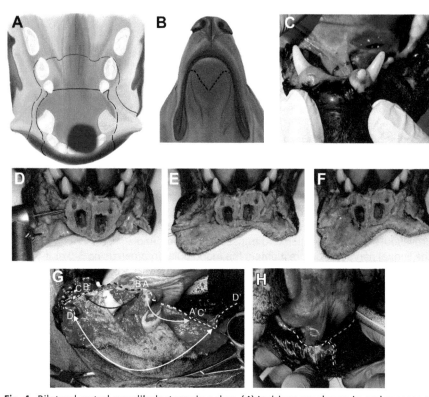

**Fig. 4.** Bilateral rostral mandibulectomy in a dog. (*A*) Incisions are shown in oral mucosa and skin for a tumor at the incisors not affecting the mandibular canines, sparing the caudal aspect of the symphysis (black *line*), and at the level or caudal to the second premolar teeth to include the entire symphysis in the resection, which may course over the ducts of the mandibular and sublingual salivary glands (purple *line*). (*B*) V-shaped incisions in the skin of the lower lip. (*C*) This dog had osteosarcoma whose soft tissue mass had been debulked during biopsy. The intended surgical margins include the salivary ducts (blue marker). Small incisions were made in sublingual mucosa on each side to access, ligate and transect the ducts (*) of the mandibular and sublingual salivary glands. (*D*), (*E*) and (*F*) Connective tissue is sutured to the edges of the cut bone after making small holes for anchorage. (*G*) Following tumor resection, reconstruction of the vestibule with a T-shape closure is performed. Each vestibular mucosal flap is sutured to the sublingual tissues in the midline (A to A'; B to B'). Then the remainder of the two vestibular mucosal flaps is sutured together in a T-shape (C to C', D to D'). Sufficient connective tissue sutures should be made to reduce tension on the mucosal suture line. (*H*) The lower lip is retracted ventrally to show the new oral vestibule after bilateral rostral mandibulectomy (resection from teeth #307–407). (© 2021 Ana C. Castejon-Gonzalez and Alexander M. Reiter.)

ligation and transection of the ducts of the mandibular and sublingual salivary glands should be completed before mandibulectomy. A small incision in the sublingual mucosa over the right and left ducts is made. The ducts are exposed, ligated, and transected. The middle mental vessels must be ligated at the level of the middle mental foramen bilaterally. If the excision is caudal to the second premolar tooth, the inferior alveolar vessels are ligated after osteotomy of the mandibular body as described for rostral mandibulectomy. Radiographic confirmation of the complete extraction of the affected teeth (roots) is recommended.

The remaining connective tissue in the mandibular symphysis (if it is spared) is used to anchor the connective tissue layer. If both mandibles are completely separated (symphysis is removed), the bone edges are covered with connective tissue that can be anchored through holes as described above. A V-shaped incision is made into the skin at the ventral chin and is removed *en block* with the tumor (even if it may not be necessary to obtain clean margins in skin) to facilitate wound closure. Right and left alveolar and labial mucosa is advanced toward the midline to close the intraoral defect in a T-shape, recreating an oral vestibule. The oral mucosa is apposed in 2 layers with 4-0 or 5-0 poliglecaprone 25 suture material. The connective tissue, subcutaneous and cutaneous layers are apposed and sutured routinely (reduction of dead space, alignment of mucocutaneous junctions, tension-free closure).

### Dorsal Marginal Mandibulectomy

This partial mandibulectomy is indicated for the treatment of tumors affecting the gingiva and alveolar mucosa caudal to the mandibular second premolar tooth in medium to large dogs with curative intent.[53,57,58] The objective is to excise the tumor, bone, and soft tissue including teeth with at least 1 cm margins in all directions, preserving the ventral mandibular border and—if possible—the contents of the mandibular canal. This technique is less suitable due to their limited height of the mandible in small dogs and cats and their extraordinary length of the roots in small dogs. It is usually performed for benign tumors (ie, plasma cell tumors, peripheral odontogenic fibroma, CAA) but in certain situations can be an appropriate treatment of MM, SCC, and papillary SCC if bone involvement is minimum, desired surgical margins can be achieved, and sufficient ventral border of the mandible will be retained.

The patient is positioned in lateral or sternal recumbency. Crescent incisions are made in the gingiva, alveolar mucosa, and buccal mucosa buccally and lingually (**Fig. 5**). These tissues are elevated away from the tumor with a periosteal elevator. The soft tissue immediately next to the tumor should not be elevated to expose the

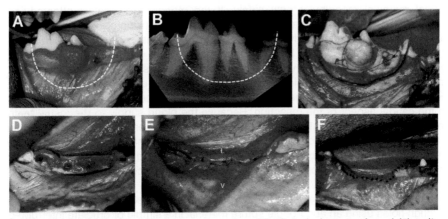

**Fig. 5.** Dorsal marginal mandibulectomy in a dog. (*A*) Clinical photograph and (*B*) radiograph of an acanthomatous ameloblastoma centered between the right mandibular fourth premolar and first molar teeth; white line shows the surgical margins. (*C*) Osteotomy; note the suture retracting mucosa so that it is not obscuring the osteotomy line. (*D*) Excision (from teeth #407–409) was completed, and any tooth segments/root remnants were removed; the mandibular canal was not exposed. Closure of the wound occurred in 2 layers, (*E*) connective tissue (L = lingual, V = vestibular) first, followed by (*F*) mucosa. (© 2021 Ana C. Castejon-Gonzalez and Alexander M. Reiter.)

bone, as that can change the perspective of the surgeon and accidently reduce surgical margins. A 700 L-702S bur is used to create a semilunar or crescent osteotomy around the tumor and through teeth, with the most ventral part of the osteotomy dorsal to or at the dorsal wall of the mandibular canal. A rectangular shape osteotomy has also been described; however, the crescent shape spares some bone and creates a smooth transition with better support for the soft tissue on wound closure. The osteotomy can be conducted full-thickness dorsally (alveolar bone) but only partial thickness on the buccal and lingual cortical bone walls if penetration into the mandibular canal is a concern. The remaining thin layer of bone around the mandibular canal will be fractured by the gentle elevation of the block of tumor tissue with a dental elevator placed at the rostral and caudal aspects of the osteotomy. Iatrogenic fracture of the ventral border of the mandible can occur if the elevation is made without enough cortical bone removed. Any root remnants (ideally the block of tumor with complete teeth were resected) are removed and the edges of the bone smoothed without iatrogenic damage to contents of the mandibular canal. Further releasing of the periosteum might be necessary to obtain a tension-free closure and recreate a gingival collar around the teeth rostral and caudal to the resection side. The oral mucosa is closed in 2 layers.

This technique maintains masticatory function and prevents malocclusion from shifting of the lower jaw as it would occur with segmental mandibulectomy.[57,58] Case selection is very important, as using excessive force during the elevation of the block of tumor or removing too much bone during osteotomy can cause intra- or postoperative fracture. An ex vivo biomechanical study showed that the fracture tends to occur through the empty alveoli in both crescent and rectangular resections.[59]

### Segmental Mandibulectomy

This type of mandibulectomy is indicated for tumors located between the third premolar and first molar teeth whereby the height of the mandible is not enough to do a dorsal marginal mandibulectomy safely. If the mandibular canal is affected, an extended subtotal or total mandibulectomy should be considered. The same principles as described earlier apply in terms of surgical margins, soft tissue manipulation, etc. Special attention should be paid to leaving sufficient soft tissue attached to the bone in all directions to achieve clean margins. When the soft tissue is dissected and the bone exposed, the rostral osteotomy is performed as described above. The inferior alveolar vessels are ligated and transected rostrally, then the process is repeated in the caudal aspect of the resection. Because the blood supply to the rostral teeth may be affected, immediate or delayed endodontic treatment might be necessary, in particular, if the teeth become discolored or nonvital on clinical and radiographic examination. It is also possible that teeth become damaged during osteotomies. If this is the case, the extraction of affected teeth should be conducted before wound closure.

Apposition of connective tissue with an anchorage at the edges of the bone is made through holes using an absorbable suture material in a simple or cruciate interrupted pattern. Care must be taken to not include the salivary ducts in the suture lines. The oral mucosa is closed in 2 layers in a simple interrupted pattern. Following surgery, the lower jaw will shift toward the treated side (mandibular drift). Secondary palatal trauma (from the opposite mandibular canine tooth) and possible upper lip entrapment with the ipsilateral mandibular canine tooth warrant crown reduction and endodontic treatment or tooth extraction. Elastic training can be used to align the opposite mandible and avoid shifting.[60]

## Total Mandibulectomy

Removal of the entire mandible is indicated for tumors affecting a large part of the mid to caudal part of the mandibular body, its mandibular canal, or the mandibular ramus. The larger the animal is, the more challenging it becomes to sever the attachments of masticatory muscles (eg, medial pterygoid muscle at the angular process and temporal muscle at the coronoid process). Also, obtaining surgical margins may become difficult for tumors located at the medial aspect of the mandible, that track inside the mandibular canal caudally (ie, peripheral nerve sheath tumor), or are situated in the mandibular ramus.[12,48,53]

The procedure can be performed by an intraoral approach (sternal recumbency), an intraoral approach combined with commissurotomy (lateral recumbency), or an extraoral ventral approach (dorsal recumbency).[12,61] If the ipsilateral regional lymph nodes are removed, the commissurotomy can be extended caudally and ventrally to get access to them. The important anatomic structures to be considered in the caudal aspect of the mandible include the maxillary artery (caudomedial to the angular process and then ventromedial to the TMJ), dorsal and ventral branches of the facial nerve and parotid salivary duct (over the masseteric aponeurosis), facial artery (coursing rostroventral to the masseter muscle toward the lip commissure), inferior alveolar nerve and vessels, and the ducts of the mandibular and sublingual salivary glands.[55] Careful manipulation of these areas is recommended to avoid life-threatening hemorrhage.

Dissection starts as described for unilateral rostral mandibulectomy (**Fig. 6**). Separation of the mandibular symphysis, lateral displacement of the mandible, and dissection of the soft tissues from rostral to caudal improve the visualization of and approach to the most caudal tissues. Skin will be included as needed in the resection, and particular attention should be paid to obtain surgical margins on the medial aspect of the mandible. Elevation of the masticatory muscles is performed by sharp and blunt dissection until the identification of the inferior alveolar neurovascular bundle whereby it enters in the mandibular canal as previously described for the extended subtotal mandibulectomy. Detaching masticatory muscles from the angular process allows ventral displacement of the lower jaw and access to the insertions of the temporal muscle in the rostral and dorsal aspects of the coronoid process. Disarticulation of the TMJ is made with blunt and sharp dissection (lateral) and rotation of the mandible. Care should be taken during dissection on the ventromedial aspect of the TMJ to avoid injury to the maxillary artery.

Following the removal of the mandible, the defect is closed by the apposition of the masticatory muscles caudally and the sublingual tissues to the remaining connective tissue in the cheek and lip with simple interrupted, cruciate, or horizontal mattress sutures. The oral mucosa is closed in 2 layers. The skin is closed routinely. Commissuroplasty with uni- or bilateral rostral advancement of the lip commissure may be beneficial after more involved mandibulectomies. If skin has not been removed during tumor resection, incisions are made in the mucocutaneous junctions of the upper and lower lip, joining at the lip commissure and extending rostrally up to the level of the second premolar teeth. Further dissection is made in the lip until exposure of the superficial muscles. The upper and lower lips are sutured together in 3 layers (mucosal, connective tissue/muscular, and cutaneous). One to 3 tension-relieving sutures through plastic tubes can be made in the rostral aspect of the new commissure, and a tape muzzle is placed to restrict the animal from opening the mouth wide during healing.[12]

## MAXILLECTOMY

The same principles apply as for mandibulectomy. Planning should be made accordingly, with CT imaging strongly recommended to identify invasion of the nasal cavity

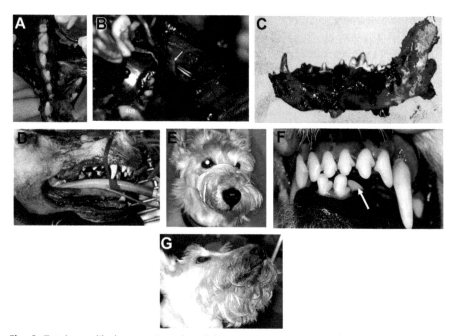

**Fig. 6.** Total mandibulectomy in a dog. (*A*) Large osteosarcoma in the right mandible. (*B*) Ligation of the inferior alveolar neurovascular bundle (*arrow*); note the use of a right-angled forceps to facilitate ligation (409 = lingual surface of the right mandibular first molar tooth). (*C*) Excised right mandible with surrounding soft tissues. (*D*) Wound before closure; note resection of some skin in the preparation of the commissuroplasty. (*E*) Patient is sent home with a tape muzzle to restrict wide mouth opening. (*F*) Displacement of the lower jaw (mandibular drift) to the right; a preemptive crown reduction and vital pulp therapy were performed on the left mandibular canine tooth (*arrow*) to avoid traumatic contact with the palate. (*G*) The patient's facial appearance at the 13-month recheck examination. (© 2021 Ana C. Castejon-Gonzalez and Alexander M. Reiter.)

and orbit. Small benign tumors located in the gingiva may be worked up with dental radiography. The excision of part of the upper jaw (incisive, maxillary, and palatine bones with surrounding soft tissue) can be accomplished with the removal of part of the nasal cavity (vomer, nasal turbinates, and nasal bones) or orbit (and its contents if necessary).[12,51,62,63] Resections of the upper jaw usually are partial maxillectomies (incisivectomy, unilateral and bilateral rostral maxillectomy, central maxillectomy, caudal maxillectomy, and palatectomy).

Depending on the extent of maxillectomy performed, traumatic occlusion with the opposing mandibular teeth may occur with subsequent ulceration of mucosa or skin, wound dehiscence, and oronasal communication. These problems can be prevented by correct surgical planning and appropriate dental treatment. Intraoperative bleeding is a concern during maxillectomies. The main vascular structures to consider during dissection and osteotomy are the infraorbital artery and vein, major palatine artery, minor palatine artery, and superior labial artery and vein. The nasolacrimal duct, sphenopalatine artery, and maxillary artery and vein should be identified as well as the papillae of the parotid and zygomatic salivary ducts in caudal maxillectomies. Healing of the maxillectomy site may result in facial asymmetry and concavity. Most upper jaw resections are partial maxillectomies, whereby part of the incisive bones, maxillae, and other facial bones with surrounding soft tissue are removed unilaterally or bilaterally. Rostral (from incisor to the second premolar teeth), central (from the canine to the fourth premolar teeth), and caudal (from the fourth premolar to the second molar teeth and beyond) maxillectomies have been described based on the location of tissue removed. Excision of small tumors affecting only the incisor region might not expose the nasal cavity if the musculature covering the nasal aperture can be preserved.[62]

### Unilateral Rostral Maxillectomy

Incisions are made in the gingiva and alveolar, labial, and palatal mucosa, followed by blunt dissection down to the bone (**Fig. 7**). Depending on the dorsal extent of the resection, the neurovascular bundle exiting the infraorbital canal at the infraorbital foramen can be preserved or is ligated. The incision in the palatal mucosa is performed after the lateral dissection because it will bleed more due to the presence of the venous plexus. If included in the maxillectomy, the major palatine artery is ligated

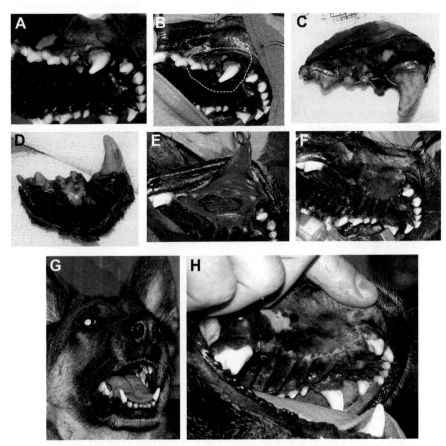

**Fig. 7.** Unilateral rostral to central maxillectomy in a dog. (A) Malignant melanoma near a supernumerary right maxillary first premolar; the tumor's soft tissue mass had been debulked at the time of biopsy. (B) Following draping, the surgical margins are determined. Labial (C) and palatal (D) views of the resected tumor (from teeth #104–107). (E) A flap is prepared, and (F) sutured closed in 2 layers (connective tissue followed by mucosa). Recheck examination in 3 weeks shows mild facial concavity (G) and appropriate flap healing (H). (© 2021 Ana C. Castejon-Gonzalez and Alexander M. Reiter.)

and transected. The palatal mucosa is elevated and reflected with stay sutures to visualize the bone.

Osteotomy is performed with the tools and techniques mentioned earlier. As the block of tumor tissue is elevated, a curved Mayo scissors is used to cut the nasal mucosa and turbinates, so that they remain attached to the tumor's nasal aspect. Hemorrhage from the nasal mucosa is controlled with cold lactated Ringer's solution, gauze sponges, and digital pressure. Hemostatic agents are rarely needed. Any major bleeders should be ligated. Osteoplasty is performed, and sectioned or injured teeth are extracted. The defect is closed with a labial mucosal flap.

The flap is elevated from the connective tissue of the upper lip (if needed up to near the mucocutaneous junction to avoid tension on the suture line). The mucosal flap should ideally include intact branches of the infraorbital neurovascular bundle. If labial mucosa is not available to close the wound without tension, advancement, rotation, or transposition flaps from the caudal and rostral aspect of the defect are harvested. Diverging releasing incisions extending beyond the mucogingival junction into alveolar and labial mucosa are made if necessary. The flap is sutured closed in 2 layers of sutures (first connective tissue, then oral mucosa).[62,64]

### Central Maxillectomy

For excisions at or caudal to the maxillary third premolar tooth, the mucosal incision and osteotomy will be made at or near the level of the infraorbital foramen (ligation of the infraorbital vessels) and lateral or dorsal to the infraorbital canal (ligation of the infraorbital vessels after the osteotomy is completed). The major palatine artery emerges from the palatine canal at the major palatine foramen, which is situated half-way between the maxillary fourth premolar tooth (more distal in dogs and more mesial in cats) and the midline. This vessel will need to be ligated depending on how far palatal the incision in the palatal mucoperiosteum is made.[12,62]

The osteotomy is made as previously described. However, only the lateral wall is cut over the infraorbital canal, carefully avoiding injury to the infraorbital neurovascular bundle. The medial wall of the infraorbital canal is fractured when the whole segment is elevated and laterally or ventrally displaced. A winged dental elevator or Seldin periosteal elevator is used to elevate the fragment. The infraorbital neurovascular bundle is ligated and transected, and the tumor is removed. Alternatively, a window on the lateral wall of the infraorbital canal can be opened with the piezotome to access and ligate the infraorbital neurovascular bundle before the osteotomy. If the caudal osteotomy is made over the maxillary first molar tooth and extended into the palatal shelf of the caudal maxilla, the area over the palatine canal should be spared and any remaining bone attachments broken during the elevation of the fragment. This will leave the major palatine artery unharmed so that it can be ligated following segment elevation.

### Caudal Maxillectomy

For excisions including the molar teeth and beyond a commissurotomy improves access to the caudal part of the oral cavity, but it should be planned accordingly in conjunction with the surgical margins needed and possible reconstruction performed. A combined dorsolateral and intraoral approach has been described to facilitate access to the most caudal part of the maxilla and orbit. It can be also modified with the ligation of the maxillary artery in the pterygoid fossa at the ventral aspect of the orbit, before performing the osteotomies.[65,66] The ducts of the parotid and zygomatic salivary glands can be included in the resection or may be damaged during the procedure. Preemptive ligation and transection of the ducts can be made to avoid sia-locele formation. The zygomatic salivary gland may also be included in the resection.

Incisions in the buccal, palatal, and caudal mucosa are made according to the surgical planning (**Fig. 8**). Following the dissection of soft tissue down to the bone, the infraorbital vessels and major palatine artery at the most rostral aspect of the resection are ligated and transected. The osteotomy is made as previously described, but the entire infraorbital canal may be included in the resection plus parts of the palatine and zygomatic bones. The cut segment is laterally and ventrally displaced to expose the maxillary vessels ventral to the eye and medial to the zygomatic salivary gland. The vessels are ligated and transected before they divide in infraorbital and descending palatine branches.[55] If the minor palatine artery is included in the excision, the maxillary artery is ligated caudal to it. The oral mucosa is closed as described previously. If a commissurotomy was per-formed, it is closed in 3 layers (oral mucosa, connective tissue, and skin).

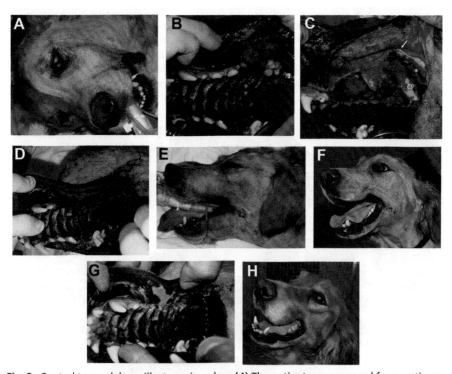

**Fig. 8.** Central to caudal maxillectomy in a dog. (*A*) The patient was prepared for aseptic sur-gery. (*B*) A squamous cell carcinoma is located buccal to the (missing) left maxillary fourth premolar and first molar teeth. (*C*) The wound following tumor resection (from teeth #206–210); note the commissurotomy which was made to gain access to the caudal aspect of the surgery site; white arrow = cut zygomatic arch, asterisk = cut masseter muscle, and CP = coronoid process of the left mandible. (*D*) The wound was closed in 2 layers (con-nective tissue and mucosa). (*E*) The patient's facial appearance before extubation. (*F*) The 2-week recheck examination shows appropriate healing of the incised skin (note a small lingual ulcer due to contact with intraoral sutures and the separate incision in the neck for the resection of regional lymph nodes) and (*G*) oral mucosa (no wound dehiscence). (*H*) The patient returned 1 year following maxillectomy; note increased plaque and calculus accumulation at the left mandibular cheek teeth due to lack of abrasive contact with opposing maxillary teeth. (© 2021 Ana C. Castejon-Gonzalez and Alexander M. Reiter.)

If sufficient buccal and caudal oral mucosa is available for wound closure, little facial distortion will be visible. Multiple flap designs (vestibular mucosa and *angular oris* axial pattern flap or bilateral vestibular mucosa flaps) may be necessary to close a defect without tension after extensive resections.[64,67] Random cutaneous pattern flaps or axial pattern flaps may be necessary for reconstruction if large amounts of skin are included in the resection. An extraoral and intraoral combined approach for excision of tumors affecting the rostral maxilla and muzzle sparing the ventral aspect has been described.[68] The superior labial artery (branch of the facial artery) must be preserved in the ventral part of the upper lip.

### Bilateral Rostral Maxillectomy

Mucosal incisions and osteotomies are made on both sides of the upper jaw, similar to when a unilateral rostral maxillectomy is performed. Following removal of the cut segment and extraction of any root remnants, transposition flaps composed of the right and left labial and buccal mucosa are sutured to palatal mucosa and connected in the midline (to maintain an oral vestibule), thus resulting in a T-shaped closure. Another option is to close the defect with 2 mucosal advancement flaps resulting in an H-shaped closure (**Fig. 9**). Direct apposition of labial mucosa ventral to the nose to palatal mucosa will result in an insufficient oral vestibule, ventral displacement of the nose, and potential dehiscence from excessive tension. Closure of the defect is

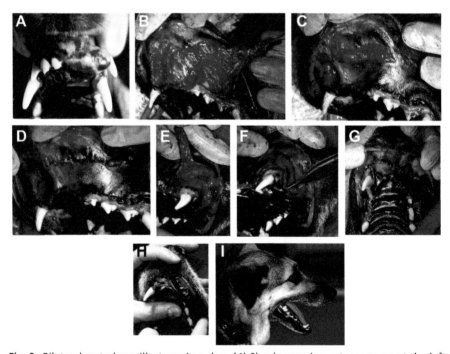

**Fig. 9.** Bilateral rostral maxillectomy in a dog. (*A*) Slowly growing osteosarcoma at the left rostral upper jaw. (*B*) Following tumor resection (from teeth #103–204), an advancement flap is prepared, and sutured (*C, D*) to the midline. (*E*) A similar flap is made on the right side, (*F*) advanced rostrally, and (*G*) sutured in the midline (H-shaped closure). (*H*) No wound dehiscence or (*I*) nose drooping was noted at the 2-week recheck examination. (© 2021 Ana C. Castejon-Gonzalez and Alexander M. Reiter.)

made in 2 layers (horizontal mattress sutures for connective tissue, simple interrupted sutures for oral mucosa).

If one maxillary canine tooth and its supporting bone can be preserved, facial distortion is minimal. Nose drooping will occur if both maxillary canine teeth with dorsal parts of maxillary and nasal bones are removed or if the ventral attachment of the nasal cartilages is lost. A cantilever suture over the bridge of the nose can be used to straighten the nose if this is needed to facilitate breathing.[69] The mandibular canine teeth may cause trauma to the mucosa or skin of the upper lips which can contribute to dehiscence of the surgical site. Crown reduction and endodontic treatment or extraction should be considered to avoid complications.

## PALATECTOMY

Excision of part of the palate is usually performed with any of the maxillectomy techniques, but it can be conducted as a sole procedure. After the mucosal incisions are made, the major palatine arteries are ligated if encountered. For palatectomies located further caudal, the major palatine artery may not be accessible because it is in the palatine canal. As described for the caudal maxillectomy, the bone over the palatine canal should be spared, and vessel ligation can be accomplished following elevation and fracture of the segment. Closure and reconstruction of the defect must be carefully planned before surgery, as failure to have enough tissue available for the creation of tension-free flaps may cause oronasal or oroantral (maxillary recess) communication. Bilateral overlapping flaps of the palatal mucosa covered by buccal mucosal advancement flaps (following the extraction of selected cheek teeth) or angular oris axial pattern flaps are suitable options.[54,67]

## MANDIBULECTOMY AND MAXILLECTOMY IN CATS

The procedures are performed as in dogs. However, clean surgical margins might be more difficult to achieve due to the small head size of the patient and the presence of a relatively larger tumor at the time of presentation. Behavior after radical mandibulectomy may be less predictable. Cats often need supportive care with feeding tubes for longer periods of times (2–3 months) with some patients not being able to regain the ability to eat, groom, or maintain a good quality of life.[70,71] Despite complications (76.3% of them persisted >4 weeks) and aggressive postoperative care, survival rates at 1 year were greater than 50% for SCC, FS, and OS, and owner satisfaction was high.[71] In the authors' experience, unilateral partial and total mandibulectomies as well as bilateral rostral mandibulectomy up to the third premolar teeth are well tolerated in the cat. Unilateral total mandibulectomy and partial mandibulectomy up to or including the third premolar tooth may still provide good quality of life in the long-term with appropriate soft tissue reconstruction (bilateral commissuroplasty). However, bilateral rostral mandibulectomy up to and including the fourth premolar teeth or unilateral total mandibulectomy and partial mandibulectomy up to or including the fourth premolar tooth may warrant life-long nutritional (feeding tube) and other support (hair coat care) (**Fig. 10**).

A recent study in cats that underwent different types of maxillectomy showed lower complication rates than for mandibulectomy and 1-year survival times in 100% and 80% of cases for benign and malignant tumors, respectively.[72] The most common postoperative complications following maxillectomy in cats were difficulty eating (20%, but all cats regained the ability to eat) and wound dehiscence (20%).[72]

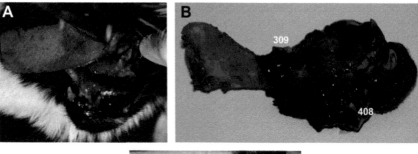

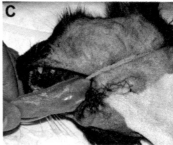

**Fig. 10.** Radical mandibulectomy in a cat. (*A*) A large squamous cell carcinoma invaded the left mandible (causing pathologic fracture) and intermandibular space. (*B*) Left total mandibulectomy and right rostral mandibulectomy up the mandibular fourth premolar tooth (#408) were performed; note the inclusion of intermandibular soft tissue to achieve clean surgical margins. (*C*) The patient's facial appearance following soft tissue reconstruction. (© 2021 Ana C. Castejon-Gonzalez and Alexander M. Reiter.)

## GLOSSECTOMY

Malignant neoplasms account for 64% of all lingual tumors, with MM, SCC, hemangiosarcoma, and FA being most common. Papillomas and plasma cell tumors are the most common benign tumors.[73] Small superficial tumors may be removed by excisional biopsy and marginal resection with an elliptical incision if the tumor is located in the dorsal or ventral surface of the tongue (consider wider surgical margins if malignant). After bleeding is controlled, the lingual mucosa is apposed and sutured in a simple interrupted or simple continuous suture pattern. A continuous suture pattern uses less suture material and potentially causes less inflammatory reaction, but better apposition and tension distribution are achieved with an interrupted pattern. For tumors located close to the edges of the tongue, a full-thickness wedge resection should be performed and the wound sutured in 3 layers (dorsal mucosa, muscle, and ventral mucosa).[74]

More invasive malignant tumors require wider surgical margins. This may not always be achievable depending on the location and size of the tumor. Postoperative lingual function and the supportive needs of the patient should be considered. Dogs adapt well even to the most aggressive resections, but thermoregulation and grooming will be impaired. They may require some assistance during feedings and need some time to learn how to eat and drink independently. Cats tend to not adapt well to large resections. Thus, removal of lingual tissue in the cat usually is restricted to wedge resections and the apex of the tongue. Esophageal feeding tubes are recommended until they can eat and drink independently.

The main arterial blood supply to the tongue is provided by the right and left lingual arteries, with anastomoses between them at the root, body, and apex of the tongue.[55] The anastomoses may not be able to provide enough vascularization to the opposite side if one artery is transected with a full-thickness wedge resection on the body of the tongue. Therefore, a full-thickness wedge resection on one side reaching close to the midline could result in necrosis of the tissue rostral to the surgery site. Transverse resection or longitudinal glossectomy may be a better option. Closure of a wedge resection is made in 3 layers (dorsal mucosa, muscle, and ventral mucosa) and that of a longitudinal glossectomy in 2 (ventral and dorsal mucosa) or 3 layers after the rotation of the long side toward the shorter side (dorsal mucosa, muscle, and ventral mucosa).[74,75]

Transverse glossectomies can be partial (only the free portion of the tongue is removed), subtotal (excision of the free part of the tongue, genioglossus and geniohyoid muscles caudal to the lingual frenulum), near total (>75% of the tongue), and total (100% tongue, ie, apex, body, and root).[76] An incision is made in the dorsal and ventral mucosa of the tongue, and sharp or blunt dissection of the intrinsic musculature is performed (**Fig. 11**). A noncrushing intestinal forceps can be placed caudal to the planned incision to control hemorrhage before the mucosal incisions are made. If the glossectomy is caudal to the lingual frenulum, the clamp is placed after creating a tunnel through the sublingual mucosa of the frenulum below the body of the tongue. Main vessels (lingual and sublingual arteries and veins) are ligated, and muscle tissue is apposed and sutured. The mucosa is sutured with a 4-0 or 5-0 polyglecaprone 25 suture material in a simple interrupted pattern.

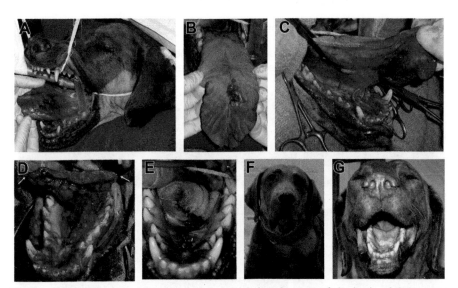

**Fig. 11.** Glossectomy in a dog. (*A*) Ventral and (*B*) dorsal aspect of the body of the tongue affected by a squamous cell carcinoma. (*C*) Two non-crushing intestinal forceps were inserted through a stab incision in sublingual mucosa to clamp the tongue. (*D*) The affection portion of tongue was removed, and important vessels were ligated; note the stay sutures on the sides of the tongue, preventing it from retracting caudally. (*E*) The wound was sutured closed. (*F*) The patient's facial appearance once recovered from anesthesia; note the bilateral incisions in the neck for regional lymph node resection and bandage material covering an esophagostomy feeding tube. (*G*) Complete healing at the 3-month recheck examination. (© 2021 Ana C. Castejon-Gonzalez and Alexander M. Reiter.)

Better outcome with glossectomy is obtained in the presence of benign tumors, tumors less than 2 cm, when the tumor is removed completely, and when no metastasis is identified (>660 days).[77,78] Complications associated with glossectomies include wound dehiscence, oral bleeding, and drooling saliva. Aspiration pneumonia can happen after radical glossectomies due to the impairment of the swallowing mechanism.[76,78]

## LIP AND CHEEK RESECTION

Small tumors affecting the skin of the lip or cheek and not invading deeper tissues can be removed with margins including the skin and deepest muscular layer. A full-thickness resection with adjacent bone resection may be needed for very invasive tumors to achieve local control. Medical and radiation oncologists should work together with the surgeon to establish the best course of action. Surgical planning is needed based on the type of tumor, size and location of the tumor, type of resection, size of resulting defect, tissue available for tension-free reconstruction, postoperative morbidity, desired masticatory function, and anticipated complications.

Wedge resection, square resection and closure in Y-shape, random pattern flaps (advancement, rotation, and transposition), and axial myocutaneous flaps (angular oris, facial, superficial temporal, superficial caudal auricular) have been described to reconstruct facial and oral defects.[64,69,74] The main complication is dehiscence, which seems to be less frequent with advancement and transposition flaps than rotational flaps.[79] Oral function is usually good, but a change of the position of the commissure can limit the range of mouth opening. Reconstruction of an oral vestibule is most desired (**Fig. 12**). Suturing skin directly to gingiva, palatal or sublingual mucosa must be avoided.[64,69]

## POSTOPERATIVE CARE AND FOLLOW-UP

Dogs have a relatively high tolerance for surgery in the OMF region and most likely will eat and drink shortly after the procedure. Some of them may need assisted feeding by

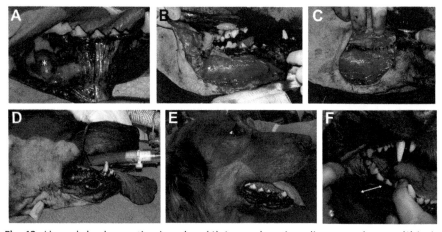

**Fig. 12.** Lip and cheek resection in a dog. (*A*) An amelanotic malignant melanoma (\*) is situated in the buccal mucosa adjacent to the right mandibular first molar tooth. (*B*) The tumor was resected with surrounding oral mucosa and skin. (*C*) Closure of oral mucosa; note the suture knots are facing the connective tissue side. (*D*) A Penrose drain was placed and the skin closed. (*E*) The patient's facial appearance at the 1-month recheck examination. (*F*) Maintenance of an oral vestibule (*double-ended arrow*) is most important to avoid drooling saliva. (© 2021 Ana C. Castejon-Gonzalez and Alexander M. Reiter.)

**Table 5**
**Complications of maxillectomy, mandibulectomy, and glossectomy**

| Complication | Procedure | Comments |
|---|---|---|
| Dehiscence | All | Use appropriate technique (avoid tension, perform osteoplasty, support soft tissue through holes in the bone, two-layer closure of oral mucosa). Preoperative RT or chemotherapy increases the likelihood of dehiscence. Small areas of dehiscence may heal by second intention. Dehiscence in the maxilla causes oronasal communication. Revision surgery is recommended. |
| Infection | All | Unlikely if appropriate surgical technique is used. Consider intraoperative antibiotics. |
| Oronasal fistula | Maxillectomy | Avoid tension and use appropriate surgical techniques. |
| Nose drooping | Unilateral or bilateral rostral maxillectomy | More likely if bone around both maxillary canine teeth is removed, nasal bones are included in the resection and nasal cartilages are excised. |
| Severe hemorrhage | Extensive mandibulectomy and maxillectomy | Higher risk in maxillectomy than mandibulectomy (particularly with caudal maxillectomy and dorsolateral and intraoral combined approach). Blood typing and cross-matching are recommended before extended subtotal, caudal and total mandibulectomy, central and caudal maxillectomy procedures. Blood transfusion may be needed. |
| Trigeminovagal reflex and asystole | All | Excessive retraction of neurovascular bundles (inferior alveolar, infraorbital, maxillary) or the tongue. Responsive to anticholinergics. |
| Dysphagia/anorexia | All | Temporary. More frequent and long-term with near-total glossectomy and extensive mandibulectomy in cats. |

*(continued on next page)*

| Complication | Procedure | Comments |
|---|---|---|

**Table 5**
**(continued)**

| Complication | Procedure | Comments |
|---|---|---|
| Drooling saliva | Mandibulectomy, glossectomy | Commissuroplasty may reduce it after mandibulectomy, but not prevent it entirely. |
| Mandibular drift and traumatic occlusion | Unilateral, subtotal, segmental, and total mandibulectomy | Preemptive extraction or crown reduction and endodontic treatment of contralateral canine tooth. As an alternative, elastic chains and buttons or brackets between maxillary fourth premolar and mandibular canine teeth. Mucosal ulceration and lip trauma can occur after maxillectomy due to traumatic contact with opposing teeth or contact of the tongue with sutures. |
| Sialocele | Mandibulectomy (ducts of sublingual or mandibular gland) and central and caudal maxillectomy (ducts of parotid or zygomatic gland). | Preemptive ligation of salivary ducts if papillae or ducts are in the surgical site or traumatized. |

*Abbreviations:* RT, radiation therapy.
   *Data from* Refs.[65,70,71,78,80–82,90]

the owner until they learn to independently eat and drink again (eg, after glossectomies or extensive mandibulectomy and maxillectomy that affect the prehension of food and intake of water). Dogs rarely need feeding tube placement, but if so, it can be placed at the time of the procedure or a couple of days after if nutritional intake is insufficient. Placement of an esophagostomy tube in cats after extensive surgery is recommended until the patient can eat and drink. A soft diet (slurry to meatball consistency) is usually given for about 2 weeks. Some patients may need soft food for longer period of times.

Restriction of mouth activity until healing is completed and minimal general activity during that time is warranted to avoid increased pressure over flaps (panting) and postoperative bleeding. Multimodal analgesia is provided during the first 5 to 7 days and continued as needed by assessing the patient needs. An Elizabethan collar during the healing period prevents accidental self-trauma. The patient should be evaluated earlier than at the scheduled 2-week recheck if there is excessive pawing, scratching or conscious self-trauma to rule out insufficient pain management, infection, wound dehiscence, or other complications.

Intraoperative antibiotics are recommended. However, the patient may only need to be discharged with postoperative antibiotics depending on health status, immunosuppression, type of surgery, tissue trauma, etc. A tape muzzle may be indicated for 1 to 2 weeks after the reconstruction of the lip commissure or unilateral partial or total mandibulectomy to provide support for the lower jaw, restrict wide mouth opening, and avoid wound dehiscence.

## COMPLICATIONS

Intraoperative bleeding and wound dehiscence are the most common complications of OMF surgery (**Table 5**).[65,78,80,81] In a recent study, 37% of dogs that underwent maxillectomy and mandibulectomy procedures had complications.[81] Despite the occurrence of complications, owner's satisfaction after wide or radical OMF surgery usually is high.[7,71]

## REFERENCES

1. Cray M, Selmic LE, Ruple A. Demographics of dogs and cats with oral tumors presenting to teaching hospitals:1996-2017. J Vet Sci 2020;21(5):e70.
2. Mikiewicz M, Paździor-Czapula K, Gesek M, et al. Canine and feline oral cavity tumours and tumour-like lesions: a retrospective study of 486 cases (2015-2017). J Comp Pathol 2019;172:80–7.
3. Wingo K. Histopathologic diagnoses from biopsies of the oral cavity in 403 dogs and 73 cats. J Vet Dent 2018;35(1):7–17.
4. Manuali E, Forte C, Vichi G, et al. Tumours in European shorthair cats: a retrospective study of 680 cases. J Feline Med Surg 2020;22(12):1095–102.
5. Tuohy J, Selmic KE, Worley DR, et al. Outcome following curative-intent surgery for oral melanoma in dogs: 70 cases (1998-2011). J Am Vet Med Assoc 2014; 245(11):1266–73.
6. Riggs J, Adams VJ, Hermer JV, et al. Outcomes following surgical excision or surgical excision combined with adjunctive, hypofractionated radiotherapy in dogs with oral squamous cell carcinoma or fibrosarcoma. J Am Vet Med Assoc 2018;253(1):73–83.
7. Sarowitz BN, Gavis GJ, Kim S. Outcome and prognostic factors following curative-intent surgery for oral tumors in dogs: 234 cases (2004 to 2014). J Small Anim Pract 2017;58(3):146–53.
8. Frazier SA, Johns SM, Ortega J, et al. Outcome in dogs with surgically resected oral fibrosarcoma (1997-2008). Vet Comp Oncol 2012;10(1):33–43.
9. Coyle VJ, Rassnick KM, Borst LB, et al. Biological behaviour of canine mandibular osteosarcoma. A retrospective study of 50 cases (1999-2007). Vet Comp Oncol 2015;13(2):89–97.
10. Boston SE, Lu X, Culp WT, et al. Efficacy of systemic adjuvant therapies administered to dogs after excision of oral malignant melanomas: 151 dogs (2001-2012). J Am Vet Med Assoc 2014;245(4):401–7.
11. Turek M, LaDue T, Looper J, et al. Multimodality treatment including ONCEPT for canine oral melanoma: a retrospective analysis of 131 dogs. Vet Radiol Ultrasound 2020;61(4):471–80.
12. Romanelli G, Lewis J. Management of oral and maxillofacial neoplasia. In: Reiter AM, Gracis M, editors. BSAVA manual of canine and feline dentistry and oral surgery. 4th edition. Gloucester, United Kingdom: BSAVA; 2018. p. 279–303.
13. Owen LN. TNM classification of tumors in domestic animals. Geneva, Switzerland: World Health Organisation; 1980.
14. Kawabe M, Tori T, Ito Y, et al. Outcomes of dogs undergoing radiotherapy for treatment of oral malignant melanoma: 111 cases (2006-2012). J Am Vet Med Assoc 2015;247(10):1146–53.
15. Carroll KA, Kuntz CA, Heller J, et al. Tumor size as a predictor of lymphatic invasion in oral melanomas of dogs. J Am Vet Med Assoc 2020;256(10):1123–8.

16. Selmic LE, Lafferty MH, Kamstock DA, et al. Outcome and prognostic factors for osteosarcoma of the maxilla, mandible or calvarium in dogs: 183 cases (1986-2012). J Am Vet Med Assoc 2014;245(8):930–8.

17. Gardner H, Fidel J, Haldorson G, et al. Canine oral fibrosarcomas: a retrospective analysis of 65 cases (1998-2010). Vet Comp Oncol 2015;13(1):40–7.

18. Bonfanti U, Bertazzolo W, Gracis M, et al. Diagnostic value of cytological analysis of tumours and tumour-like lesions of the oral cavity in dogs and cats: a prospective study on 114 cases. Vet J 2015;205(2):322–7.

19. Arzi B, Verstraete FJM. Clinical staging and biopsy of maxillofacial tumors. In: Verstraete FJM, Lommer MJ, Arzi B, editors. Oral and maxillofacial surgery in dogs and cats. 2nd edition. St. Louis, MO: Elsevier; 2020. p. 415–22.

20. Reiter AM. Equipment for oral surgery. Vet Clin North Am Small Anim Pract 2013; 43(3):587–608.

21. Mendez SE, Drobatz K, Duda L, et al. Treating the locoregional lymph nodes with radiation and/or surgery significantly improves outcome in dogs with high grade mast cell tumors. Vet Com Oncol 2020;18(2):239–46.

22. Congiusta M, Lawrence J, Rendahl A, et al. Variability in recommendations for cervical lymph node pathology for staging of canine oral neoplasia: a survey study. Front Vet Sci 2020;7:506.

23. Williams LE, Packer RA. Association between lymph node size and metastasis in dogs with oral malignant melanoma: 100 cases (1987-2001). J Am Vet Med Assoc 2003;222(9):1234–6.

24. Herring ES, Smith MM, Robertson JL. Lymph node staging of oral and maxillofacial neoplasms in 31 dogs and cats. J Vet Dent 2002;19(3):122–6.

25. Ghisleni G, Roccabianca P, Ceruti R, et al. Correlation between fine-needle aspiration cytology and histopathology in the evaluation of cutaneous and subcutaneous masses from dogs and cats. Vet Clin Pathol 2006;35(1):24–30.

26. Grimes JA, Mestrinho LA, Berg J, et al. Histologic evaluation of mandibular and medial retropharyngeal lymph nodes during staging of oral malignant melanoma and squamous cell carcinoma in dogs. J Am Vet Med Assoc 2019;254(8):938–43.

27. Odenweller PH, Smith MM, Taney KG. Validation of regional lymph node excisional biopsy for staging oral and maxillofacial malignant neoplasms in 97 dogs and 10 cats (2006-2016). J Vet Dent 2019;36(2):97–103.

28. Green K, Boston SE. Bilateral removal of the mandibular and medial retropharyngeal lymph nodes through a single ventral midline incision for staging of head and neck cancers in dogs: a description of surgical technique. Vet Comp Oncol 2017;15(1):208–14.

29. Wainberg SH, Oblak ML, Giuffrida MA. Ventral cervical versus bilateral lateral approach for extirpation of mandibular and medial retropharyngeal lymph nodes in dogs. Vet Surg 2018;47(5):629–33.

30. Smith MM. Surgical approach for lymph node staging of oral and maxillofacial neoplasms in dogs. J Vet Dent 2002;19(3):170–4.

31. Chiti LE, Stefanello D, Manfredi M, et al. To map or not to map the cN0 neck: Impact of sentinel lymph node biopsy in canine head and neck tumours. Vet Comp Oncol 2021. https://doi.org/10.1111/vco.12697.

32. Wan J, Oblak ML, Ram A, et al. Determining agreement between preoperative computed tomography lymphography and indocyanine green near infrared fluorescence intraoperative imaging for sentinel lymph node mapping in dogs with oral tumours. Vet Comp Oncol 2021;19(2):295–303.

33. Randall EK, Jones MD, Kraft SL, et al. The development of an indirect computed tomography lymphography protocol for sentinel lymph node detection in head

and neck cancer and comparison to other sentinel lymph node mapping techniques. Vet Comp Oncol 2020;18(4):634–44.

34. Townsend KL, Milovancev M, Bracha S. Feasibility of near-infrared fluorescence imaging for sentinel lymph node evaluation of the oral cavity in healthy dogs. Am J Vet Res 2018;79(9):995–1000.

35. Grimes JA, Secrest SA, Northrup NC, et al. Indirect computed tomography lymphangiography with aqueous contrast for evaluation of sentinel lymph nodes in dogs with tumor of the head. Vet Radiol Ultrasound 2017;58(5):559–64.

36. Skinner OT, Boston SE, Giglio RF, et al. Diagnostic accuracy of contrast-enhanced computed tomography for assessment of mandibular and medial retropharyngeal lymph node metastasis in dogs with oral and nasal cancer. Vet Comp Oncol 2018;16(4):562–70.

37. Thierry F, Longo M, Pecceu E, et al. Computed tomographic appearance of canine tonsillar neoplasia: 14 cases. Vet Radiol Ultrasound 2018;59(1):54–63.

38. Carozzi G, Zotti A, Alberti M, et al. Computed tomographic features of pharyngeal neoplasia in 25 dogs. Vet Radiol Ultrasound 2015;56(6):628–37.

39. Armbrust LJ, Biller DS, Bamford A, et al. Comparison of three-view thoracic radiography and computed tomography for detection of pulmonary nodules in dogs with neoplasia. J Am Vet Med Assoc 2012;240(9):1088–94.

40. Nemanic S, London CA, Wisner ER. Comparison of thoracic radiographs and single breath-hold helical CT for detection of pulmonary nodules in dogs with metastatic neoplasia. J Vet Intern Med 2006;20(3):508–15.

41. Alexander K, Joly H, Blond L, et al. A comparison of computed tomography, computed radiography, and film-screen radiography for the detection of canine pulmonary nodules. Vet Radiol Ultrasound 2012;53(3):258–65.

42. Ghirelli CO, Villamizar LA, Pinto AC. Comparison of standard radiography and computed tomography in 21 dogs with maxillary masses. J Vet Dent 2013; 30(2):72–6.

43. DuPont GA, DeBowes L. Atlas of dental radiography in dogs and cats. St. Louis, MO: Saunders Elsevier; 2009.

44. Kuntsi H, Schwarz T, Mai W, et al. Dental and oral diagnostic imaging and interpretation. In: Reiter AM, Gracis M, editors. BSAVA manual of canine and feline dentistry and oral surgery. 4th edition. Gloucester, United Kingdom: BSAVA; 2018. p. 49–88.

45. Amory JT, Reetz JA, Sánchez MD, et al. Computed tomographic characteristics of odontogenic neoplasms in dogs. Vet Radiol Ultrasound 2014;55(2):147–58.

46. Goldschmidt S, Bell C, Waller K, et al. Biological behavior of canine acanthomatous ameloblastoma assessed with computed tomography and histopathology: a comparative study. J Vet Dent 2020;37(3):126–32.

47. Gendler A, Lewis JR, Reetz JA, et al. Computed tomographic features of oral squamous cell carcinoma in cats: 18 cases (2002-2008). J Am Vet Med Assoc 2010;236(3):319–25.

48. Lommer MJ, Verstraete FJM, Arzi B. Principles of oral oncologic surgery. In: Verstraete FJM, Lommer MJ, Arzi B, editors. Oral and maxillofacial surgery in dogs and cats. 2nd edition. St. Louis, MO: Elsevier; 2020. p. 469–77.

49. Farese JP, Liptak JM, Withrow SJ. Surgical oncology. In: Vail D, Thamm DH, Liptak JM, editors. Withrow and macewen's small animal clinical oncology. 6th edition. St. Louis, MO: Elsevier; 2020. p. 164–73.

50. Goldschmidt SL, Bell CM, Hetzel S, et al. Clinical characterization of canine acanthomatous ameloblastoma (CAA) in 263 dogs and the influence of postsurgical histopathological mrgin on local recurrence. J Vet Dent 2017;34(4):241–7.

51. AVDC Nomenclature. American Veterinary Dental College. Available at: https://avdc.org/avdc-nomenclature/. Accessed September 4, 2021.
52. Fiani N, Peralta S. Extended subtotal mandibulectomy for the treatment of oral tumors invading the mandibular canal in dogs - A novel surgical technique. Front Vet Sci 2019;6:339.
53. Verstraete FJM, Arzi B, Lanz GC. Mandibulectomy techniques. In: Verstraete FJM, Lommer MJ, Arzi B, editors. Oral and mxillofacial surgery in dogs and cats. 2nd edition. St. Louis, MO: Elsevier; 2020. p. 515–28.
54. Zacher AM, Manfra Marretta S. Oral and maxillofacial surgery in dogs and cats. Vet Clin North Am Small Anim Pract 2013;43(3):609–49.
55. Evans HE, de Lahunta A. Miller's anatomy of the dog. 4th edition. St. Louis, MO: Elsevier; 2013.
56. Arzi B, Verstraete FJM, Garcia TC, et al. Kinematic analysis of mandibular motion before and after mandibulectomy and mandibular reconstruction in dogs. Am J Vet Res 2019;80(7):637–45.
57. Arzi B, Verstraete FJ. Mandibular rim excision in seven dogs. Vet Surg 2010;39(2):226–31.
58. Walker KS, Reiter AM, Lewis JR. Marginal mandibulectomy in the dog. J Vet Dent 2009;26(3):194–8.
59. Linden D, Matz BM, Farag R, et al. Biomechanical comparison of two ostectomy configurations for partial mandibulectomy. Vet Comp Orthop Traumatol 2017;30(1):15–9.
60. Bar-Am Y, Verstraete FJ. Elastic training for the prevention of mandibular drift following mandibulectomy in dogs: 18 cases (2005-2008). Vet Surg 2010;39(5):574–80.
61. De Mello Souza CH, Bacon N, Boston S, et al. Ventral mandibulectomy for removal of oral tumours in the dog: Surgical technique and results in 19 cases. Vet Comp Oncol 2019;17(3):271–5.
62. Arzi B, Verstraete FJM, Lantz GC. Maxillectomy techniques. In: Verstraete FJM, Lommer MJ, Arzi B, editors. Oral and maxillofacial surgery in dogs and cats. 2nd edition. St. Louis, MO: Elsevier; 2020. p. 499–514.
63. Thomson AE, Rigby BE, Geddes AT, et al. Excision of extensive orbitozygomaticomaxillary complex tumors combining an intra- and extraoral approach with transpalpebral orbital exenteration. Front Vet Sci 2020;7:569747.
64. Guzu M, Rossetti D, Hennet P. Locoregional flap reconstruction following oromaxillofacial oncologic surgery in dogs and cats: a review and decisional algorithm. Front Vet Med 2021;21(8):685036.
65. Carroll KA, Mathews KG. Ligation of the maxillary artery prior to caudal maxillectomy in the dog- A description of the technique, retrospective evaluation of blood loss, and cadaveric evaluation of maxillary artery anatomy. Front Vet Sci 2020;7:588945.
66. Lascelles BD, Thomson MJ, Dernell WS, et al. Combined dorsolateral and intraoral approach for the resection of tumors of the maxilla in the dog. J Am Anim Hosp Assoc 2003;39(3):294–305.
67. Tuohy JL, Worley DR, Wustefeld-Janssens BG, et al. Bilateral caudal maxillectomy for resection of tumors crossing palatal midline and use of the angularis oris axial pattern flap for primary closure or dehiscence repair in two dogs. Vet Surg 2019;48(8):1490–9.
68. Thomson AE, Soukup JW. Composite resection of tumors of the rostral maxilla and dorsolateral muzzle utilizing an upper lip-sparing, combined approach in dogs. Front Vet Sci 2018;5:54.

69. Pavletic MM. Atlas of small animal wound management and reconstructive surgery. 4th edition. Hoboken, NJ: Wiley; 2018.
70. Boston SE, van Stee LL, Bacon NJ, et al. Outcome of eight cats with oral neoplasia treated with radical mandibulectomy. Vet Surg 2020;49(1):222–32.
71. Northrup NC, Selting KA, Rassnick KM, et al. Outcomes of cats with oral tumors treated with mandibulectomy: 42 cases. J Am Anim Hosp Assoc 2006;42(5): 350–60.
72. Liptak JM, Tatcher GP, Mestrinho LA, et al. Outcomes of cats treated with maxillectomy: 60 cases. A Veterinary Society of Surgical Oncology retrospective study. Vet Comp Oncol 2020. https://doi.org/10.1111/vco.12634.
73. Dennis MM, Ehrhart N, Duncan CG, et al. Frequency of and risk associated with lingual lesions in dogs. 1,196 cases (1995-2004). J Am Vet Med Assoc 2006; 228(10):1533–7.
74. Séguin B. Surgical treatment of tongue, lip and cheek tumors. In: Verstraete FJM, Lommer MJ, Arzi B, editors. Oral and maxillofacial surgery in dogs and cats. 2nd edition. St. Louis, MO: Elsevier; 2020. p. 478–98.
75. Montinaro V, Boston SE. Tongue rotation for reconstruction after rostral hemiglossectomy for excision of a liposarcoma of the rostral quadrant of the tongue in a dog. Can Vet J 2013;54(6):591–4.
76. Dvorak L, Beaver D, Ellison GW, et al. Major glossectomy in dogs: a case series and proposed classification system. J Am Anim Hosp Assoc 2004;40(4):331–7.
77. Culp WTN, Ehrhart N, Withrow SJ, et al. Results of surgical excision and evaluation of factors associated with survival time in dogs with lingual neoplasia: 97 cases (1995-2008). J Am Vet Med Assoc 2013;242(10):1392–7.
78. Syrcle JA, Bonczynski JJ, Monette S, et al. Retrospective evaluation of lingual tumors in 42 dogs: 1999-2005. J Am Anim Hosp Assoc 2008;44(6):308–19.
79. Jones CA, Lipscomb VJ. Indications, complications, and outcomes associated with subdermal plexus skin flap procedures in dogs and cats: 92 cases (2000-2017). J Am Vet Med Assoc 2019;255(8):933–8.
80. MacLellan RH, Rawlinson JE, Rao S, et al. Intraoperative and postoperative complications of partial maxillectomy for the treatment of oral tumors in dogs. J Am Vet Med Assoc 2018;252(12):1538–47.
81. Cray M, Selmic LE, Kindra C, et al. Analysis of risk factors associated with complications following mandibulectomy and maxillectomy in dogs. J Am Vet Med Assoc 2021;259(3):265–74.
82. van der Steen F, Zandvliet M. Treatment of canine oral papillary squamous cell carcinoma using definitive-intent radiation as a monotherapy-a case series. Vet Comp Oncol 2021;19(1):152–9.
83. Soukup JW, Snyder CJ, Simmons BT, et al. Clinical, histologic, and computed tomographic features of oral papillary squamous cell carcinoma in dogs: 9 cases (2008- 2011). J Vet Dent 2013;30(1):18–24.
84. Mas A, Blackwood L, Cripps P, et al. Canine tonsillar squamous cell carcinoma - a multi-centre retrospective review of 44 clinical cases. J Small Anim Pract 2011; 52(7):359–64.
85. Grant J, North S. Evaluation of the factors contributing to long-term survival in canine tonsillar squamous cell carcinoma. Aust Vet J 2016;94(6):197–202.
86. Sharma S, Boston SE, Skinner OT, et al. Survival time of juvenile dogs with oral squamous cell carcinoma treated with surgery alone: a Veterinary Society of Surgical Oncology retrospective study. Vet Surg 2021;50(4):740–7.

87. Esplin DG. Survival of dogs following surgical excision of histologically well-differentiated melanocytic neoplasms of the mucous membranes of the lips and oral cavity. Vet Pathol 2008;45(6):889–96.

88. Tjepkema J, Bell CM, Soukup JW. Presentation, diagnostic imaging, and clinical outcome of conventional ameloblastoma in dogs. J Vet Dent 2020;37(1):6–13.

89. Blackford Winders C, Bell CM, Goldschmidt S. Case report: Amyloid-producing odontogenic tumor with pulmonary metastasis in a Spinone Italiano - Proof of malignant potential. Front Vet Sci 2020;7:576376.

90. Vezina-Audette R, Benedicenti L, Castejon-Gonzalez A, et al. Anesthesia case of the month: recurrent asystole and severe bradycardia during surgical repair of cleft palate in a dog. J Am Vet Med Assoc 2017;250(10):1104–6.

# Patient Triage, First Aid Care, and Management of Oral and Maxillofacial Trauma

Christopher J. Snyder, DVM[a],*, Charles Lothamer, DVM[b]

## KEYWORDS

- Maxillofacial trauma • Repair • Craniomaxillofacial • Dog • Cat

## KEY POINTS

- Patients younger than 12 months are overly represented.
- Computed tomography provides the most accurate evaluation of the extent and number of injuries.
- The largest advantage for use of noninvasive repair techniques is preservation of dental structures and their use for anchorage.
- The largest advantage for use of invasive repair techniques is the opportunity to apply rigid fixation and achieve primary bone healing.

Maxillofacial trauma management is a frequent occurrence in general and emergency practice. The occurrence of trauma has been reported to have seasonal, etiologic, and particular demographic associations.[1–3] Patients younger than 12 months have repeatedly been overrepresented as those presenting injured as well as small breed dogs.[1,3–6] Etiologic associations with craniomaxillofacial (CMF) injuries include animal altercations, falls, motor vehicle accidents, blunt force trauma, and unknown causes.[1,3,6]

Patterns of CMF trauma are becoming better understood in veterinary medicine.[3,7] Mandibular injuries are common, with the mandibular first molar location being overrepresented as a frequent location for jaw fracture occurrence.[4,6,8,9] Mandibular fractures are more easily diagnosed and commonly prioritized for treatment and repair compared with maxillary fractures that may be less displaced or may seem to have less of a negative impact on function/prehension. Accurate assessment and patient management are essential for maintenance of occlusion and quick return to function. Reasons for fracture occurrence at the mandibular first molar tooth include buccal cortical bone thinning over the mesial root, decreased mandibular bone height over the distal root, and chronic periodontal disease. It has also been noted that the mandibular first molar tooth

---

[a] University of Wisconsin-Madison, School of Veterinary Medicine, 2015 Linden Drive, Madison, WI 53706, USA; [b] University of Tennessee, College of Veterinary Medicine, 2407 River Drive, Knoxville, TN 37996, USA
* Corresponding author.
*E-mail address:* Christopher.snyder@wisc.edu

Vet Clin Small Anim 52 (2022) 271–288
https://doi.org/10.1016/j.cvsm.2021.09.006
0195-5616/22/© 2021 Elsevier Inc. All rights reserved.
vetsmall.theclinics.com

does not get proportionally larger with the supporting mandibular bone.[10,11] It has been shown that as the patient's weight goes down, the proportionality of the mandibular first molar tooth root length gets closer to a 1:1 ratio.[10] This phenomenon was not unique to just the first molar tooth roots but also was noted to occur in the mandibular canine teeth as well. Similar studies do not exist in the maxilla; however, tooth crowding and missing teeth are more common in smaller breed patients.[12]

## PATIENT TRIAGE AND INITIAL MANAGEMENT

It is important to not lose site of the fact that patients with maxillofacial trauma can present with a variety of confounding injuries. Recognizing that the full extent of maxillofacial trauma cannot be determined without general anesthesia, a thorough physical examination and general parameters should be evaluated before considering heavy sedation or general anesthesia. Instances of unknown trauma should include thoracic radiographs and basic bloodwork to ensure suitability and safety for general anesthesia. Patients presenting with obvious maxillofacial trauma should also pay particular attention to mentation, including a cranial nerve examination before sedation or heavy use of analgesics. In addition, other components of a conscious examination can begin to bolster evidence that other injuries exist. Testing a patient's ability to perform ocular tracking (left to right, top to bottom) can be helpful at determining fracture of the orbital rim or extraocular muscle damage. Evidence of changes in mentation, epistaxis, or abnormalities in ocular tracking support the need for critical evaluation of the patients with head trauma and assessing their suitability for general anesthesia.

Patients suffering trauma resulting in temporomandibular joint (TMJ) luxation,[13–15] intractable bleeding, and tooth avulsion (in instances where clients wish to replant the tooth) must all be identified and treated acutely. Life-threatening bleeding is rarely a complication following facial trauma. When TMJ luxation is suspected, prompt workup and reduction, once the patient is stable for general anesthesia, is recommended to improve the likelihood of reduction being maintained.[13,16,17] Tooth luxation/avulsion also requires immediate intervention if the client's wishes to restore the tooth to the normal location. Presence of dentoalveolar trauma resulting from maxillofacial trauma can be difficult to definitively determine; however, it has been noted to occur in 72% of patients with maxillofacial trauma and thus should be carefully evaluated for.[8]

## NUTRITIONAL SUPPORT

Nutritional support needs of the traumatized patient should be considered on a per-patient basis. Animals sustaining chronic injury may present after a protracted period where they have been functionally unable or too painful to eat. The nature of CMF injury may dictate methods of providing nutritional support because major oronasal communications may necessitate bypassing the oral cavity with placement of a nasoesophageal tube, temporary esophagostomy tube, or intravenous total parenteral nutrition until repair can be performed. Because patients with many maxillofacial trauma do not necessitate immediate general anesthesia and repair, patients should receive appropriate analgesics, antibiotics for grossly contaminated wounds, and then be fasted in preparation for general anesthesia to facilitate diagnostics and repair. Neonatal ($\geq$6 weeks of age) and pediatric patients (6–12 weeks of age) present additional challenges with stabilization, support, and repair, considering that they demonstrate altered metabolism of anesthetic drugs and risk for hypothermia and hypoglycemia.[18]

## ALTERNATIVE METHODS OF INTUBATION

Aside from typical principles of fracture repair (fracture reduction, apposition, and stabilization), restoration of a normal function and occlusion are particular issues with fracture repair that are unique to maxillofacial trauma. Intraoperative assessment of occlusion can become challenging when an endotracheal tube is in place that prevents complete closure of the mouth. Alternative methods for maintaining inhalant general anesthesia, without interfering with assessment of a closed mouth occlusion, include tracheostomy or pharyngotomy intubation[19,20] and transmylohyoid intubation.[21] An advantage to these techniques is that following placement of these alternative methods to maintain anesthesia, the mouth can be secured closed, in normocclusion, with something as simple as a gauze muzzle. Once normal occlusion is restored, freedom for patient draping and extraoral approach to repair is easily facilitated. Knowing the patient's occlusion is maintained, this provides confidence that the repair will optimally return the patient to preinjury occlusion and does not disrupt the surgery with intermittent checking of how the repair is affecting occlusion. The primary disadvantage to alternative intubation techniques is that closure of the alternative access for the endotracheal tube requires surgical closure once the patient is returned to traditional *per os* intubation.

## DIAGNOSTIC IMAGING OF THE TRAUMA PATIENT

When presented with maxillofacial trauma, the use of common and advanced diagnostic imaging is invaluable for diagnosis, providing treatment options, and determining prognosis. The modalities of head radiographs, dental radiographs, conventional computed tomography (CT) or cone-beam CT (CBCT), and MRI are now readily available to many veterinarians, especially those associated with specialty practices or in large metropolitan areas. Each modality has its own pros and cons to be aware of, and it is the practitioner's responsibility to be familiar with these differences when determining which form of imaging to pursue. Often multiple modalities are used in the same case.

Head radiographs are widely available and can be used to confirm gross pathology. The biggest downside to them is that it is difficult to acquire 2-dimensional (2D) images that do not have superimposition of bony structures over areas of potential injury or disease; this creates problems with clearly identifying fracture lines or determining which is left or right, unless the image is clearly labeled. Along with lateral and ventrodorsal or dorsoventral images, lateral oblique views can help to mitigate the superimposition of bone structures[22]; this is especially valuable for the mandibles, where clear fracture lines can often be seen on such views (**Fig. 1**). Areas that are particularly difficult to image with head radiography and produce a valuable image include the maxilla, the cranium, and the TMJ. Although the dentition can be viewed on head radiographs, the detail is poor and superimposition common, compared with intraoral dental radiographs.[23] Head radiography is best used to confirm gross pathology before pursuing more advanced imaging that will provide more detailed information.[24]

Dental radiographs are useful when evaluating trauma that has occurred in the dentate areas, the maxilla, incisive bone, body of the mandible, and mandibular symphyseal region. The intraoral placement of the sensor pad or phosphor plate for dental radiography eliminates superimposition that occurs with head radiography; this allows for a more diagnostic image for gross pathology as well as for evaluation of the dental and periodontal structures that may be involved with the trauma (**Fig. 2**), and this aids in recognition of potential pathology that may have predisposed the patient to trauma, such as periodontal disease in an area of the mandible resulting in pathologic fracture.[9] Dental radiographs also allow for evaluation of whether a tooth needs to be extracted from a facture or if it can be salvaged and aid in the fixation of the injury.[24] Dental radiographs

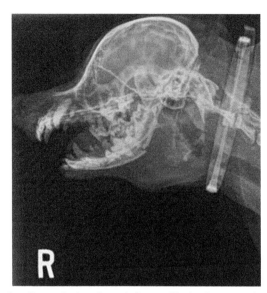

**Fig. 1.** Lateral head radiograph showing a left mandibular fracture along the distal aspect of the left mandibular first molar tooth 309. Although the radiograph is labeled, it is not obvious which side is fractured. Periodontal health is not easily assessed. Compare with **Figs. 2** and **3**.

can be produced quickly and close to the table where the repair of the trauma is taking place. These radiographs easily allow imaging to be used during the procedure to ensure that the surgical repair and/or apposition of bones is proceeding as desired.

The gold standard for evaluation of maxillofacial trauma is CT.[25] There are 2 forms of CT available to veterinarians, conventional helical CT or cone-beam CT. Because of the cost of equipment, the availability of these modalities is generally limited to specialty practices. Both modalities offer excellent evaluation of hard tissue structures of the head.

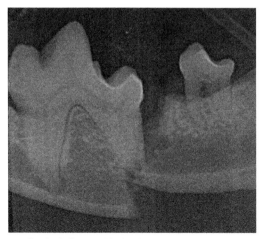

**Fig. 2.** Dental radiograph of a left mandibular fracture along the distal aspect of tooth 309. Horizontal bone loss is noted for tooth 310. Compare with **Figs. 1** and **3**.

Conventional CT is required to evaluate other areas of the body, such as the thorax or abdomen, and is also the better option when the evaluation of soft tissues is important.[26] CBCT seems comparable to conventional CT when evaluating bone and may be more sensitive in the evaluation of dental and periodontal pathology.[27–31] Compared with radiography, CT revealed almost twice the number of injuries when evaluating maxillofacial trauma in dogs and cats.[25] CT allows for elimination of the superimposition that occurs with head radiographs, allowing for clearer visualization of areas that are difficult to view with that modality. Software can be used to create 3D reconstructions of CT scans that increase the viewer's ability to comprehend anatomy and pathology (**Fig. 3**). In addition, 3D printers now give the ability to use CT information to create models that can be used in treatment planning or fabrication of fixation devices or jigs.[32] MRI is also available to veterinarians, typically in larger specialty practices, and is most useful for evaluation of soft tissue structures such as the brain, eyes, ligaments, or tendons.[33]

## NONINVASIVE AND MINIMALLY INVASIVE MAXILLOFACIAL FRACTURE REPAIR

The maxilla and mandibles have features that allow for different repair techniques compared with other areas of the body. The teeth can be used as anchors for attachment of various materials or devices to aid in fracture stabilization.[34] On the mandible, fractures generally result in tension forces occurring along the dorsal (alveolar) aspect of the bone due to pull from the muscles of mastication, the effect of gravity, and mechanical force placed by a food bolus; these same forces create compression on the ventral aspect of the mandible[35] — this means that fractures of the mandible can often be treated with fixation techniques that focus on neutralizing the tension forces at the dorsal aspect of the bone, and the ventral aspect will naturally compress requiring less direct efforts for stabilization. The techniques considered in the noninvasive and minimally invasive category are those that require little manipulation of the fractured bones to achieve alignment, resulting in immobility that allows the tissue to heal. Benefits of these techniques include preservation of the periosteum and any callus or hematoma that has started to form, less surgical pain, minimal cost, and prioritization of occlusion. Negatives of noninvasive techniques include creating a less ridged fixation compared with more invasive techniques, thereby the potential for a larger callus to form. Also, the less invasive a technique is, the more potential there is for prolonged healing times, and there is more potential for variation in the final occlusion of the

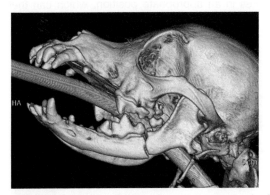

**Fig. 3.** Three-dimensional reconstruction from a computed tomography (CT) scan of a dog with a left mandibular fracture along the distal aspect of tooth 309. The reconstruction allows for easy comprehension of the fracture for clinicians and clients. Compare with **Figs. 1** and **2**.

teeth, which could result in traumatic malocclusion. The noninvasive and minimally invasive techniques include the use of maxillomandibular apposition (muzzle coaptation, sutures through buttons), maxillomandibular fixation (interarch splinting), and interdental wiring and composite splinting.

### Maxillomandibular Apposition

There are 2 possibilities, muzzling and sutures through buttons. Muzzles are cheap and readily available. Muzzles use the dental interlock of the canine teeth to provide alignment while allowing minor movement of the jaws (**Fig. 4**).[36] This technique is best used with caudal mandibular fractures with minimal displacement, in juvenile patients who generally heal quickly, and as a support device with other fixation techniques or when waiting for more definitive treatment.[37] Various materials are available as are prefabricated muzzles. Size 1″ or 2″ surgical tape can be used to create custom tape muzzles. The goal for sizing a tape muzzle is to have a device that allows for some opening of the mouth, so that the patient can lap up soft food and water, and keeps the canine teeth aligned in normal occlusion. As tape muzzles do restrict some movement of the TMJ, they should only be used for 3 to 5 weeks to prevent fibrosis of the TMJ from occurring. Supplying multiple muzzles is useful, as the devices often become soiled after eating, and switching to a clean dry muzzle can help prevent dermatitis from occurring. Because this technique provides the least amount of stabilization it also carries the greatest risk for nonunion or malunion, which may result in malocclusion. If a traumatic malocclusion occurs with healing, the teeth causing trauma should be treated appropriately.[37]

An alternative to muzzling includes the sutures through buttons technique and the use of anchors to attach orthodontic elastic bands between maxillary and mandibular teeth (**Fig. 5**).[38] This technique maintains occlusion while allowing restricted range of motion of the mouth, without the use of an external muzzle, that some patients will not tolerate or may have a head conformation that makes use of a muzzle difficult. The sutures through buttons technique use materials that are found in most general practices, making it a good option for practitioners without specialty dental materials or training.

### Maxillomandibular Fixation

Maxillomandibular fixation is a technique in human oral surgery in which the patient is placed in normal occlusion and the maxilla and mandible are connected via various devices preventing movement of the jaws.[39] Placement in normal occlusion will often help to align fractures in an appropriate position, which can then heal via closed

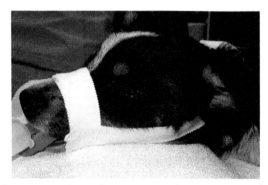

**Fig. 4.** Example of a tape muzzle used to support and restrict range of motion in a young patient with a mandibular fracture.

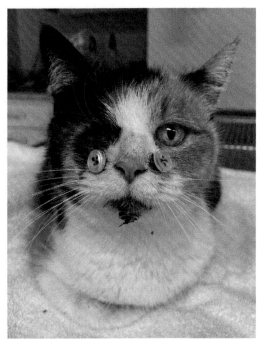

**Fig. 5.** Example of the sutures through buttons technique to achieve nonrigid maxilloman-dibular apposition (MMA).

reduction or can be used with more invasive open reduction techniques. This same principle can be applied to veterinary patients. If the patient is placed in normal occlusion, then the fracture fragments may be in reasonable alignment for healing. Because there are dangers with keeping veterinary patients in a closed mouth position, such as aspiration of vomit or regurgitation, and difficulty in maintaining proper temperature control (inhibition of thermoregulating panting), veterinary patients are placed into MMF with the mouth slightly opened.

Interarch splinting is a technique that uses bis-acryl composite material to bridge from the maxillary canine (or other) teeth to the mandibular canine (or other) teeth.[40] This technique creates a fixed position of the jaws, which can be sufficient for healing fractures with minimal displacement, such as caudal mandibular fractures in which the muscles of mastication help to keep the fractures aligned, in small patients in which use of more invasive techniques is difficult due to the size of available materials being inappropriate or in those with TMJ injuries in which stabilization is desired after repair. With this treatment, the canine (or other) teeth are bonded so that the patient's tongue can still be used for eating soft foods and drinking (**Fig. 6**). This technique should be used for 3 to 5 weeks to reduce development of ankyloses of the TMJ, as it restricts movement. Thought needs to be put into removal of this form of fixation, as intubation is made difficult by the restricted mouth movement, and dental trauma can also occur with removal so the owner must be made aware of these risks before selection of this treatment.[41] For removal, intubation can be performed blindly, with the help of a rigid endoscope, or the bonding material may need to be quickly broken, freeing the mouth to open. Quickly breaking the bonding increases the risk for dental trauma. Variations of this technique include the use of orthodontic brackets bonded to the canine (or other) teeth and connected with wire and/or composite materials or the use of MMF screws implanted into the surrounding bone to be used as attachment points for fixation materials. An alternative to interarch splinting is the bi-gnathic encircling retaining device (BEARD technique).[42]

### Interdental Wiring and Composite Splinting

Interdental wiring techniques use teeth on either side of a jaw fracture to form a semi-rigid fixation device along the alveolar margin. Twisting of the wire on itself or with the use of secondary wires will create compression or resist tension along the tension band of the alveolar margin. The interdental wiring techniques should be combined with an acrylic or bis-acryl composite interdental splint, as the splint will supply rigid support to the wire and will cover the sharp ends of the wire to prevent iatrogenic trauma. The combination of wire and composite has been shown to supply a stronger and stiffer apparatus compared with either technique alone.[43] Ideally, 2 teeth on either side of a simple fracture are the minimum used for stabilization. Compound fractures may be too unstable to be suitable for these techniques. Often, surrounding teeth are not in an ideal state of health, may be missing, or could have a difficult shape or size to work with. In these cases, combining other fixation techniques with interdental wiring and splinting, such as MMA, MMF, or interfragmentary wires, can provide adequate stabilization, if not then rigid fixation should be pursued. Using diagrams or illustrations is helpful for understanding interdental wiring techniques. Needles can be useful to act as guides for wires through gingiva or in between teeth. An 18 G needle, or appropriate size can be placed through gingiva in the interproximal space between teeth, and the end of a wire can then be fed into the needle tip. Because the wire needs to fit into the interdental spaces, sizes 22 to 26 G are generally used.

Techniques using a single wire include the Ivy loop and Stout loop techniques (**Fig. 7**).[44] The main difference in these techniques is that the Ivy loop incorporates 1 tooth on either side of a jaw fracture, whereas the Stout loop incorporates multiple teeth. When possible, the Stout loop technique should be used. These techniques are best used in the areas of the canine, premolar, and molar teeth. Techniques using a primary wire and secondary wires include the Risdon (**Fig. 8**) and Essig techniques (**Fig. 9**).[44] The Risdon technique is best used for rostral jaw fractures, and the Essig technique is best used in the area of the incisor teeth.

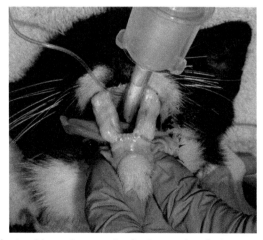

**Fig. 6.** Example of using bis-acryl composite for interarch splinting.

Self- and dual-cure bis-acryl composite materials can be bonded to teeth to create an interdental splint that will resist tension forces at the alveolar margin and create a load-sharing rigid apparatus (**Fig. 10**). The strength of the splint depends on the amount of material used (the thickness of the splint). Bis-acrylic splints should always be combined with an underlying interdental wiring technique.[43] The composite adds rigidity to the apparatus and covers the sharp wire twists. Composite bonds to the crown's surface, which necessitates removal of plaque and calculus. Tooth crowns must also be acid etched to achieve successful micromechanical bond between tooth and composite.[45] Following application, composite can be shaped with high-speed or low-speed dental burs to achieve the desired final shape. As with wiring techniques, at least 2 teeth on either side of the fracture should be incorporated into the interdental splint. A proper relationship between maxillary and mandibular arches can be maintained by placement of the composite on nonoccluding surfaces of the teeth. With maxillary teeth sitting buccal to mandibular teeth, composite placement on the buccal surface of maxillary teeth will not impede mouth closure; the opposite relationship exists for placement of composite on mandibular teeth.[45] Care to minimize contact between composite with periodontal soft tissues is important because it may be associated with irritation. Contact irritation commonly resolves within days of splint removal. Owners should be warned that dental trauma may be associated with composite removal, which is treated accordingly.

## INVASIVE MAXILLOFACIAL FRACTURE REPAIR

Invasive forms of fracture fixation require exposure of the fracture site and/or involve applying an apparatus to the bone. Interfragmentary (intraosseous) wiring, external skeletal fixation, and plates and screws techniques are the most commonly used. External skeletal fixation is rarely indicated except for caudal and highly comminuted fractures.[46,47] Interfragmentary wiring is performed using 18 to 20 G orthopedic wire in dogs and 20 to 24 G in cats and affords flexibility of pilot hole placement to avoid tooth roots and neurovascular structures. However, it is considered only a semirigid form of fixation with poor compression. Two sets of pilot holes with wires are typically used and placed perpendicular to the fracture plane to prevent telescoping.[48,49]

Titanium miniplates are commonly used in maxillofacial trauma and reconstruction in humans, with veterinary-specific sets becoming readily available. Veterinary-specific applications for CMF repair are increasingly reported clinically in patients[50,51] and experimentally[52,53] (biomechanically) in the literature. Titanium miniplates accepting 2.4 mm screws and smaller are increasingly applied for fixation and stabilization (**Fig. 11**).

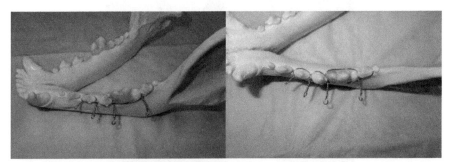

**Fig. 7.** Example of the Stout multiloop wiring technique. Note that the Ivy wiring technique is similarly applied with the difference being that only 2 teeth are included within the wire. Clinically, smaller loops that are pushed flush with the crowns of the teeth would be used.

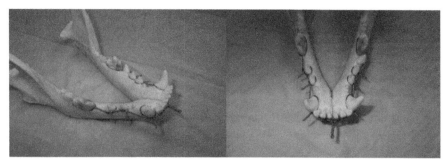

**Fig. 8.** Example of the Risdon wiring technique. Clinically, wire twists could be cut shorter and pushed flush with the crowns of the teeth.

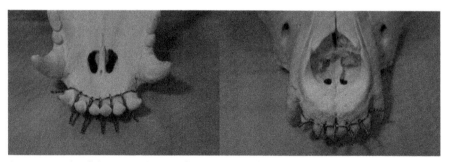

**Fig. 9.** Example of the Essig wiring technique. Clinically, wire twists could be cut shorter and pushed flush with the crowns of the teeth.

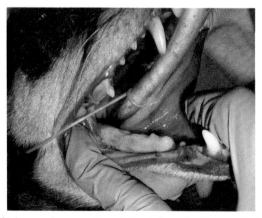

**Fig. 10.** Example of a bis-acryl composite splint reinforced with interdental wire (covered by the composite) used to stabilize a right caudal mandibular fracture.

Mechanical properties of how miniplates stabilize fractures are affected by plate position, screw number, plate thickness, plate size, and metallurgy. Miniplate constructs can also be categorized based on the type of plate and the screw-plate relationship. Adaptation plates, locking plates, and reconstruction plates vary in their biomechanical properties and warrant specific surgeon training and familiarity to select optimal constructs. Use of 3D printed models can aid in the presurgical planning[32,54] and 3D printed constructs for fixation.[55] The widespread investigation into 3D printing applications has also resulted in exploration into patient-specific custom printed fixation devices.[55]

When using an osteotomy model in cats, use of 2 plates was not stronger than 1; however, the use of 2 plates was associated with a significant increase in instances of tooth damage.[56] Tooth structure damaged by implant placement offers limited capacity for healing.[57] In efforts to optimize healing, recombinant human bone morphogenetic protein 2,[58–62] various scaffolds, allografts,[63–65] and autograft[66] procedures have been experimentally and clinically used in veterinary medicine. However, access to materials or surgical expertise limits widespread use.

## TEMPOROMANDIBULAR JOINT LUXATION

Luxation of the TMJ most commonly occurs in a rostrodorsal direction,[67] and this creates a clinical picture where the patient cannot close its mouth and has a shift of the lower jaw away from the affected joint. The injury can be confirmed with oblique radiographs of the TMJ or ideally with CT (**Fig. 12**).[68,69] Closed reduction is accomplished by placing a wooden dowel rod between maxillary and mandibular carnassial teeth, and the mouth is slowly closed on the dowel, which will allow the condylar process of the mandible to move back into the mandibular fossa of the temporal bone.[17] A hexagonal wooden pencil can be used in small dogs and cats; larger dogs will take a thicker dowel rod. If the injury is acute and reduction was easily accomplished, then the patient can be discharged with instructions for restricted use of its mouth and a soft food diet for several weeks. If reduction is accomplished but was difficult, injury was chronic, or if reluxation occurs easily, then the patient can be sent home with a MMA device to restrict movement for 2 to 3 weeks.[67] In patients in which closed reduction is unsuccessful, open reduction can be performed followed by use of a MMA or MMF. Condylectomy or gap arthroplasty are options when reduction is not possible or repeatedly fails.

Another reason for difficulty closing the mouth would be open-mouth jaw locking due to lateralization of the coronoid process of the mandible to the zygomatic arch, and this can

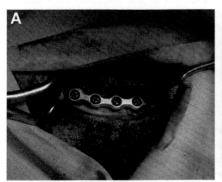
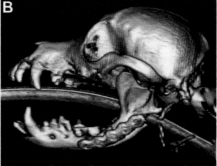

**Fig. 11.** (*A*) Locking titanium miniplate is applied to an edentulous area of the caudal mandible in a dog. (*B*) CT 3D reconstruction demonstrates plate placement and accuracy of the repair.

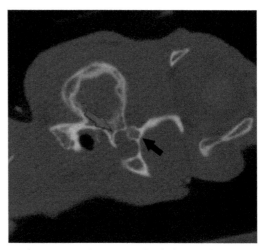

**Fig. 12.** Sagittal view of a computed tomography (CT) scan showing the temporomandibular joint with rostrodorsal displacement of the condylar process of the mandible (*black arrow*) from the mandibular fossa of the temporal bone (*red arrow*).

present as an animal that cannot close its mouth and potentially has a visible or palpable swelling over the zygomatic arch on the affected side. Causes include TMJ dysplasia, pterygoid muscles spasticity, abnormal confirmation of the zygomatic arch, or laxity of the mandibular symphysis.[70] Often with heavy sedation, the mouth can be fully opened and the coronoid process dislodged from the zygomatic arch. Manual reduction will only provide temporary relief, as locking usually recurs with wide mouth opening (eg, during yawning). Thus, surgical treatment will be necessary such as partial coronoidectomy, partial zygomectomy, or a combination of these procedures. Symphysiotomy, symphysiectomy, and intermandibular arthrodesis have also been reported to be successful in a cat with open-mouth jaw locking and increased laxity in the mandibular symphysis.[70,71]

Trauma to the area of the TMJ can result in callus formation over time that prevents normal joint range of motion. Fractures of the temporal bone, mandibular condylar process, zygomatic arch, and maxilla can have exuberant callus formation that abnormally bridges these bones to each other (**Fig. 13**). Treatment is aimed at removing a portion of the affected mandible allowing movement of the uninjured contralateral side. Surgical options include condylectomy, gap arthroplasty, or caudal mandibulectomy depending on the size and location of the callus formation.[72] Complications of any of these options can include mandibular drift with potential resultant trauma from abnormal occlusion, and redevelopment of a callus again resulting in progressive inability to open the mouth or never regaining full range of motion.[73]

## SOFT TISSUE TRAUMA

Soft tissue trauma often accompanies hard tissue injuries or can happen independently. Lacerations, soft tissue avulsions, and thermal injuries are frequently encountered. Injuries from trauma should be considered contaminated, and wounds should be cleaned and debrided before primary closure. Lip avulsions are seen most commonly in young and smaller patients.[74,75] Surgical correction has a high success rate.[74] The avulsed tissue is cleaned, freshened, and then apposed to where it tore off with a tension-free closure. To relieve tension on soft tissues, mattress sutures can be passed from the soft tissue

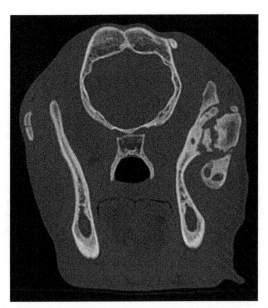

**Fig. 13.** Computed tomography (CT) scan of a 6-month-old German shepherd dog that sustained bite wound trauma to the temporomandibular joint and zygomatic arch 2 months back. CT revealed a bone density callus incorporating the bones of the mandibular ramus and zygomatic arch. The patient presented for inability to open the mouth. The other side shows normal distance between the zygomatic arch and mandibular ramus.

and then around the crowns of teeth. In edentulous areas, small holes can be created through the bone near the alveolar margin. A needle is passed through the edge of the avulsed tissue, through the created bony tunnel, and then through the apposing soft tissue and tied off. Thermal injuries can create intermediate problems, as the full extent of necrosis often takes days to weeks to manifest. Owners should be warned that tissue necrosis may continue. If underlying bone has been damaged and becomes nonvital, overlying soft tissue may initially seem to have healed only to necrose later and reveal an underlying bony defect. For soft tissue thermal wounds, once adequate time has passed so that the tissue can declare vitality or nonvitality, the wound is debrided of necrotic tissue and the soft tissue closed. Mucosal flaps may be required to create good apposition. Bone necrosis may continue for some time, so the patient needs to be monitored for the occurrence of nonvital soft tissues or the formation of bone defects.

Symphyseal separation is the most commonly described CMF trauma in cats.[76] Actually, the mandibular symphysis is a fibrocartilaginous joint. Symphyseal separation can be a component of cats suffering from "high-rise syndrome," which can also be associated with, but not limited to, hard palate fracture and epistaxis.[77] Separations can be treated by closing soft tissue lacerations and stabilization of the rostral lower jaw by mandibular cerclage wire, figure-of-eight wiring of the canine teeth ± composite splinting. Because these injuries are primarily soft tissue in nature, they commonly heal without the protracted stabilization necessary for bony healing. Symphyseal separations frequently occur concomitantly with other CMF injuries. Maxillary fractures commonly involve injury to other structures including the TMJ and skull base.[7]

Ballistic injuries in dogs and cats occasionally occur, and wounds should be considered contaminated.[78–80] Generalized patient stabilization, analgesia, and assessment for systemic organ involvement are important components of patient management before general anesthesia.[81] Historically, ballistic injury management has been managed from 1 of 2 different perspectives. On one hand, the idea of early intervention, debridement, repair, and closure may improve a quick return to function. However, delayed declaration of tissue health may result in sloughing, necrosis, and dehiscence requiring revision surgery. The alternative approach of stabilization of the patient and supportive care for several days while allowing tissues to declare their nonvitality may improve the chances for a single surgery and minimize dehiscence. Risks for infection and tissue contracture increase with time.[81,82] There has been no evidence in the veterinary literature suggesting acute versus delayed management is best for ballistic injuries.[81]

## SUMMARY

Patients with maxillofacial trauma commonly present with multiple injuries. Attention should be paid to the patient to determine the severity of injuries and comorbidities that may affect general anesthetic safety. A thorough oral examination to identify dentoalveolar trauma should accompany 3D diagnostic imaging for most patients. Repair of injuries should focus on reduction of bony fragments and return to normal occlusion. Considerations should be made for the selection of the fracture repair technique's impact on teeth and remaining structures.

## CLINICS CARE POINTS

- Imaging using computed tomography demonstrates a greater number of injuries than radiographs alone.
- Dental radiographs are useful for evaluation of dental and periodontal structures and can be used intra-operatively.
- Invasive forms of stabilization risk greater risk for tooth damage.
- Invasive (miniplates) and non-invasive (interdental wiring) forms of fixation in dentate locations should include at least 2-3 anchorage locations on either side of the fracture.
- Due to the natural forces exerted on the mandible, mandibular fractures can often be stabilized with neutralization of tension forces primarily focused on the dorsal crest of the bone.
- Healing outcomes of trauma patients rarely ends with confirmation of bone healing. Long term monitoring for tooth vitality should be considered for most every maxillofacial trauma patient, regardless of the location of injury.

## REFERENCES

1. Mulherin BL, Snyder CJ, Soukup JW, et al. Retrospective evaluation of canine and feline maxillomandibular trauma cases; a comparison of signalment with non-maxillomandibular traumatic injuries (2003-2012). Vet Comp Orthop Traumatol 2014;27:192–7.
2. Mulherin BL, Snyder CJ, Soukup JW, et al. Retrospective evaluation of canine and feline maxillomandibular trauma cases. Comparison of lunar cycle and seasonality with non-maxillomandibular traumatic injuries (2003-2012). Vet Comp Orthop Traumatol 2014;27:198–203.
3. De Paolo MH, Arzi B, Pollard RE, et al. Craniomaxillofacial trauma in dogs—Part I: Fracture location, morphology and etiology. Front Vet Sci 2020;7.
4. Lopes FM, Gioso MA, Ferro DG, et al. Oral fractures in dogs of Brazil—a retrospective study. J Vet Dent 2005;22:86–90.

5. Umphlet RC, Johnson AL. Mandibular fractures in the dog a retrospective study of 157 cases. Vet Surg 1990;19:272–5.
6. Kitshoff AM, de Rooster H, Ferreira SM, et al. A retrospective study of 109 dogs with mandibular fractures. Vet Comp Orthop Traumatol 2013;26:1–5.
7. De Paolo MH, Arzi B, Pollard RE, et al. Craniomaxillofacial trauma in dogs—Part II: Association between fracture location, morphology and etiology. Front Vet Sci 2020;7.
8. Soukup JW, Mulherin BL, Snyder CJ. Prevalence and nature of dentoalveolar injuries among patients with maxillofacial fractures. J Small Anim Pract 2013;54:9–14.
9. Scherer E, Hetzel S, Snyder CJ. Assessment of the role of the mandibular first molar tooth in mandibular fracture patterns of 29 dogs. J Vet Dent 2019;36:32–9.
10. Gioso MA, Shofer F, Barros PS, et al. Mandible and mandibular first molar tooth measurements in dogs: relationship of radiographic height to body weight. J Vet Dent 2001;18:65–8.
11. Scherer E, Snyder CJ, Malberg J, et al. A volumetric assessment using computed tomography of canine and first molar roots in dogs of varying weight. J Vet Dent 2018;35:131–7.
12. Kim CG, Lee SY, Kim JW, et al. Assessment of dental abnormalities by full-mouth radiography in small breed dogs. J Am Anim Hosp Assoc 2013;49:23–30.
13. Somrak AJ, Marretta SM. Management of temporomandibular join luxation in a cat using custom-made tape muzzle. J Vet Dent 2015;32:239–46.
14. Lantz GC, Verstraete FJM. Fractures and luxations involving the temporomandibular joint. In: Verstraete FJM, Lommer MJ, Bezuidenhout AJ, editors. Oral and maxillofacial surgery in dogs and cats. Edinburgh: Saunders/Elsevier; 2012. p. 321–32.
15. Gemmill T. Conditions of the temporomandibular joint in dogs and cats. Practice 2008;30:36–43.
16. Schulz K. Diseases of the joints. In: Fossum TW, editor. Small animal surgery. 3rd edition. St. Louis, MO: Mosby; 2007. p. 1145–315.
17. Thatcher G. Temporomandibular joint luxation in the cat: diagnosis and management. Can Vet J 2017;58:989–93.
18. Grubb TL, Perez Jimenez TE, Pettifer GR. Neonatal and pediatric patients. In: Grimm KA, Lamont LA, Tranquilli WJ, et al, editors. Veterinary anesthesia and analgesia. Ames, IA: Wiley Blackwell; 2015. p. 983–7.
19. Smith MM. Pharyngostomy endotracheal tube. J Vet Dent 2004;21:191–4.
20. Hartsfield SM, Genfreau CL, Smith CW, et al. Endotracheal intubation by pharyngotomy. J Am Anim Hosp Assoc 1977;13:71–4.
21. Soukup JW, Snyder CJ. Transmylohyoid orotracheal intubation in surgical management of canine maxillofacial fractures: an alternative to pharyngotomy endotracheal intubation. Vet Surg 2015;44:432–6.
22. Morgan JP. Radiography of the head. In: Techniques of veterinary radiography. 5th edition. Ames, IA: Iowa State Press; 1993. p. 121–33.
23. Buelow ME, Marretta SM. Diagnostic imaging in veterinary dental practice. Mandibular fractures diagnosed by radiography. J Am Vet Med Assoc 2011;239:931–3.
24. Schloss AJ, Marretta SM. Prognostic factors affecting teeth in the line of mandibular fractures. J Vet Dent 1990;7(4):7–9.
25. Bar-Am Y, Pollard RE, Kass PH, et al. The diagnostic yield of conventional radiographs and computed tomography in dogs and cats with maxillofacial trauma. Vet Surg 2008;37:294–9.
26. Lechuga L, Weidlich GA. Cone beam CT vs fan beam CT: A comparison of image quality and dose delivered between two differing CT imaging modalities. Cureus 2016;8(9). https://doi.org/10.7759/cureus.778.

27. Döring S, Arzi B, Hatcher DC, et al. Evaluation of the diagnostic yield of dental radiography and cone-beam computed tomography for the identification of dental disorders in small to medium-sized brachycephalic dogs. Am J Vet Res 2018;79:62–72.

28. Heney CM, Arzi B, Kass PH, et al. The diagnostic yield of dental radiography and cone-beam computed tomography for the identification of dentoalveolar lesions in cats. Front Vet Sci 2019;6(42). https://doi.org/10.3389/fvets.2019.00042.

29. Heney CM, Arzi B, Kass PH, et al. Diagnostic yield of dental radiography and cone-beam computed tomography for the identification of anatomic structures in cats. Front Vet Sci 2019;6(58). https://doi.org/10.3389/fvets.2019.00058.

30. Roza MR, Silva LAF, Barriviera M, et al. Cone beam computed tomography and intraoral radiography for diagnosis of dental abnormalities in dogs and cats. J Vet Sci 2001;12:387–92.

31. Soukup JW, Drees R, Koenig LJ, et al. Comparison of the diagnostic image quality of the canine maxillary dentoalveolar structures obtained by cone beam computed tomography and 64-multidetector row computed tomography. J Vet Dent 2015;32:80–6.

32. Winer J, Verstraete F, Cissell D, et al. The application of 3-dimensional printing for preoperative planning in oral and maxillofacial surgery in dogs and cats. Vet Surg 2017;46:942–51.

33. Macready DM, Hecht S, Craig LE, et al. Magnetic resonance imaging features of the temporomandibular joint in normal dogs. Vet Radiol Ultrasound 2010;51:436–40.

34. Legendre L. Intraoral acrylic splints for maxillofacial fracture repair. J Vet Dent 2003;20:70–8.

35. Boudrieau R, Arzi B, Verstraete F. Principles of maxillofacial trauma repair. In: Verstraete F, Lommer M, Arzi B, editors. Oral and Maxillofacial Surgery in Dogs and Cats. 2nd edition. Saunders (Elsevier): St. Louis, MO; 2020. p. 252–61.

36. Howard PE. Tape muzzle for mandibular fractures. Vet Med Small Anim Clin 1981; 76:517–9.

37. Castejon-Gonzalez AC, Buelow ME, Reiter AM. Management and outcome of maxillofacial trauma in a 9-week-old dog. J Vet Dent 2018;35:167–77.

38. Goodman AE, Carmichael DT. Modified labial button technique for maintaining occlusion after caudal mandibular fracture/temporomandibular joint luxation in the cat. J Vet Dent 2016;33:47–52.

39. Oikarinen KS. Clinical management of injuries to the maxilla, mandible, and alveolus. Dent Clin North Am 1995;39:113–31.

40. Bennett JW, Kapatkin AS, Marretta SM. Dental composite for the fixation of mandibular fractures and luxations in 11 cats and 6 dogs. Vet Surg 1994;23:190–4.

41. Hoffer M, Manfra Marretta S, Kurath P, et al. Evaluation of composite resin materials for maxillomandibular fixation in cats for treatment of jaw fractures and temporomandibular joint luxations. Vet Surg 2011;40:357–68.

42. Nicholson I, Wyatt J, Radke H, et al. Treatment of caudal mandibular fracture and temporomandibular joint fracture-luxation using a bi-gnathic encircling and retaining device. Vet Comp Orthop Traumatol 2010;23:102–8.

43. Lothamer C, Snyder CJ, Duenwald-Kuehl S, et al. Crown preservation of the mandibular first molar tooth impacts the strength and stiffness of three non-invasive jaw fracture repair constructs in dogs. Front Vet Sci 2015;2:18.

44. Taney K, Smithson C. Oral surgery – Fracture and trauma repair. In: Lobrise H, Dodd J, editors. Wigg's veterinary Dentistry principles and practice. 2nd edition. Hoboken, NJ: Wiley Blackwell; 2018. p. 265–88.

45. Legendre L. Maxillofacial fracture repairs. Vet Clin North Am Small Anim Pract 2005;35:985–1008.
46. Owen MR, Hobbs SL, Moores AP, et al. Mandibular fracture repair in dogs and cats using epoxy resin and acrylic external skeletal fixation. Vet Comp Orthop Traumatol 2004;17:189–97.
47. Woodbridge N, Owen M. Feline mandibular fractures: A significant surgical challenge. J Feline Med Surg 2013;15:211–8.
48. Boudrieau RJ. Fractures of the mandible. In: Johnson AL, Houlton JEF, Vannini R, editors. AO principles of fracture management in the dog and cat. Davos (Switzerland): AO Publishing; 2005. p. 99–116.
49. Snyder CJ, Soukup JW, Gengler WR. Imaging and management of a caudal mandibular fracture in an immature dog. J Vet Dent 2009;26:97–105.
50. Boudrieau RJ. Miniplate reconstruction of severely comminuted maxillary fractures in two dogs. Vet Surg 2004;33:154–63.
51. Arzi B, Verstraete FJ. Internal fixation of severe maxillofacial fractures in dogs. Vet Surg 2015;44:437–42.
52. Sverzut CE, Lucas MA, Sverzut AT, et al. Bone repair in mandibular body ostetolomy after using 2.0 miniplate system-histological and histometric analysis in dogs. Int J Exper Path 2008;89:91–7.
53. Freitag V, Landau H. Healing of dentate or edentulous mandibular fractures treated with rigid or semirigid plate fixation- an experimental study in dogs. J Cranio-Maxillofacial Surg. 1996;24:83–7.
54. Southerden P, Barnes DM. Caudal mandibular fracture repair using three-dimensional printing, presurgical plate contouring and a preformed template to aid anatomical fracture reduction. J Feline Med Surg Open Rep 2018;4(2). 2055116918798875.
55. Liptak JM, Thatcher GP, Bray JP. Reconstruction of a mandibular segmental defect with a customized 3-dimensional–printed titanium prosthesis in a cat with a mandibular osteosarcoma. J Am Vet Med Assoc 2017;250:900–8.
56. Greiner CL, Verstraete FJ, Stover SM, et al. Biomechanical evaluation of two plating configurations for fixation of a simple transverse caudal mandibular fracture model in cats. Am J Vet Res 2017;78:702–11.
57. Cornelis MA, Tepedino M, Cattaneo PM, et al. Root repair after damage due to screw insertion for orthodontic miniplate placement. J Clin Exp Dent 2019; 11(12). https://doi.org/10.4317/jced.56472.
58. Boudrieau RJ, Mitchell SL, Seeherman H. Mandibular reconstruction of a partial hemimandibulectomy in a dog with severe malocclusion. Vet Surg 2004;33:119–30.
59. Boudrieau RJ. Initial experience with rhBMP-2 delivered in a compressive resistant matrix for mandibular reconstruction in 5 dogs. Vet Surg 2015;44:443–58.
60. Lewis JR, Boudrieau RJ, Reiter AM, et al. Mandibular reconstruction after gunshot trauma in a dog by use of recombinant human bone morphogenetic protein-2. J Am Vet Med Assoc 2008;233:1598–604.
61. Arzi B, Verstraete FJ, Huey DJ, et al. Regenerating mandibular bone using rhBMP-2: Part 1—Immediate reconstruction of segmental mandibulectomies. Vet Surg 2015;44:403–9.
62. Verstraete FJ, Arzi B, Huey DJ, et al. Regenerating mandibular bone using rhBMP-2: part 2—treatment of chronic, defect non-union fractures. Vet Surg 2015;44:410–6.
63. Bauer TW, Muschler GF. Bone graft materials: an overview of the basic science. Clin Orthop Rel Res 2000;371:10–27.

64. Snyder CJ, Bleedorn JA, Soukup JW. Successful treatment of mandibular nonunion with cortical allograft, cancellous autograft, and locking titanium miniplates in a dog. J Vet Dent 2016;33:160–9.
65. Messora MR, Nagata MJ, Fucini SE, et al. Effect of platelet-rich plasma on the healing of mandibular defects treated with fresh frozen bone allograft: a radiographic study in dogs. J Oral Implantol 2014;40:533–41.
66. Boudrieau RJ, Tidwell AS, Ullman SL, et al. Correction of mandibular nonunion and malocclusion by plate fixation and autogenous cortical bone grafts in two dogs. J Am Vet Med Assoc 1994;204:744–50.
67. Klima LJ. Temporomandibular joint luxation in the cat. J Vet Dent 2007;24:198–201.
68. Schwarz T, Weller R, Dickie AM, et al. Imaging of the canine and feline temporomandibular joint: A review. Vet Radiol Ultrasound 2002;43:85–97.
69. Arzi B, Cissell DD, Verstraete FJM, et al. Computed tomographic findings in dogs and cats with temporomandibular joint disorders: 58 cases (2006-2011). J Am Vet Med Assoc 2013;242:69–75.
70. Soukup JW, Snyder CJ, Gengler WR. Computed tomography and partial coronoidectomy for open-mouth jaw locking in two cats. J Vet Dent 2009;26:226–33.
71. Reiter AM. Symphysiotomy, symphysiectomy, and intermandibular arthrodesis in a cat with open-mouth jaw locking–case report and literature review. J Vet Dent 2004;21:147–58.
72. Villamizar-Martinez LA, Chia H, Robertson JB, et al. Comparison of unilateral rostral, middle and caudal segmental mandibulectomies as an alternative treatment for unilateral temporomandibular joint ankylosis in cats: an ex vivo study. J Feline Med Surg 2020. https://doi.org/10.1177/1098612X20977134.
73. Strøm PC, Arzi B, Cissell DD, et al. Ankylosis and pseudoankylosis of the temporomandibular joint in 10 dogs (1993-2015). Vet Comp Orthop Traumatol 2016;29:409–15.
74. Saverino KM, Reiter AM. Clinical presentation, causes, treatment, and outcome of lip avulsion injuries in dogs and cats: 24 cases (2001-2017). Front Vet Sci 2018;5:144.
75. White TL. Lip avulsion and mandibular symphyseal separation repair in an immature cat. J Vet Dent 2010;27:228–33.
76. Wiggs RB, Loprise HB. Oral fracture repair. In: Veterinary Dentistry Principals and practice. Philadelphia, PA: Lippincott-Raven; 1997. p. 261–2.
77. Bonner SE, Reiter AM, Lewis JR. Orofacial manifestations of high-rise syndrome in cats: a retrospective study of 84 cases. J Vet Dent 2012;29:10–8.
78. Kim Y, Lee D, Heo S, et al. The treatment of gunshot wounds with maxillofacial fracture in a dog. J Vet Clin 2018;35:215–7.
79. Tian HM, Deng GG, Huang MJ, et al. Quantitative bacteriological study of the wound track. J Trauma 1988;28:S215–6.
80. Pavletic MM. A review of 121 gunshot wounds in the dog and cat. Vet Surg 1985;14:61–2.
81. Pavletic MM, Trout NJ. Bullet, bite, and burn wounds in dogs and cats. Vet Clin North Am Small Anim Pract 2006;36:873–93.
82. Melugin MB. Maxillofacial firearm injuries. In: Fonseca RJ, Walker RV, Betts NJ, et al, editors. Oral and maxillofacial trauma. 3rd edition. St Louis (MO): Elsevier-Saunders; 2005. p. 931–48.

# *Moving?*

## *Make sure your subscription moves with you!*

To notify us of your new address, find your **Clinics Account Number** (located on your mailing label above your name), and contact customer service at:

**Email: journalscustomerservice-usa@elsevier.com**

**800-654-2452** (subscribers in the U.S. & Canada)
**314-447-8871** (subscribers outside of the U.S. & Canada)

**Fax number: 314-447-8029**

**Elsevier Health Sciences Division**
**Subscription Customer Service**
**3251 Riverport Lane**
**Maryland Heights, MO 63043**

*To ensure uninterrupted delivery of your subscription, please notify us at least 4 weeks in advance of move.

Printed and bound by CPI Group (UK) Ltd, Croydon, CR0 4YY

14/10/2024

01773715-0003